PRACTICAL PHYSIOLOGY
A Student's Workbook

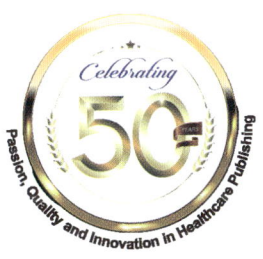

PRACTICAL PHYSIOLOGY
A Student's Workbook

VP Varshney MBBS MD
Director-Professor and Head
Department of Physiology
Maulana Azad Medical College
New Delhi, India

Mona Bedi MBBS MD
Director-Professor
Department of Physiology
Maulana Azad Medical College
New Delhi, India

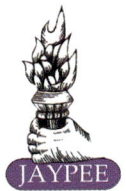

JAYPEE BROTHERS MEDICAL PUBLISHERS
The Health Sciences Publisher

New Delhi | London | Panama

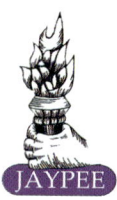

Jaypee Brothers Medical Publishers (P) Ltd

Headquarters
Jaypee Brothers Medical Publishers (P) Ltd
4838/24, Ansari Road, Daryaganj
New Delhi 110 002, India
Phone: +91-11-43574357
Fax: +91-11-43574314
Email: jaypee@jaypeebrothers.com

Overseas Offices
J.P. Medical Ltd
83 Victoria Street, London
SW1H 0HW (UK)
Phone: +44 20 3170 8910
Fax: +44 (0)20 3008 6180
Email: info@jpmedpub.com

Jaypee-Highlights Medical Publishers Inc
City of Knowledge, Bld. 235, 2nd Floor
Clayton, Panama City, Panama
Phone: +1 507-301-0496
Fax: +1 507-301-0499
Email: cservice@jphmedical.com

Jaypee Brothers Medical Publishers (P) Ltd
Bhotahity, Kathmandu, Nepal
Phone: +977-9741283608
Email: kathmandu@jaypeebrothers.com

Website: www.jaypeebrothers.com
Website: www.jaypeedigital.com

© 2019, Jaypee Brothers Medical Publishers

The views and opinions expressed in this book are solely those of the original contributor(s)/author(s) and do not necessarily represent those of editor(s) of the book.

All rights reserved. No part of this publication may be reproduced, stored or transmitted in any form or by any means, electronic, mechanical, photocopying, recording or otherwise, without the prior permission in writing of the publishers.

All brand names and product names used in this book are trade names, service marks, trademarks or registered trademarks of their respective owners. The publisher is not associated with any product or vendor mentioned in this book.

Medical knowledge and practice change constantly. This book is designed to provide accurate, authoritative information about the subject matter in question. However, readers are advised to check the most current information available on procedures included and check information from the manufacturer of each product to be administered, to verify the recommended dose, formula, method and duration of administration, adverse effects and contraindications. It is the responsibility of the practitioner to take all appropriate safety precautions. Neither the publisher nor the author(s)/editor(s) assume any liability for any injury and/or damage to persons or property arising from or related to use of material in this book.

This book is sold on the understanding that the publisher is not engaged in providing professional medical services. If such advice or services are required, the services of a competent medical professional should be sought.

Every effort has been made where necessary to contact holders of copyright to obtain permission to reproduce copyright material. If any have been inadvertently overlooked, the publisher will be pleased to make the necessary arrangements at the first opportunity. The **CD/DVD-ROM** (if any) provided in the sealed envelope with this book is complimentary and free of cost. **Not meant for sale**.

Inquiries for bulk sales may be solicited at: jaypee@jaypeebrothers.com

Practical Physiology: A Student's Workbook

First Edition: **2019**

ISBN 978-93-89188-32-5

Printed at: Samrat Offset Pvt. Ltd.

Dedicated to

*Our students,
the teaching fraternity
and
our parents.*

Preface

The need for a comprehensive book on practical physiology that encompasses all the aspects of Medical Council of India (MCI) syllabus and is easy for the students made us undertake this venture. It has been a difficult but beautiful journey, right from the time this book was conceived to the time we had the published book in our hands.

The book follows the scope and sequence of most human physiology courses. This book is written for medical students as well as for dental and nursing graduates, physiotherapy students as well as teachers. The text offers a complete yet concise knowledge of the major physiology practicals. The whole text has been divided into four sections for easy understanding. Each practical is discussed under the following headings: *Aim*, *Theory*, *Principle*, *Apparatus*, *Procedure*, *Precautions*, *Sources of Error* and *Physioclinical Significance*. At the end of each practical, *Questions and Answers* are given, which will help the students in self-assessment. The students are required to write the *Observation* and *Result* in the space designated for it. At the end of each chapter, the students are supposed to write their *Interpretation* of the *Result* obtained. Some other highlights of the book are:

- Important terms are highlighted in bold.
- Key concepts are given in the form of text boxes as a separate *Note*.
- *Physioclinical Significance* is integrated throughout the text.
- Graphs and charts, colored diagrams and flowcharts have been incorporated to illustrate the essential concepts.
- Actual photographs of instruments and clinical examination have been added.
- Bullets and numbers have been used to simplify the text.
- Study questions and answers are provided at the end of each chapter.
- Objective Structured Practical Examination (OSPE) and Objective Structured Clinical Examination (OSCE) have been added wherever applicable.
- Text has been updated as per recent MCI guidelines.

The development choices for this book were made with the guidance of our faculty, residents and last but not the least our students. With their inputs we have endeavored to bring out a practical student's workbook which would clarify the concepts and help in the skill-based learning of practical physiology.

But how so much we try, there is always scope for improvement. We welcome suggestions from our readers to help us improve the book in further editions.

VP Varshney
Mona Bedi

Acknowledgments

The completion of this workbook would not have been possible without the participation and assistance of so many people whose names may not all be enumerated.

We are immensely appreciative of M/s Jaypee Brothers Medical Publishers (P) Ltd, New Delhi, India for believing in us and providing us with an opportunity to put forth this practical workbook. This was just like a dream coming true. We are highly obliged to Shri Jitendar P Vij (Group Chairman), Mr Ankit Vij (Managing Director), Mr MS Mani (Group President) for their vision and the Wwhole publishing team for their effort.

We would especially like to thank Dr Madhu Choudhary (Publishing Head–Education), Dr Priyanka Manchanda (Development Editor), Ms Pooja Bhandari (Production Head), Ms Sunita Katla (Executive Assistant to Group Chairman and Publishing Manager), Ms Seema Dogra (Cover Visualizer) and Ms Samina Khan (Executive Assistant to Publishing Head–Education) of M/s Jaypee Brothers Medical Publishers for their guidance and help.

We are highly obliged to our faculty, residents and technical staff for their generous, friendly and helping attitude.

We are deeply indebted to Dr Aprajita and Dr Amina Sultan Zaidi, Senior Residents, Department of Physiology, Maulana Azad Medical College, New Delhi, India. This work would not have been possible without the continuous support and hard work put in by them. Their dedication and willingness to work was commendable and their contribution unmatched. Their knowledge and untiring effort eased the difficult task of successfully completing this venture.

Most importantly, we wish to thank all those who provided us unending inspiration…especially our students, who are our educators as well.

Above all, we would like to thank the Almighty for giving us the power to believe in our passion and pursue our dreams.

Last but not the least, we would like to thank our families with immense gratitude. Nobody has been more important to us in the pursuit of this project than them. Their constant support and love has been extensively helpful in focusing on what has been an extremely enriching and fulfilling process.

Contents

Section 1: Hematology

1.1:	The Compound Microscope	3
1.2:	Collection of Blood Sample	9
1.3:	Estimation of Hemoglobin	15
1.4:	Hemocytometry	22
1.5:	Total Red Blood Cell Count	28
1.6:	Total Leukocyte Count	34
1.7:	Preparation of a Peripheral Blood Smear and Determination of Differential Leukocyte Count	39
1.8:	Arneth Count (Cooke-Arneth Count)	49
1.9:	Determination of Blood Groups (A, B, O and Rh System)	53
1.10:	Bleeding Time and Clotting Time	60
1.11:	Erythrocyte Sedimentation Rate and Packed Cell Volume	66
1.12:	Red Blood Cell Indices	73
1.13:	Platelet Count	76
1.14:	Absolute Eosinophil Count	80
1.15:	Reticulocyte Count	83
1.16:	Osmotic Fragility of Red Blood Cells	87
1.17:	Specific Gravity of Blood	92

Section 2: Amphibian (Frog) Experiments

2.1:	Introduction to Amphibian Experiments	99
2.2:	Study of Apparatus	102
2.3:	Dissection of Gastrocnemius Muscle-Sciatic Nerve Preparation of Frog	111
2.4:	Simple Muscle Twitch	114
2.5:	Effect of Temperature on Simple Muscle Twitch	118
2.6:	Conduction Velocity of Sciatic Nerve of Frog	121
2.7:	Effect of Two Successive Stimuli (of Same Strength) on Skeletal Muscle Contraction	124
2.8:	Effect of Increasing Strength of Stimulus on Skeletal Muscle Contraction	128

2.9: Genesis of Tetanus	132
2.10: Genesis of Fatigue	136
2.11: Effect of Load on Skeletal Muscle Contraction (Freeload and Afterload)	140
2.12: Recording of a Normal Cardiogram of Frog's Heart and Effect of Temperature on it	145
2.13: Properties of Cardiac Muscle	149
2.14: Effect of Stimulation of Vagosympathetic Trunk and White Crescentic Line on Frog's Cardiogram	154
2.15: Effect of Variables on Intact Frog's Heart	158
2.16: Perfusion of Isolated Frog's Heart	162

Section 3: Human Experiments

Unit 1: Cardiovascular System

3.1: Examination of Arterial (Radial) Pulse	167
3.2: Recording of Systemic Arterial Blood Pressure	172
3.3: Effect of Posture on Blood Pressure and Heart Rate	180
3.4: Effect of Exercise on Blood Pressure and Heart Rate	184
3.5: Recording and Interpretation of an Electrocardiogram	188
3.6: Cardiac Efficiency Tests	197

Unit 2: Respiratory System

3.7: Stethography	200
3.8: Spirometry: Lung Volumes and Capacities	206
3.9: Vitalography and Effect of Posture on Vital Capacity	216
3.10: Cardiopulmonary Resuscitation	220
3.11: Basal Metabolic Rate	228

Unit 3: Special Senses

3.12: Perimetry	231

Unit 4: Nervous System

3.13: Reaction Time (Visual and Auditory)	237
3.14: Electroencephalography	240
3.15: Electroneurodiagnostic Tests	245
A: Nerve Conduction Study *246*	
B: Electromyography *249*	
C: Evoked Potentials *251*	
3.16: Study of Human Fatigue by Mosso's Ergograph and Handgrip Dynamometer	255
3.17: Autonomic Function Tests	260

Unit 5: Reproductive System

3.18:	Semen Analysis	267
3.19:	Pregnancy Diagnostic Tests	270
3.20:	Birth Control Methods	274

Section 4: Clinical Examination

4.1:	History Taking and General Physical Examination	281
4.2:	Clinical Examination of the Respiratory System	288
4.3:	Clinical Examination of the Cardiovascular System	296
4.4:	Clinical Examination of the Abdomen	305
4.5:	Clinical Examination of the Nervous System	315
	A: Examination of Higher Functions *316*	
	B: Examination of the Cranial Nerves *316*	
	C: Examination of the Motor System *333*	
	D: Reflexes *339*	
	E: Examination of the Sensory System *348*	

Appendix: Units and Measures Employed in Physiology — *357*

Index — *365*

Instructions to Candidates

1. Every student has to maintain a record of the experiments performed and demonstrations attended.
2. The record should be neatly written as follows:
   a. Write the date of the experiment on the top left-hand side of the experiment
   b. The results should be presented in the form of tables and graphs, and findings are to be interpreted.
   c. Answer the questions given at the end of each chapter.
3. Signatures should be obtained at the end of each chapter from the respective teacher-in-charge after the completion of each experiment.
4. Index page to be filled in and signatures to be obtained in time period specified by the teacher-in-charge.

Index of Experiments

Sl. No.	Date	Experiment	Remarks	Teacher's Signature

Sl. No.	Date	Experiment	Remarks	Teacher's Signature

Suggested Evaluation of Practicals

1. OSPE/Spotting
2. Graphs and charts from amphibian and heart experiments
3. Problem solving question
4. Hematology experiment
5. Human experiment
6. Clinical exercise
7. Assessment of practical workbook.

Competency Table

No.	COMPETENCY The student should be able to:	Core (Y/N)	Chapter number	Page number
Topic: Haematology	**Number of competencies: (08)**		**Number of procedures that require certification: (NIL)**	
PY2.4	Describe RBC formation (erythropoiesis & its regulation) and its functions	Y	1.5	31
PY2.5	Describe different types of anaemias & Jaundice	Y	1.12, 4.1	74, 282
PY2.7	Describe the formation of platelets, functions and variations.	Y	1.13	76-78
PY2.8	Describe the physiological basis of hemostasis and, anticoagulants. Describe bleeding & clotting disorders (Hemophilia, purpura)	Y	1.2, 1.10	11-13, 61, 63
PY2.9	Describe different blood groups and discuss the clinical importance of blood grouping, blood banking and transfusion	Y	1.9	53-58
PY2.11	Estimate Hb, RBC, TLC, RBC indices, DLC, Blood groups, BT/CT	Y	1.3, 1.5, 1.6, 1.7, 1.9, 1.10	15-20, 28-31, 34-37, 39-46, 53-58, 60-63, 73-74,
PY2.12	Describe test for ESR, Osmotic fragility, Hematocrit. Note the findings and interpret the test results etc	Y	1.11, 1.17	66-71, 70, 87-90
PY2.13	Describe steps for reticulocyte and platelet count	Y	1.13, 1.15	76-78, 83-85
Topic: Nerve and Muscle Physiology	**Number of competencies: (04)**		**Number of procedures that require certification: (NIL)**	
PY3.14	Perform Ergography	Y	3.16	255-257
PY3.15	Demonstrate effect of mild, moderate and severe exercise and record changes in cardiorespiratory parameters	Y	3.4	184-186
PY3.16	Demonstrate Harvard Step test and describe the impact on induced physiologic parameters in a simulated environment	Y	3.4	185
PY3.18	Observe with Computer assisted learning (i) amphibian nerve - muscle experiments (ii) amphibian cardiac experiments	Y	2.1-2.16	99-162
Topic: Gastro-intestinal Physiology	**Number of competencies: (01)**		**Number of procedures that require certification: (NIL)**	
PY4.10	Demonstrate the correct clinical examination of the abdomen in a normal volunteer or simulated environment	Y	4.4	305-309
Topic: Cardiovascular Physiology (CVS)	**Number of competencies: (05)**		**Number of procedures that require certification: (03)**	
PY5.12	Record blood pressure & pulse at rest and in different grades of exercise and postures in a volunteer or simulated environment	Y	3.2	172-178
PY5.13	Record and interpret normal ECG in a volunteer or simulated environment	Y	3.5	188-195
PY5.14	Observe cardiovascular autonomic function tests in a volunteer or simulated environment	N	3.17	260-265
PY5.15	Demonstrate the correct clinical examination of the cardiovascular system in a normal volunteer or simulated environment	Y	4.3	296-301
PY5.16	Describe and discuss arterial pulse tracing	N	3.1	167–170

Contd...

Contd...

No.	COMPETENCY The student should be able to:	Core (Y/N)	Chapter number	Page number
Topic: Respiratory Physiology	*Number of competencies: (03)*	*Number of procedures that require certification: (01)*		
PY6.8	Demonstrate the correct technique to perform & interpret Spirometry	Y	3.8	209-214
PY6.9	Demonstrate the correct clinical examination of the respiratory system in a normal volunteer or simulated environment	Y	4.2	288-293
PY6.10	Demonstrate the correct technique to perform measurement of peak expiratory flow rate in a normal volunteer or simulated environment	Y	3.8	211, 214
Topic: Reproductive Physiology	*Number of competencies: (03)*	*Number of procedures that require certification: (NIL)*		
PY9.6	Enumerate the contraceptive methods for male and female. Discuss their advantages & disadvantages	Y	3.20	274-276
PY9.9	Interpret a normal semen analysis report including (a) sperm count, (b) sperm morphology and (c) sperm motility, as per WHO guidelines and discuss the results	Y	3.18	267-268
PY9.10	Discuss the physiological basis of various pregnancy tests	Y	3.19	270-272
Topic: Neurophysiology	*Number of competencies: (04)*	*Number of procedures that require certification: (09)*		
PY10.11	Demonstrate the correct clinical examination of the nervous system: Higher functions, sensory system, motor system, reflexes, cranial nerves in a normal volunteer or simulated environment	Y	4.5	315-348
PY10.12	Identify normal EEG forms	Y	3.14	271
PY10.19	Describe and discuss auditory & visual evoke potentials	Y	4.5	317-322, 327-330
PY10.20	Demonstrate (i) Testing of visual acuity, colour and field of vision and (ii) hearing (iii) Testing for smell and (iv) taste sensation in volunteer/simulated environment	Y	4.5	315-348
Topic: Integrated Physiology	*Number of competencies: (03)*	*Number of procedures that require certification: (NIL)*		
PY11.11	Discuss the concept, criteria for diagnosis of Brain death and its implications	Y	4.5	340
PY11.13	Obtain history and perform general examination in the volunteer / simulated environment	Y	4.1	281
PY11.14	Demonstrate Basic Life Support in a simulated environment	Y	3.10	220-221

Section 1

Hematology

CHAPTERS

- 1.1 The Compound Microscope
- 1.2 Collection of Blood Sample
- 1.3 Estimation of Hemoglobin
- 1.4 Hemocytometry
- 1.5 Total Red Blood Cell Count
- 1.6 Total Leukocyte Count
- 1.7 Preparation of a Peripheral Blood Smear and Determination of Differential Leukocyte Count
- 1.8 Arneth Count (Cooke-Arneth Count)
- 1.9 Determination of Blood Groups (A, B, O and Rh System)
- 1.10 Bleeding Time and Clotting Time
- 1.11 Erythrocyte Sedimentation Rate and Packed Cell Volume
- 1.12 Red Blood Cell Indices
- 1.13 Platelet Count
- 1.14 Absolute Eosinophil Count
- 1.15 Reticulocyte Count
- 1.16 Osmotic Fragility of Red Blood Cells
- 1.17 Specific Gravity of Blood

Date ....

CHAPTER 1.1

The Compound Microscope

AIM

To study the compound microscope.

THE COMPOUND MICROSCOPE

Antonie van Leeuwenhoek (1632–1723) invented the compound microscope.

The compound microscope magnifies the image of an object that is not visible to the naked eye to an extent where it can be seen clearly. These are of two types:
1. **Monocular microscope:** It has only one eyepiece (Fig. 1.1.1A).
2. **Binocular microscope:** It is a compound bright-field microscope but having two eyepieces instead of one, so that both eyes can be used simultaneously. This prevents eyestrain (Fig. 1.1.1B).

PARTS OF A COMPOUND MICROSCOPE

The Support System

It acts as a framework to which various functional units are attached (Fig. 1.1.2):
1. **Base:** It is a heavy metallic, U-shaped or horseshoe-shaped base or foot, which supports the microscope on the work table to provide maximum stability.

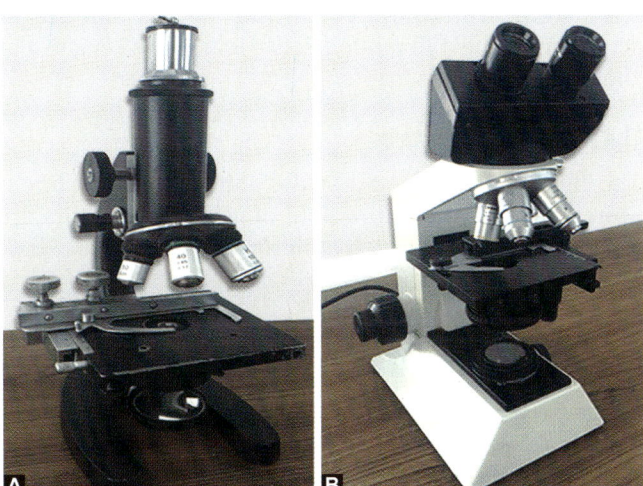

Figs. 1.1.1A and B: (A) Monocular microscope; (B) Binocular microscope.

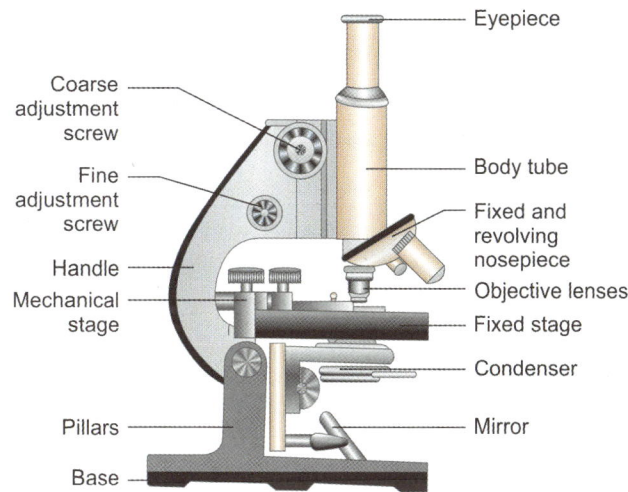

Fig. 1.1.2: Compound microscope.

2. **Pillars:** Two upright pillars project up from the base and are attached to the C-shaped handle. The hinge joint allows the microscope to be tilted at a suitable angle for comfortable viewing.

> **NOTE**
> The microscope is never tilted when counting cells in a chamber or when examining a blood film under oil immersion. It can be tilted for viewing histology slides.

3. **Handle (the arm or limb):** The curved handle, which projects up from the hinge joint, supports the focusing and magnifying systems.

Optical (Magnifying) System

It is mounted on the body tube which is in two parts:
1. **External tube:** There is a revolving nosepiece at its lower end in which are fitted three interchangeable objective lenses of different magnifications (Fig. 1.1.3).
   a. Low power objective (LP) (10x)
   b. High power objective (HP) (40x)
   c. Oil immersion objective (OI) (100x)
2. **Inner draw tube:** It has an eyepiece fitted on its top which has a magnification of 10x.

> **NOTE**
> "x" is the sign of multiplication. The magnifying power of each objective, as that of the eyepiece, is etched on it.

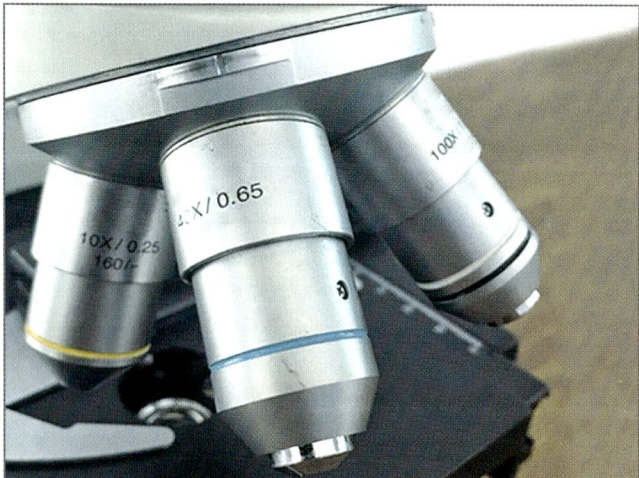

Fig. 1.1.3: Objective lenses.

> **NOTE**
> *Parfocal system:* The objectives these days are so constructed that when one lens (LP, for example) is in focus, the others are more or less in focus. Thus, switching from one lens to another (e.g. from LP to HP) requires only a little turn of fine adjustment to bring the image into sharp focus. This arrangement of lenses is called "parfocal system".

The Stage

It has three components:
1. **Fixed stage:** It is a square platform on which the slide is placed. There is an aperture in the center through which light enters to reach the object. It is fitted to the limb below the objective lens.
2. **Mechanical stage:** It is a calibrated metal frame fitted on the right edge of the fixed stage. There is a spring-mounted clip to hold the slide or the counting chamber in position. Two screw heads are present that help to move the slide from side to side or forward/backward.
3. **Substage:** It is fitted with a **condenser** and **iris diaphragm.**
   - **Condenser:** It consists of two convex lenses which condense the light rays on the object. It can be raised or lowered with the help of a screw so as to focus the light on the object. Each time the objective is changed, a corresponding adjustment must be performed on the condenser to provide proper light.
   - **The iris diaphragm:** It is fitted immediately below the condenser. It can control the amount of light reaching the object.

> **NOTE**
> In a compound microscope proper illumination includes a combination of position of light source, regulation of light intensity, position of condenser and regulation of the size of field of view.

Position of the condenser and the iris diaphragm according to the different objective lenses used is given in Table 1.1.1.

The Illumination System

The illumination system provides uniform, soft and bright illumination of the entire field of view. Two factors are involved in providing such uniform illumination:
1. Position of the condenser.
2. Size of the iris diaphragm.

Table 1.1.1: Important features of compound microscope.

Objective lens	Numerical aperture	Mirror (simple microscope)	Position of condenser	Iris diaphragm
Low power (LP) (10x)	0.25	Concave	Lowest position	Slightly open
High power (HP) (40x)	0.65	Concave	Midway	Half open
Oil Immersion (OI) (100x)	1.25	Plane	Highest position	Fully open

The illumination system consists of:
1. **Source of light:** In most microscopes, there is a built-in light source. This unit has frosted tungsten lamp to provide uniform white light. Natural light may also be used.
2. **The mirror:** A double-sided mirror, which is plane on one side and concave on the other is located below the condenser.
   - The plane mirror is used with a distant source of light (natural or daylight). The parallel rays of light remain parallel when they enter the iris diaphragm.
   - The concave mirror is employed when the light source is from a bulb. The divergent rays of light are reflected as parallel rays and directed into the iris diaphragm.

PHYSICAL BASIS OF MICROSCOPY

Resolving Power (Resolution)
- Resolving power is the ability to show closely located structures as separate and distinct from each other.
- Generally, the resolving power of the unaided human eye is said to be between 0.15 mm and 0.25 mm.
- The resolving power of a lens depends on its numerical aperture (NA) as well as the wavelength of light.
- The resolving power of a microscope is expressed in terms of **limit of resolution (LR)**.

Numerical Aperture
The NA of a microscope objective is a measure of its ability to gather light and resolve fine specimen detail at a fixed object distance. The NA of a lens is an index of its power of resolution. As the NA increases, the resolving power of the lens increases.

> **NOTE**
> 1 nanometer (nm) = 0.001 micrometer (μm) = 0.000001 mm

Magnification
The total magnification of a compound microscope is calculated by multiplying the power of objective with that of eyepiece.

Calculation of Total Magnification
With an eyepiece of 10x, the magnifications with the three objectives will be:
1. **Low power objective (10x)** = 10 × 10 = 100 times.
2. **High power objective (40x)** = 40 × 10 = 400 times.
3. **Oil immersion objective (100x)** = 100 × 10 = 1,000 times.

Image Formation in the Compound Microscope
It is the objective that starts the process of magnification. It forms a **real, inverted and enlarged** image (primary image: A′ B′) (Fig. 1.1.4) in the upper part of the body tube.

The field lens of the eyepiece collects the divergent rays of light of the primary image and passes these through the eye lens, which therefore the image seen by the eye is— virtual, inverted and highly magnified image. The light rays reaching the observer's eye are divergent and about 25 cm in front of the eye. Figure 1.1.4 shows the ray diagram of a compound microscope.

Working Distance
The working distance is the distance between the objective and the slide under study. This distance decreases with increasing magnification. It is 8–13 mm in LP, 1–3 mm in HP and 0.5–1.5 mm in OI lenses, respectively. Figure 1.1.5 shows the approximate working distances for each lens.

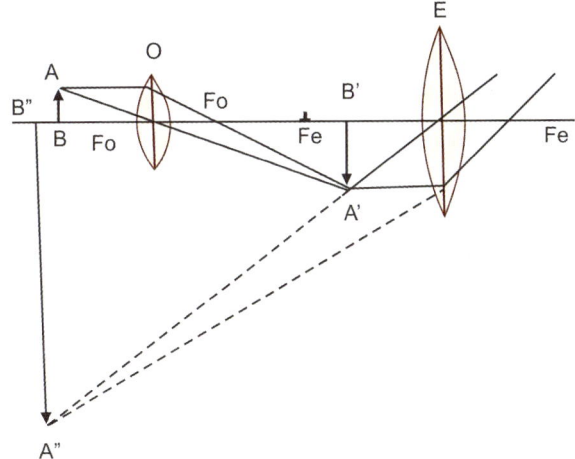

Fig. 1.1.4: The ray diagram of a compound microscope. AB = object; A′ B′ = real, inverted and magnified image; A″ B″ = virtual, inverted and magnified image; O = objective lens; E = Eyepiece; Fo = Focus of objective; Fe = Focus of eyepiece.

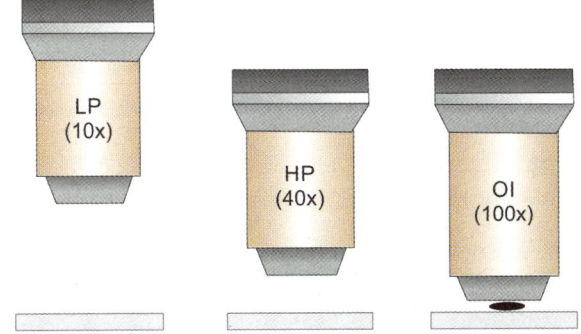

Fig. 1.1.5: Diagram to show the working distances of low power (LP), high power (HP) and oil immersion (OI) lenses.

FOCUSING OF AN OBJECT UNDER MICROSCOPE

Focusing Under Low Power (10x)

1. Place the microscope on your worktable in an upright position and raise the body tube 7–8 cm above the stage. Put the slide on the stage and, using the mechanical stage, bring the specimen over the central aperture.
2. Select and adjust the mirror (plane or concave) so that the light shines on the specimen.
3. Under LP before focusing the object, the condenser is brought to the lowest position and the iris diaphragm is slightly opened to cut down excess light.
4. Looking from the side and using the coarse adjustment, bring the body tube down so that the LP lens is about 1 cm above the slide. Now look into the eyepiece and gently raise the tube till the specimen comes into focus. When the image comes into focus, scan the entire field, racking the fine adjustment all the time.

Focusing Under High Power (40x)

1. For focusing under high magnification, simply rotate the nosepiece so that the HP lens clicks into position.
2. The iris diaphragm is partially opened.
3. The condenser has to be slightly raised midway to get maximum clarity in focusing. Use fine adjustment as required.
4. Look from the side and bring the lens down to about 1–2 mm above the slide. Now look into the microscope and raise the tube slowly and gently till the image comes into focus.

Focusing Under Oil Immersion (100x)

1. Place a drop of cedar wood oil on the slide.
2. Rotate the nosepiece so that the oil immersion lens comes above the slide. It will automatically dip into the oil drop.
3. The condenser has to be raised to its highest position and iris diaphragm should be fully opened.
4. Use the fine adjustment for focusing. When you move the slide, the oil will move with it.

> **NOTE**
> **"Racking the Microscope"**
> The cells and their constituents are three-dimensional structures and lie at different levels. Therefore, it is important not to keep a fixed focus but **to continuously "rack" the microscope by using fine adjustment** after the specimen has been brought under focus under any magnification.

COMMON DIFFICULTIES ENCOUNTERED BY STUDENTS

1. **The material cannot be focused or the image is very faint:**
   a. The slide may not be near the focus of the objective or there may be no visible material under it. Check this out and start with coarse adjustment once again.
   b. The slide bearing the material may have been placed upside down on the stage. The thickness of the glass slide does not allow the OI lens to reach down to its working distance. Reversing the slide will solve the problem.
2. **There may be a dark shadow in the field:** If the shadow rotates when the eyepiece is rotated, remove it and clean it or there may be an air bubble in the cedar wood oil.
3. **The field of view appears oval instead of round:** This problem arises when the objective has not been properly "clicked" into position.
4. **The illumination of the image is poor:** Check the source of light, angle of the mirror, the position of the condenser and iris diaphragm.
5. **The image does not come into focus even when the objective is in the lowest position and the fine adjustment cannot move down any further:** This happens when the fine adjustment screw reaches the end of its thread (turn) before the image is brought to its focus. To overcome this problem, turn the adjustment screw in the opposite direction for several turns and then use the coarse adjustment screw to regain the focus once again (It is therefore, best to keep the fine adjustment screw near the middle of its turning range).

PRECAUTIONS

1. Students using glasses should put on their glasses while using the microscope.
2. While using one eye with the monocular microscope, do not close the other eye as this will cause lot of strain on that eye.
3. Ensure that all the lenses are clean and free from dust.
4. Check the position of the objective, condenser and diaphragm to ensure optimal illumination.
5. Never lower the optical tube while looking into the microscope.
6. Once a specimen has been focused, continuously "rack" the microscope.
7. Clean all the lenses after using the microscope. Never leave cedar wood oil on the OI lens.
8. Carefully use the fine adjustment screw to obtain the exact focus while using high power and oil immersion lenses.

9. Use xylene swab to clean the objectives after using the microscope.

OTHER TYPES OF MICROSCOPES

Various types of microscopes have been specially introduced for particular purposes over the past many decades. Some of these are:

1. **Dissection microscope:** It is a binocular microscope used for microdissection under magnification.
2. **Dark-field microscope:** It employs a special condenser that causes light waves to cross on the material under study rather than passing through it. As a result the field of view appears dark (hence called "dark-field" in contrast to "bright-field" microscopy) against which the object appears bright.
3. **Phase-contrast microscope:** In this microscope, a special phase plate is inserted into the condenser, which can retard the speed of some light waves. Since the tissue cells and organisms have different refractive indices, this microscope uses these differences to produce an image with good contrast of light and shade.
4. **Interference-contrast microscope:** A special prism that can split a beam of light is added to the condenser to produce a three-dimensional image.
5. **Polarizing microscope:** It has a polarizer (filter), which is usually placed between the light source and the specimen and an analyzer, which is located between the objective and the eyepiece.
6. **Fluorescence microscope:** A fluorescent dye is used to stain tissues which are then studied under this microscope.
7. **Transmission electron microscope (TEM):** TEM uses a strong beam of electrons instead of light and electromagnetic fields in place of glass lenses.
8. **Scanning electron microscope (SEM):** This microscope, which achieves a resolution of about 30 Å, has been developed for three-dimensional study of surface topography of cells and object.

Objective Structured Practical Examination

Aim: To focus a given slide of blood film under LP/HP/OI lens.
Procedural steps: See text above.
Checklist:
1. Raise the body tube, put the slide on the stage and use mechanical stage to bring the object over the central aperture.
2. Choose the light source and correctly bring the different objective lenses into position.
3. Adjust the position of the condenser and iris diaphragm for:
   a. LP   b. HP   c. OI
4. Look from the side while lowering the body tube.
5. Adjust the light and use coarse and fine adjustment screws.
6. Rack the microscope constantly.

QUESTIONS

Q.1. Why is the microscope called a compound microscope? What type of image is produced by it?

Q.2. When will we use a plane mirror or a concave mirror in a light microscope?

Q.3. What is the total magnification of a compound microscope and how will you calculate it?

Q.4. What is meant by the term numerical aperture? What is its significance?

Q.5. How will you identify oil immersion objective lens? Why is cedar wood oil used with this lens and not with others?
There is a thin layer of air between this objective and the glass slide when the lens is in focus. When light passes from a denser medium (glass of the slide) into a rarer medium (the thin layer of air), they are refracted away from the normal. As a result, when light rays emerge from the slide, many of them are refracted away from the aperture of the objective and very few enter it and a faint image results. Cedar wood oil, which has the same refractive index as that of glass, i.e. 1.55 (air = 1.00; water = 1.33), removes this layer of air so that the glass of the slide and the objective lens become a continuous column (thus avoiding refraction) and allow enough light to enter the objective. **Other mediums that can be used are glycerin and paraffin, their refractive indexes being 1.35–1.40. However, cedar wood oil, though costly, gives best results.**

Q.6. Will you see any image with the oil immersion lens without the cedar wood oil?

Q.7. Why does the oil immersion lens have pinhole-sized aperture?
The aperture being very small, it allows only the central cone of light to pass through and form the image. Had the diameter been large, excessive refraction would have caused spherical and chromatic aberrations, thus making the image indistinct.

Q.8. Why should the position of the condenser be low with the LP lens and highest with oil immersion lens?
Since the aperture of the LP lens is wide, a high condenser would allow too much light to enter the microscope and cause glare. The position of the condenser with the oil immersion lens has to be highest to allow enough light to enter it through its pin-hole aperture.

Q.9. What are the factors affecting illumination when using a microscope and why?
The clarity of an image depends on an optimal (ideal) amount of light available. The illumination (the process of providing light) can be altered by raising or lowering the condenser and opening or closing the diaphragm. A proper combination of the two has to be selected under different conditions. In general, we require less illumination when viewing a clear, unstained object and greater illumination when viewing a stained preparation.

Q.10. What is meant by racking the microscope and what is its importance?
Since the cells and their components are three-dimensional entities and situated at different levels, the focus has to be constantly changed to see all these structures.

Q.11. What are the other types of microscopes?

STUDY NOTES

Date ....

CHAPTER 1.2

Collection of Blood Sample

AIM

Collection of blood sample.

INTRODUCTION

Two types of blood samples are used. When small quantity of blood is required for investigations, capillary blood is used. When the large quantity of blood is required venous blood is used.

ASEPSIS

The term asepsis refers to the condition of being free from septic or infectious material—bacteria, viruses, etc. Puncturing the skin always poses the danger of infection. In order to achieve asepsis, the following aspects need to be kept in mind.

Sterilization of Equipment

All the instruments to be used for collecting blood—syringes, needles, lancets and cotton and gauze swabs—should preferably be sterilized in an autoclave. Disposable sterile needles and lancets are now in common use.

Cleaning/Sterilization of Skin

At least 2–3 sterile cotton/gauze swabs soaked in 70% alcohol, methylated spirit or ether should be used to clean and scrub the area.

> **NOTE**
> After cleaning the skin, allow the alcohol to dry by evaporation (do not blow on it), because sterilization with alcohol is effective only after it has dried.

Prevention of Contamination

Any material used for skin puncture or the operator's hands may cause contamination. Therefore, once the site has been cleaned and dried, it should not be touched again.

COLLECTION OF BLOOD SAMPLE

Capillary Blood

The skin and other tissues are richly supplied with capillaries, so when a drop or a few drops of blood are required, as for estimation of Hb, cell counts, bleeding time (BT) and clotting time (CT), blood films, microchemical tests, etc., blood from a skin puncture (skin-prick) with a lancet or needle is adequate. Capillary blood is also called **"peripheral blood"** as it comes out of the peripheral vessels (capillaries) in contrast to venous blood (Table 1.2.1).

In adults and older children, capillary blood is generally obtained from a skin puncture made on the tip of the middle or ring finger or on the lobe of the ear. In infants and young children in whom the fingers are too small for a prick, the medial or lateral side of the pad of the big toe or heel is used. The site for skin-prick should be clean and free from edema, infection, skin disease, callus or circulatory defects.

Table 1.2.1: Differences between venous and capillary blood.

Venous blood	Capillary blood
It is obtained from a superficial vein by venepuncture	It is obtained from a skin puncture, usually over a finger, ear lobe/or the heel of a foot
A clean venepuncture provides blood without any contamination with tissue fluid	Blood from a skin prick comes from punctured capillaries and from smallest arterioles and venules
There is less risk of contamination since sterile syringe and needle are used	There is greater risk of contamination and transmission of disease as one may be careless about sterilization since skin prick is considered a harmless procedure
Cell counts, Hb and PCV values are generally higher	These values are likely to be on the lower side since some tissue fluid is bound to dilute the blood even when it is free-flowing
Venous blood is preferable when normal blood standards are to be established or when two samples from the same person are to be compared at different times	Capillary blood is not suitable for these purposes

(PCV: packed cell volume)

Apparatus

1. **Blood lancet/Pricking needle:** Disposable, sterile, one-time use blood lancets are commercially available and should be preferred.
2. Sterile gauze/cotton moist with 70% alcohol/methylated spirit.
3. Glass slides, pipettes, etc. according to requirements.

Procedure

1. All aseptic precautions must be taken. Clean the finger with the spirit swab.
2. Allow the alcohol to dry by evaporation for the following reasons:
   - Sterilization with alcohol/spirit is effective only after it has dried by evaporation.
   - The thin film of alcohol can cause the blood drop to spread sideways along with alcohol so that it will not form a satisfactory round drop.
     ◆ The alcohol may cause hemolysis of blood.
3. Prick the finger sharply and quickly to a depth of 3–4 mm. The blood should start to flow slowly, spontaneously and freely (without any squeezing)—if a good prick has been given.

> **IMPORTANT**
> Do not squeeze or press the finger as the tissue fluid squeezed out will dilute the blood and give false low values. The forearm or the hand may be squeezed or milked toward the fingers to facilitate blood flow. If all efforts fail, a fresh prick may be required.

4. Wipe away the first drops of blood with dry, sterile gauze as it may be contaminated with tissue fluid.
5. Allow a fresh drop of blood of sufficiently large size (about 3–4 mm diameter) to well up from the wound and make a blood smear or fill a pipette as the case may be.
6. Clean the area of the prick with a fresh swab and ask the subject to keep the swab pressed on the wound with his/her thumb till the bleeding stops, which occurs in a minute or so.

Precautions

1. The selected site should be clean, free from infection, edema or skin disease.
2. The site should be cleaned with sterile gauze and alcohol.
3. The lancet/needle should be sterile.
4. The puncture should be deep enough to give free-flowing blood but not so deep that it takes inordinately long time for the bleeding to stop.
5. Do not press or squeeze the finger to increase the blood flow.

Earlobe Prick

With the use of a sterile needle or corner edge of a sterile blade give a 2-mm deep prick (The skin here is usually thinner than at the fingertip). Wipe away the first drop and allow a new one to form.

Pricking the Heel

In infants and young children, blood can be collected from the cleaned medial or lateral areas of the heel.

> **NOTE**
> The central plantar and the posterior curvature areas of the heel should be avoided as the prick may cause injury to the underlying tarsal bones which lie near the surface.

Venous Blood

When larger amount of blood are needed as for complete hematological and biochemical investigations, venous blood is obtained with a syringe and needle by puncturing a superficial vein.

> **NOTE**
> Venous blood is always preferred for clinical tests.

Apparatus

Keep the following equipment ready before venepuncture:
1. Disposable gloves.
2. Sterile, disposable, 10 mL syringe with side nozzle.
3. 10 mL test tubes/vials with or without anticoagulant.
4. Sterile gauze pieces moist with 70% alcohol/methylated spirit.
5. Tourniquet: A 2-3 cm wide elastic bandage with Velcro strips to keep it securely in place can be used. An inflated BP cuff can also be used.

Procedure

1. Compress the upper arm to make the veins prominent. The antecubital vein is embedded in subcutaneous fat and is usually sufficiently large to take a wide-bore needle. It also runs straight for about 3 cm and is usually palpable—even in obese subjects.
2. Apply the tourniquet about 2-3 cm above the elbow to obstruct the venous return. The subject may open and close the fist to increase the venous return and make the veins engorged (filled) with blood.
3. Clean the skin over the selected vein with gauze and alcohol and allow it to dry.
4. Puncture the skin and push in the needle under the skin with a firm and smooth thrust, at an angle of 15-20° to the skin.
5. Slightly pull the plunger back with your thumb and little finger to produce a little negative pressure in the syringe. Advance the needle gently along the vein and puncture it from the side, a few milliliters ahead of the skin puncture. This prevents counterpuncture of the opposite wall of the vein and formation of a hematoma (local leakage of blood).
6. As the vein is punctured, all resistance will suddenly cease and blood will start to enter the syringe. Do not withdraw blood faster than the punctured veins is filling; as too much pressure applied to the plunger is likely to cause mechanical injury and hemolysis of red cells. The subject may open and close the fist to enhance venous return.
7. When enough blood has been collected, release the tourniquet and press a fresh swab over the skin puncture. Withdraw the needle gently but keep the swab in position. Ask the subject to flex the arm and keep it so as to maintain pressure on the puncture site till the bleeding stops.

    Expel the blood gently into the container; do not apply force as it may cause mechanical injury to red cells. Gently shake or swirl the container between your palms so that the anticoagulant (if used) mixes well with the blood without frothing.

> **IMPORTANT**
> The entire process of withdrawing blood should be completed within 2 minutes of applying the tourniquet because stagnation of blood in the vein is likely to increase the cell counts.

Precautions

1. All aseptic precautions must be observed and disposable gloves, syringe and needles must be used.
2. The tourniquet (or the BP cuff) must be removed before taking the needle out of the vein to avoid formation of hematoma.
3. The blood from the syringe should be transferred to the container without delay to prevent clotting.
4. Ask the subject to keep the swab in position till the bleeding from the puncture site stops.

Arterial Blood

When arterial blood is needed for special tests, such as blood pH, gas levels, etc. an artery, such as radial or femoral is punctured with a syringe and needle. This, however, is not a routine procedure.

For a sample of whole blood or plasma: The blood is transferred to a container containing a suitable anticoagulant. This is to prevent clotting of blood.

COMMONLY USED ANTICOAGULANTS

Anticoagulants are substances employed to delay, suppress or prevent clotting of blood.

Anticoagulants for In Vitro Use

Ethylenediamine Tetraacetic Acid (EDTA)

Both the potassium and sodium salts of EDTA are strong anticoagulants. The dry (anhydrous) dipotassium salt of EDTA, being more readily soluble than the sodium salt, is the anticoagulant of choice. The tripotassium salt of EDTA causes some shrinkage of RBCs that results in 2-3% decrease in packed cell volume.

Mode of action: EDTA prevents clotting by removing ionic calcium (which is an essential clotting factor) from the blood sample by **chelation**. The platelets appear clear and are neither aggregated nor destroyed.

Preparation: EDTA is used in a concentration of 1 mg/mL of blood. 0.2 mL of 2.5% solution of the salt placed in a container and dried in gentle heat in an oven is sufficient for 5 mL of blood. This provides 1 mg of EDTA/mL of blood (a number of containers can be prepared from the stock solution at a time).

> **NOTE**
> Excess of EDTA (more than 2 mg/mL blood) affects all blood cells. Red cells shrink, thus reducing packed cell volume (PCV), while WBCs show degenerative changes. Platelets break up into large enough fragments to be counted as normal platelets. Care should, therefore, be taken to use correct amount of EDTA and blood should be thoroughly mixed with the anticoagulant.

Uses: Except for coagulation studies EDTA is used for most hematological tests.

Trisodium Citrate

Trisodium citrate is the anticoagulant of choice in blood tests for disorders of coagulation.
Mode of action: Acts as a chelating agent (inactivates calcium ions).
Preparation: 3.8% solution is prepared in distilled water and then sterilized.
Uses: Citrate and blood in the ratio of 1:9, is used for coagulation studies and for ESR test by the Westergren's method in the ratio of 1:4. Along with other components, sodium citrate is used for storing donated blood in blood banks (*Refer* Chapter 1.9), since it can be safely given intravenously. Oxalates are toxic and cannot be given intravenously.

Double Oxalate Mixture

This is a mixture of ammonium oxalate and potassium oxalate in the ratio of 3:2. It is thus called double oxalate. It is an effective anticoagulant.
Mode of action: Oxalates prevent clotting by forming insoluble calcium salts, thus removing ionic calcium.
Preparation: A large number of containers can be prepared at a time by placing 0.2 mL of oxalate mixture (3.0 g of ammonium oxalate and 2.0 g of potassium oxalate in 100 mL of distilled water) in each container and drying in gentle heat in an oven. This amount is sufficient for 8–10 mL of blood. Too much oxalate is hypertonic and damages all blood cells, while too little will not prevent clotting.
Uses: Though each oxalate by itself can prevent clotting, a mixture is used. Sodium oxalate should not be used since it causes crenation of red cells. Ammonium salt should not be used in urea and nonprotein nitrogen tests. It is used in the tests where the cell volume should remain unaffected, e.g. erythrocyte sedimentation rate (ESR), PCV.

Sodium Fluoride

A mixture of 10 mg of sodium fluoride and 1 mg thymol is an anticoagulant as well as a preservative when a blood sample has to be stored for a few days. Since fluoride inhibits glycolytic enzymes (thus preventing loss of glucose), it is employed when plasma glucose is to be estimated.

Heparin

Heparin, a highly charged mixture of sulfated polysaccharides and related to chondroitin, has a molecular weight ranging from 15,000 to 18,000 and is a naturally occurring powerful anticoagulant. It is normally secreted by mast cells that are present in many tissues, especially immediately outside many of the capillaries in the body. Both mast cells and basophils release heparin directly into blood. Heparin is also a cofactor for the lipoprotein lipase—the clearing factor.

Commercial heparin is extracted from many different tissues and is available in almost pure form (it was first extracted from the liver—hence the name "heparin"). Low molecular weight fragments (5,000 units) have been produced from unfractionated heparin and are being used clinically since they have a longer half-life and produce more predictable results.
Mode of action and uses: Heparin by itself has no anticoagulant activity. However, when it combines with **antithrombin III,** the ability of the latter to remove thrombin (as soon as it is formed) increases hundreds of times. The complex of these two substances removes many other activated clotting factors—IX, X, XI and XII.
Preparation: Theoretically, heparin is an ideal anticoagulant since no foreign substance is introduced into the blood. The required amount of stock solution is taken in a number of containers and dried at low heat. At a concentration of 10–20 IU/mL blood, it does not change red cell size and their osmotic fragility. It is, however, inferior to EDTA for general use. It should not be used for leukocyte counts, as these cells tend to clump. It also imparts a blue tinge to the background of blood films.
Uses: It is used for estimation of blood gases, pH assay and osmotic fragility. Clinically, it is used to prevent intravascular clotting of blood.

Acid-citrate-dextrose and Citrate-phosphate-dextrose-adenine

Acid-citrate-dextrose (ACD) and citrate-phosphate-dextrose-adenine (CPD-A) are the anticoagulants of choice for storing donated blood in blood banks (*Refer* Chapter 1.9). The CPD-A mixture is preferred as it preserves 2, 3-diphosphoglycerate (2, 3-DPG) better.

Anticoagulants for In Vivo Use

The two in vivo anticoagulants are heparin and coumarins. Patients at increased risk of forming blood clots in their blood vessels, e.g. leg veins during prolonged confinement to bed or during long flights, are sometimes put on these drugs (e.g. warfarin) to prevent thromboembolism. Their bleeding time, clotting time and prothrombin time (PT) are checked from time to time to adjust the dosage of the drug.

Dicoumarol and Warfarin

The coumarin derivatives are vitamin K antagonists and thus inhibit the action of this vitamin that is essential as a cofactor for the synthesis of six glutamic acid-containing proteins—namely, factors II (prothrombin), VII, IX and X, protein C and protein S. The action of this anticoagulant is, however, slower than that of heparin.

Heparin

It is particularly used during open-heart surgery in which the blood has to be passed through a heart-lung machine; or the dialysis machine during hemodialysis in kidney failure and then back into the patient.

> **IMPORTANT**
> Anticoagulant therapy should not be confused with thrombolytic agents employed for dissolving blood clots (*Refer* Chapter 1.10).

QUESTIONS

- Q.1. What measures are taken to prevent infection during venepuncture and skin-pricking?
- Q.2. What are the sources and main differences between venous blood and capillary blood? Why is capillary blood called peripheral blood?
- Q.3. What is the difference between plasma and serum? How will you get a sample of each?
- Q.4. What precautions will you observe to prevent hemolysis of venous blood sample?
- Q.5. What are anticoagulants? What is meant by *in vivo* and *in vitro* anticoagulants?
- Q.6. Why are the thumb and little finger not pricked?
- Q.7. What are the sites for collecting capillary blood in infants?
- Q.8. Why should the pricked finger not be squeezed? What is meant by free-flowing blood and why should it be preferred over squeezed blood?

Section 1: Hematology

STUDY NOTES

Teacher's Signature

Date ....

CHAPTER 1.3

Estimation of Hemoglobin

AIM

To estimate hemoglobin by Sahli's hemoglobinometer.

PRINCIPLE

The hemoglobin (Hb) present in a measured amount of blood is converted by dilute hydrochloric acid into acid hematin, which is golden brown in color. The intensity of color depends on the concentration of acid hematin which, in turn, depends on the concentration of Hb. The color of the solution, after dilution with water, is matched with the color of the comparator by direct vision. The readings are obtained in g%.

NORMAL VALUES

- Newborns : 18–22 g/dL
- At 3 months : 14–16 g/dL
- 3 months to 1 year : 13–15 g/dL
- Adult males : 14.5 g/dL (14–18 g/dL)
- Adult females : 12.5 g/dL (12–15 g/dL).

APPARATUS

1. Sahli's hemoglobinometer (Figs. 1.3.1A to C)
   a. **Comparator:** It is a rectangular plastic box with a slot in the middle which accommodates the calibrated Hb tube. Nonfading, standardized, golden brown glass rods are fitted on each side of the slot for matching the color. An opaque white glass (or plastic) is fitted behind the slot to provide uniform illumination during direct visual color matching.
   b. **Hemoglobinometer tube:** The square or round glass tube is calibrated in gram percent (2–24 g%) in yellow color on one side and in percentage Hb (20–160%) in red color on the other side (Fig. 1.3.1B).
   c. **Hemoglobinometer pipette:** It is a glass capillary pipette with only a single calibration mark—0.02 mL (20 mm^3 or 20 µL) (Fig. 1.3.1C). There is no bulb in this pipette (as compared to blood cell pipettes) as no dilution of blood is done.

   > **NOTE**
   > The calibration mark 20 mm^3 indicates a definite, measured volume and not an arbitrary volume.

   d. **Stirrer:** It is a thin glass rod with a flattened end which is used for stirring and mixing the blood and dilute acid.
   e. **Glass dropper**.
   f. **Distilled water**.
2. N/10 hydrochloric acid (HCl)
3. Pricking apparatus.

SAHLI'S ACID HEMATIN METHOD

Procedure

1. Using a dropper, place N/10 HCl in the Hb tube, up to the lowest mark (20% or 2 g%).
2. Make a bold finger prick under aseptic conditions, wipe away the first drop of blood. When a large drop of

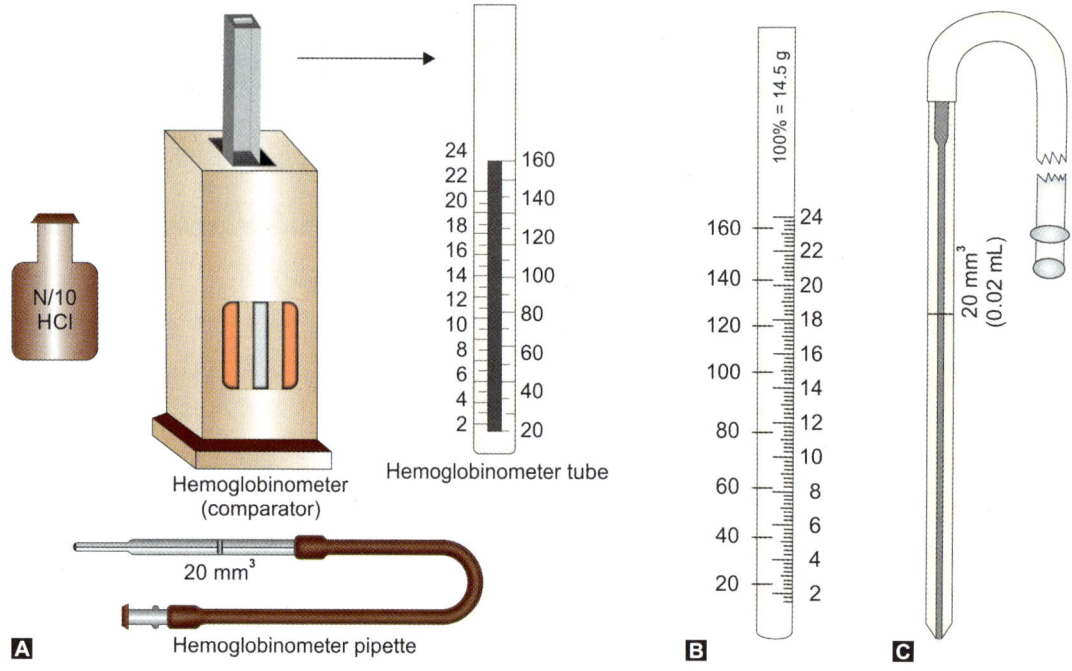

Figs.1.3A to C: (A) Sahli's hemoglobinometer; (B) Graduated hemoglobinometer tube; (C) Hemoglobinometer pipette.

free-flowing blood has formed, hold the pipette horizontally, apply its tip to the drop and then draw blood up to the 20 μL mark, taking care that no air bubbles are formed. Carefully wipe the blood sticking to the tip of the pipette, but avoid touching the bore or else blood will be drawn out by capillary action.

> **NOTE**
> If any blood remains sticking to the outside of the pipette, it will be that much extra blood in addition to 20 mm³.

3. Immediately immerse the tip of the pipette to the bottom of the acid solution and expel the blood gently. Rinse the pipette three to four times by drawing up the acid solution till all the blood has been washed out from it. Avoid frothing of the mixture.
4. Withdraw the pipette from the tube ensuring that no mixture is carried out of the tube. Mix the blood with the acid solution with the flat end of the stirrer.
5. Put the Hb tube back in the comparator and let it stand for 10 minutes. During this time, the acid ruptures the red cells, releasing their Hb into the solution (hemolysis). The acid acts on the Hb and converts it into **acid hematin**, which is deep golden brown in color.
6. **Diluting and matching the color:** Then dilute the acid hematin solution by adding distilled water (preferably by buffered water) drop by drop stirring the mixture each time till its color matches the color of the standard tinted glass rods in the comparator (Fig. 1.3.2).

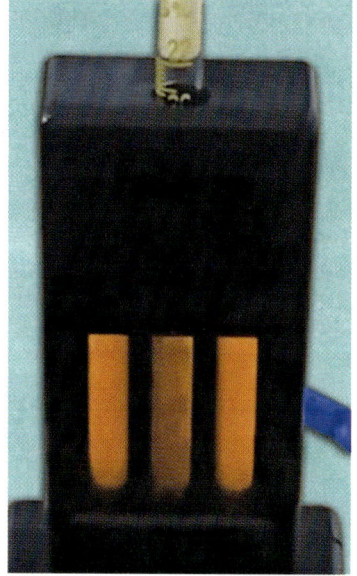

Fig. 1.3.2: Comparator.

> **NOTE**
> Each time you compare the color, lift and hold the glass stirrer against the side of the Hb tube above the solution (**rather than taking it out completely**) thus allowing it to drain fully back into the tube. If the stirrer is left in the solution, it will lighten the color (since it is translucent) and thus matching will occur earlier. This will give a false low value. If, however, it is taken out every time the color is matched, it is bound to take away some of the solution out of the tube, thus, again giving a low value.

7. Hold the comparator at eye level, away from your face, against bright natural light. Read the **lower meniscus (lower meniscus is read in colored transparent solutions)**.

> **NOTE**
> The color of acid hematin does not develop fully immediately, but its intensity increases with time, reaching a maximum, after which it starts to decrease. An adequate time, usually 10 minutes, must be allowed before its dilution is started. In less time, all Hb may not be converted into acid hematin.

8. Compare the color of the solution in the tube with that of the standard and record the observations in your workbook.
   Take two readings, one just darker and other just lighter.
   Take the average of two readings as shown here and report your result as: Hb- ....g/dL.

Advantages of Sahli's Method
1. The method is simple, fairly quick and accurate.
2. It does not require any costly apparatus, since it needs only direct color matching.
3. Its cost is minimal and therefore can be used in mass surveys.

Disadvantages of Sahli's Method
1. Since the acid hematin is not in true solution, some turbidity may occur.
2. The method estimates only the oxyHb and reduced Hb, other forms, such as carboxyhemoglobin (carboxyHb) and metHb are not estimated.
3. Also the **degree of error (10–15%)** is high.
4. The color of the standard may not always be reliable, especially if an old apparatus is used.

Sources of Error
False results with this method may be due to:
1. **Technical error:** It may be due to not taking exactly 20 mm^3 blood, not giving enough time for formation of acid hematin or using an old comparator that has faded glass rods.
2. **Personal error:** Generally, it is not difficult to match color but since it is a visual method, color matching may vary from person to person.

Precautions
1. All precautions mentioned for blood collection and filling of the pipette must be observed.
2. The finger should not be squeezed and there should not be any blood sticking to the outside of the pipette tip.
3. To prevent clotting of the blood in the pipette, blood should be transferred immediately into the tube containing N/10 HCl.
4. Only the recommended time should be allowed for the formation of acid hematin by the action of acid on Hb.
5. When diluting the color of acid hematin solution, avoid overdilution by adding distilled water drop by drop.
6. The color matching should be done against the natural source of light.
7. The stirrer should never be taken out of the tube.
8. When matching the color, the solution should be uniformly golden brown throughout the solution.
   Dark color near the bottom of the tube indicates poor mixing.
9. During color matching, two readings should be taken to reduce the personal error.

PHYSIOCLINICAL SIGNIFICANCE

Increased level of Hb may be due to:
1. **Experimental error:**
   a. Blood taken more than 20 mm^3
   b. Blood sticking to the outside of the pipette tip
   c. Fading of colored glass standards.
2. **High red cell count:**
   a. *Physiological:*
      - Males
      - Newborns
      - High altitude.
   b. *Pathological:*
      - Polycythemia
      - Hypoxia due to heart or lung diseases.

Decreased level of Hb may be due to:
1. **Experimental error:**
   a. Blood sample diluted with tissue fluid
   b. Blood taken is less than 20 mm^3
   c. Less than the required quantity of N/10 HCl is taken for hemolysis purpose
   d. Color of acid hematin is not allowed to develop fully.
2. **Decreased red cell count:**
   a. *Physiological:* Females during pregnancy (hemodilution)
   b. *Pathological:* All causes of **anemia.**

Section 1: Hematology

> **Objective Structured Practical Examination**
>
> **Aim:** To convert a known volume of blood sample into acid hematin using the apparatus provided.
> **Procedural steps:** See text above.
> **Checklist:**
> 1. Select the Hb pipette and tube and check that they are clean and dry. (Y/N)
> 2. Take N/10 HCl in the Hb tube up to the mark 20% or 2 g%. (Y/N)
> 3. Shake the container of blood and draw blood into the pipette exactly to the mark 20 µL. (Y/N)
> 4. Wipe off blood from the tip of the pipette and blow out the blood into acid solution. (Y/N)
> 5. Rinse the pipette several times into acid solution. Note the time. (Y/N)

QUESTIONS

Q.1. What is meant by the term "normality" of a solution?
The normality (N) of a solution is the number of gram equivalents in 1 liter of water. In a normal (N) solution, 1 g equivalent weight of a substance is dissolved in 1 liter of solvent.

Q.2. What is the underlying principle of this experiment?

Q.3. Can strong acids (such as nitric, sulfuric and hydrochloric acids) or alkalis be used in place of N/10 HCl?
- The strong acids which are very strong oxidizing agents and alkalis will cause disruption of Hb and thus cannot be used.
- Only N/10 HCl is used because standardization has been done for acid hematin.

Q.4. How would estimation of hemoglobin be affected if less or more than 8–10 drops of N/10 HCl is taken in the hemoglobin tube?
- If less acid is taken, the blood may not mix well and/or may clot. All the Hb will not be converted into acid hematin. This will result in false low value.
- If much more acid is taken, the final color developed in a case of anemia would be much lighter than the standard. Color matching will then not be possible, because the color of the solution cannot be concentrated.

Q.5. Can tap water be used for diluting and color matching?
No, it cannot be used because its salt content and impurities may cause turbidity which will interfere with the color matching.

Q.6. Can N/10 HCl be used (if distilled water is not available) for diluting and color matching?
Yes, it can be used because it being transparent, it cannot further deepen the color once all the Hb has been converted into acid hematin.

Q.7. Why is it necessary to wait for 10 minutes after adding blood to N/10 HCl solution?

Q.8. While matching the color, why is it important to lift the stirrer above the solution and not leave it there or take it out?

Q.9. Which of the two scales given on the hemoglobin tube are preferred over the other and why?
The scale which gives the Hb concentration in a blood sample directly in gram percent is used. The scale in percentages is of no value as there is no standard single value of Hb which can be taken as 100%.

Q.10. What are the normal levels and ranges of hemoglobin at different ages?

Q.11. Compared to males, why are the hemoglobin levels lower in females?
- It is the estrogen in the females which has an inhibitory effect on the secretion of erythropoietin (EP) which is the main stimulant of red cell production.
- Also, the androgens (mainly testosterone) has a stimulatory effect on EP secretion. Both these factors tend to keep the red cell count higher in males.

Q.12. Why is the hemoglobin level high in the newborns?
The Hb may be as high as 20–22 g/dL at the time of birth due to the high red cell count (>6 million/mm^3). The newborn has been living in state of relative hypoxia which is a very potent stimulus for the secretion of EP. As age advances, the Hb levels decrease and adult levels are reached in a few years.

Q.13. What would happen if hemoglobin were present freely in the plasma instead of in the red cells?
- Increase in viscosity of blood.
- Hemoglobin might get excreted out by getting filtered through the kidney. This would cause severe damage to the kidneys.

Q.14. What are the common causes of increased and decreased hemoglobin readings?

Q.15. What are the different types of hemoglobin?
Different types of hemoglobin are:
1. **Normal hemoglobin**
   a. **Adult hemoglobin (HbA):**
      i. Hemoglobin A: $\alpha_2\beta_2$
      ii. Hemoglobin A$_2$: $\alpha_2\delta_2$
   b. **Fetal hemoglobin (HbF):** $\alpha_2\gamma_2$
   c. **Embryonic hemoglobin:** $\zeta_2\varepsilon_2$
   d. HbA1c is characterized by α_2 and β_2 globin chains. It is formed by the covalent binding of glucose to HbA. The levels of HbA1c increase in poorly controlled diabetes mellitus.
2. **Abnormal hemoglobin**
   a. *Hemoglobin S (HbS):* In sickle cell anemia, the alpha chains are normal but in each beta chain, one glutamic acid residue has been replaced by a valine residue.
   b. The abnormal HbS are associated with two types of inherited anemias:
      i. Hemoglobinopathies: These are due to abnormal chains.

ii. **Thalassemias:** The chains are normal, but are less in amount or even absent. The α- and β-thalassemias are defined by decreased or even absent α- and β-polypeptides.

Q.16. What are the differences between adult and fetal hemoglobin?

Differences between adult and fetal hemoglobin.	
Adult hemoglobin	Fetal hemoglobin
Contains four polypeptide chains (two alpha and two beta chains)	The two beta chains replaced by gamma chains
Appears in red cells of the fetus in 5th month. At birth, 20% of total Hb is HbA	HbF at birth makes up 80% of total Hb. Disappears by 5th month after birth
Lifespan long—120 days	Lifespan short—about 2 weeks
It has the usual affinity for oxygen	It has greater affinity for oxygen as it binds 2,3-BPG less avidly
Percentage saturation at a pO_2 of 20 mm Hg = 30–35%	Percentage saturation at a pO_2 of 20 mm Hg = 70%

Q.17. What are the derivatives of hemoglobin?
1. **Oxyhemoglobin (HbO_2):** Hb contains four iron atoms, each molecule of Hb carries four molecules of oxygen.
2. **Reduced (deoxygenated) hemoglobin:** It is hemoglobin from which O_2 has been removed.
3. **Carbaminohemoglobin:** In this, CO_2 is attached to the globin part of Hb. The affinity of Hb for CO_2 is about 20 times that for oxygen.
4. **Carboxyhemoglobin:** Carbon monoxide is attached to Hb where O_2 is normally attached. The affinity of Hb for CO is 200–300 times that for O_2.
5. **Methemoglobin (MetHb):** When blood is exposed to some drugs or oxidizing agents in vitro or in vivo, the ferrous iron of Hb is converted into ferric iron forming metHb which is dark in color.
6. **Sulfhemoglobin:** It is formed by the action of some drugs and chemicals (e.g. sulfonamides), the reaction being irreversible.
7. **Cyanmethemoglobin (cyanmetHb):** It is formed by the action of cyanide on Hb.

Q.18. What are the other methods of estimating hemoglobin?
1. **Spectrophotometric methods:** In these methods, a photoelectric colorimeter is employed to measure the amount of light absorbed by a derivative of Hb.
   a. *Oxyhemoglobin method:* The blood is treated with ammonium hydroxide or sodium carbonate. The red cells are hemolyzed and the Hb is converted immediately and quickly into oxyHb. The solution is then compared with a standard gray screen in photoelectric colorimeter.
   b. *Cyanmethemoglobin method:* All forms of Hb normally present in blood (i.e. oxyHb, reduced Hb, carboxyHb and metHb) are converted into a stable compound—cyanmetHb. The sample of blood is treated with modified Drabkin's reagent (it contains potassium cyanide, potassium ferricyanide and potassium phosphate—the last replacing sodium bicarbonate of Drabkin's reagent). This method is the most accurate method of estimating Hb.
2. **Alkaline hematin method:** The blood is treated with N/10 NaOH, which converts all forms of Hb into alkaline hematin which is in true solution. There are two methods: (1) the standard method and (2) acid alkaline method.
3. **Haldane's carboxyhemoglobin method:** The red cells are hemolyzed in distilled water to release Hb. Carbon monoxide is then passed through the solution to form carboxyHb that is bright red in color. The color is then compared with that of the standard.
4. **Tallquist method:** A drop of blood absorbed on a white filter paper is allowed to spread over the paper to form an even spot. As soon as the blood spot loses its shine (gloss), but before it dries, it is matched against a scale of increasingly dark red-colored round spots printed on a card. The method, though quick, is rather inaccurate due to personal error. It is sometimes used in mass surveys for anemia.
5. **Copper sulfate falling drop method:** It is a rapid method for estimating the approximate level of Hb and is used in large surveys.

Q.19. How can oxygen-carrying capacity be calculated if you know the Hb concentration?
Knowing your Hb concentration and that 1 g of Hb can carry 1.34 mL of O_2, calculate its oxygen-carrying capacity = Hb content × 1.34 = …….mL O_2/dL.
Normal values: Males: 21 mL/dL
Females: 18 mL/dL

Q.20. What do you understand by 100% saturation of hemoglobin with oxygen?
When blood is equilibrated with pure (100%) oxygen at a pO_2 of 120 mm Hg, the Hb gets 100% saturated.

Q.21. What is the physioclinical significance of this experiment?

Q.22. Define anemia. How will you grade its severity based on Hb content?
Anemia is defined as the decrease in number of RBCs less than 4 million/mm³ or hemoglobin content less than 12 g/dL or both.
Depending on Hb concentration grading of severity of anemia may be:
- **Mild:** Hb = 9–11 g/dL
- **Moderate:** Hb = 7–9 g/dL
- **Severe:** Hb = Below 7 g/dL

Q.23. What are the common causes of anemia in India?
1. Chronic loss of blood, e.g. worm infestation
2. Deficiency of nutrients—deficiency of iron, vitamin B_{12} and folic acid.

Normally, about 1% of RBCs are destroyed daily (cells present in about 50 mL of blood) and equal numbers (about 3 million/second) enter the circulation. It may be caused when more cells are lost or when less cells are produced or both. It will develop if:

- Red cell production is normal but loss is increased.
- Red cell production is decreased but loss remains normal.
- Red cell production is decreased and loss is also increased.

Q.24. How do you classify anemia?

1. **Morphological causes:**
   a. Normochromic microcytic anemia
   b. Hypochromic microcytic anemia—iron deficiency anemia
   c. Normochromic normocytic anemia
   d. Macrocytic anemia—B_{12} and folic acid deficiency anemia **(there can be no hyperchromic anemia because the saturation of red cells with Hb cannot exceed the normal upper limit of 36%).**

2. **Etiological causes:**
   a. *Excessive blood loss:* The anemia is usually normocytic. The common causes include: Large wounds, bleeding piles, peptic ulcer, hookworm infestation, malarial parasites or heavy menstruation. Excessive RBC loss or destruction.
   b. *Inadequate RBC production.*
   c. *Nutritional (deficiency) anemias:* These are due to lack of essential nutrients, such as iron, vitamin B_{12}, folic acid, etc. Iron deficiency anemia: This is the most common type of anemia.
   d. *Hemolytic anemias:* The red cell plasma membranes (cell membranes) rupture prematurely and pour their Hb into the plasma (hemolysis).
      It may be inherited or acquired:
      i. Inherited: This can be due to **structural abnormalities** (hereditary spherocytosis and hereditary elliptocytosis), **defects in hemoglobin production** (thalassemia, sickle cell anemia) and **defective enzyme production**.
      ii. Acquired: The hemolysis of red cells may result from parasites (malaria), bacterial toxins, snake venom, adverse drug reactions (aspirin), autoimmunity, etc.
   e. *Aplastic anemia:* There is suppression or destruction of red bone marrow due to overexposure to ionizing radiations (gamma rays, X-rays); adverse drug reactions that inhibit enzymes needed for erythropoiesis (drugs, such as chloramphenicol, sulfonamides and cytotoxic drugs used in treatment of cancers may cause this anemia). The anemia is usually normocytic.
   f. *Anemias due to chronic diseases:* Tuberculosis, chronic infections, cancers, lung diseases, etc. frequently cause anemia.

OBSERVATION

S. No.	Just darker (g/dL)	Just lighter (g/dL)	Average (g/dL)

RESULT

The Hb content of my blood is..........

....

....

....

....

....

INTERPRETATION

....

....

....

....

....

STUDY NOTES

CHAPTER 1.4

Hemocytometry

INTRODUCTION

Hemocytometry is the procedure of counting the number of cells in a sample of blood; the red cells, the white cells and the platelets being counted separately. The apparatus used for this is known as **Hemocytometer**.

PRINCIPLE

Since the number of blood cells is very high, it is difficult to count them even under the microscope. This difficulty is partly overcome by diluting the blood to a known degree with suitable diluting fluid and then counting the blood cells.

APPARATUS

1. The counting chamber (Improved Neubauer's chamber)
2. The diluting pipettes: A. RBC pipette, B. WBC pipette
3. Cover slips
4. Red blood cell (RBC) and white blood cell (WBC) diluting fluids.
5. Watch glasses, spirit swabs, blood lancet/needle, etc.

Counting Chamber

Improved Neubauer's chamber is used in hemocytometry nowadays (Table 1.4.1).
1. The counting chamber (Figs. 1.4.1A to C) is a solid thick glass slide with a central platform divided by a short transverse gutter in two partitions. Each partition has a ruled area called the counting grid.
2. The central platform on each side is bounded by a groove called **moat**.

Table 1.4.1: Comparison between Neubauer's chamber (old) and improved Neubauer's chamber.

Neubauer's chamber (Old)	Improved Neubauer's chamber
Total ruled area is 3 mm × 3 mm	Total ruled area is 3 mm × 3 mm
Central ruled area is 1 mm × 1 mm which consists of **16 groups** of 16 small squares separated by triple lines	Central ruled area is 1 mm × 1 mm which consists of **25 groups** of 16 small squares separated by triple lines

3. The two lateral platforms can support a cover slip which, when in position provides a capillary space of 0.1 mm between the undersurface of the cover slip and the upper surface of the central platform.
4. Identically ruled areas called **"counting grids"**, consisting of squares of different sizes, are etched on each central platform.

The ruled area on each platform, the counting grid has the following dimensions:
- Each counting grid (Fig. 1.4.2) measures 9 mm^2 (3 mm × 3 mm).
- It is divided into nine large squares, each 1 mm^2 (1 mm × 1 mm).
- Of these nine squares, the four large corner squares (WBC squares) are lightly etched and each is divided by single lines into 16 medium-sized squares.
- Each of which has a side of 1/4 mm and an area of 1/16 mm^2 (1/4 mm × 1/4 mm) (Fig. 1.4.2).
- The central densely etched large square (1 mm × 1 mm), called the RBC square are divided into 25 medium-sized squares, each of which has a side of 1/5 mm.

- Each of these medium squares is separated from its neighbors by very closely placed triple lines. These triple lines extend in all directions beyond the boundaries of the 9 mm² ruling, i.e. in between all the WBC squares around the central RBC square.
- Each of the 25 medium squares (side = 1/5 mm), bounded by triple lines is further divided into 16 smallest squares by single lines. Thus, each smallest square has a side of $1/5 \times 1/4 = 1/20$ mm and an area of 1/400 mm² (1/20 mm × 1/20 mm).
- Since the depth of the chamber is 1/10 mm.

Diluting Pipettes

1. RBC pipette
2. WBC pipette.

Parts of a Diluting Pipette

- **The stem:** The long narrow stem has a capillary bore and a well-grounded conical tip. It is divided into 10 equal parts (graduations) but has only two numbers etched on it—0.5 in the middle of the stem and 1.0 (or 1) at the junction of stem and the bulb.
- **The bulb:** The stem widens into a bulb which contains a free-rolling bead—red in the RBC pipette and white in the WBC pipette (Figs. 1.4.3A and B). **The bead serves the following purposes**:
    - It aids mixing the blood with the diluent.
    - It helps in identifying the pipette.
    - It tells whether the pipette is dry or not. In a dry pipette, the bead rolls freely without sticking to the inside of the bulb which would happen if the bulb were wet.
- **Rubber tube and mouthpiece:** The bulb narrows again into a short stem to which a long, narrow and soft-rubber tube bearing a mouthpiece (red in RBC pipette and white in WBC pipette) is attached. The rubber tube is 25–30 cm long to facilitate filling of the pipette by gentle suction.

Just beyond the bulb, the number 101 is etched on the RBC pipette and 11 on the WBC pipette.

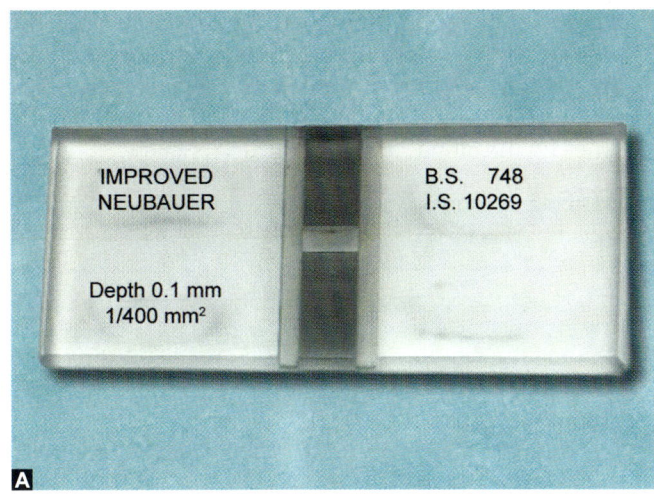
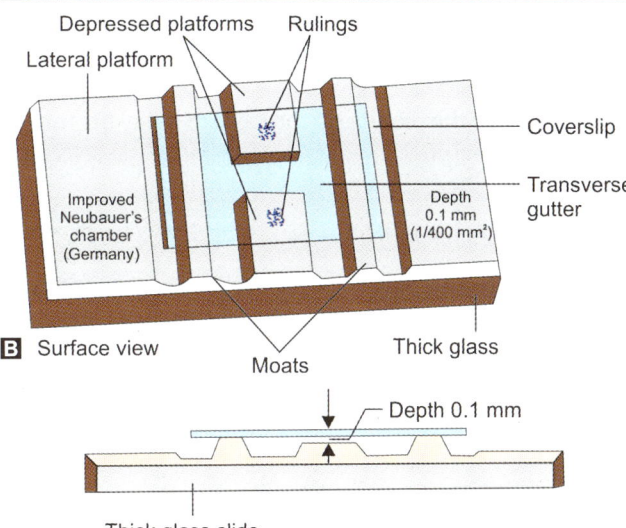

Figs. 1.4.1A to C: Improved Neubauer's chamber.

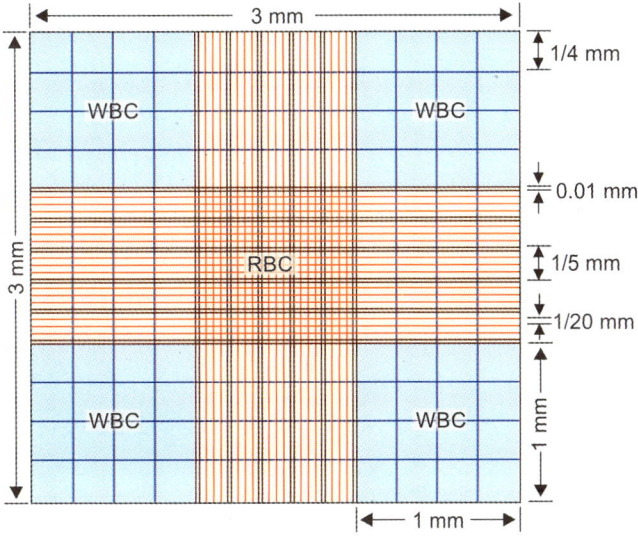

Fig. 1.4.2: The counting grid.

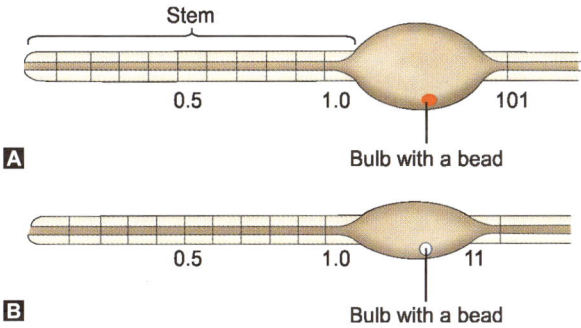

Figs. 1.4.3A and B: The diluting pipettes. (A) RBC pipette and (B) WBC pipette.

> **NOTE**
> The markings etched on the pipette refer to relative values rather than absolute values.

Differences Between Red Blood Cell Pipette and White Blood Cell Pipette

RBC pipette	WBC pipette
Calibrations are 0.5 and 1.0 below the bulb and 101 above the bulb	Calibrations are 0.5 and 1.0 below the bulb and 11 above it
The capillary bore is narrow, thus it is a **slow-speed pipette**	The capillary bore is wider, hence it is a **fast-speed pipette**
Bulb is larger and has a red bead	Bulb is smaller and has a white bead
The volume of the bulb is 100 times the volume contained in stem	The volume of the bulb is 10 times the volume of the stem

Filling the Pipette (Fig. 1.4.4)

- Under aseptic precautions give a bold prick to the finger. Wipe off the first drop of blood.
- Holding the mouthpiece of the pipette between your lips and keeping the pipette (with its graduations facing you) at an angle of about 40° to the horizontal, place its tip within the edge of the drop. Gently suck on the mouthpiece and draw blood upto the mark 0.5 (capillary action cannot fill the pipette when it is kept at 40° angle).
- The blood drop should be of adequate size (say 3–4 mm in diameter).
- Remove the pipette from the blood drop and clean its outer surface with a nonabsorbent material by wiping it toward the tip.
- If more than required amount of blood is drawn into the pipette, then by keeping the pipette horizontal all the time, bring the blood in the stem to the exact mark 0.5 by wiping the tip on your palm (or on a paper) a couple of times till the blood recedes to the exact mark.

> **NOTE**
> Do not use filter paper for this purpose as it will absorb a large amount of blood and neither should you try to blow out the extra blood.

- Holding the pipette, immerse its tip in the diluting fluid taken in a watch glass and suck the diluent to the mark 11 in WBC pipette or 101 in RBC pipette.
- The dilution of blood should not be delayed otherwise it is likely to clot in the stem.
- Once the diluent has been taken to the appropriate mark, keep the pipette horizontal so that the fluid does not run out by gravity.
- Do not place the pipette on the table or delay the mixing because it becomes impossible to dislodge the cells from the walls of the bulb once they settle down.

Mixing the Blood with the Diluting Fluid

Once the diluting fluid has been sucked up, remove the rubber tube. Holding the short stem above the bulb between your thumb and first two fingers and pressing the tip of the pipette against the palm of the other hand, rotate it to and fro for 3–4 minutes so that the blood and diluent get thoroughly mixed.

Charging the Chamber

Once the blood and the diluent have been mixed well, "charge" the chamber (Fig. 1.4.5).

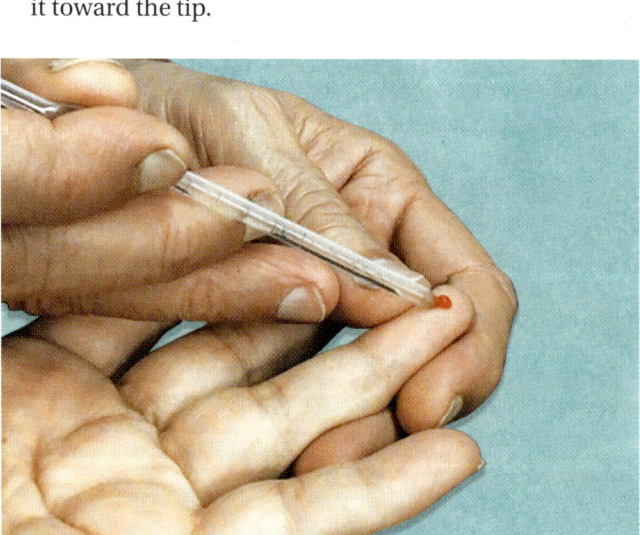

Fig. 1.4.4: Filling the pipette.

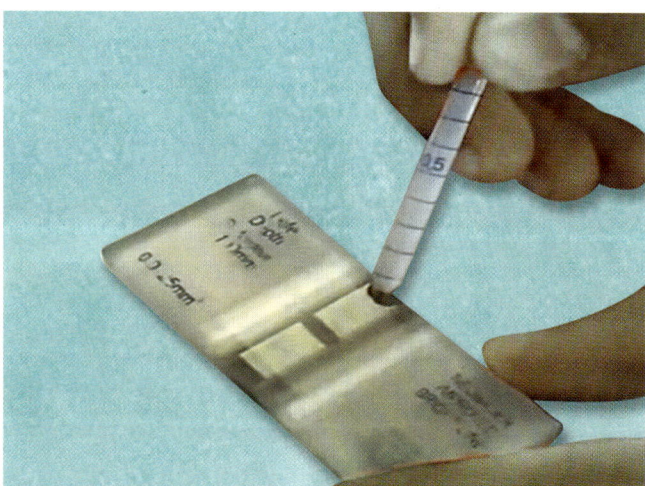

Fig. 1.4.5: Charging a chamber.

- Clean the Neubauer's chamber and place the clean coverslip on the central platform of the Neubauer's chamber.
- After the blood is mixed well with the diluents, discard the first few drops.
- Make an adequate sized drop at the tip of the pipette.
- Place the tip of the pipette on the surface of the chamber at the edge of the coverslip at the suitable angle. The diluted blood drop is allowed to flow by capillary action evenly and slowly under the coverslip.
- Allow the cells to settle down for 2–3 minutes.
- Charged chamber is then placed under the stage of microscope for counting.

> **NOTE**
> **High-speed pipette:** Since the bore of the WBC pipette is wider, a drop will form more quickly at its tip and it will be larger, as compared to the RBC pipette. This requires that this pipette should be held more horizontally say, at an angle of 10–20° and for a shorter time.
> **Slow-speed pipette:** The bore of the RBC pipette being narrow, it will take a longer time for a suitable drop to form. It should, therefore, be held at a steeper angle—say, 60–70°.

Ideally charged chamber: An ideally charged chamber is completely filled with diluted blood. If any blood flows into the trenches, it is called "overcharging". If the fluid is insufficient to cover the platform or if there are air bubbles it is called "undercharging" (air bubbles are formed if the coverslip or the platform is dirty with grease or is moist).

Effects of overcharging: When the chamber is overcharged the fluid will overflow into the gutters. This may give **false low results** as the cells will enter the gutter and settle there.

Effects of undercharging: In an undercharged chamber fluid does not cover the entire central platform. There may be no cells in the peripheral squares thus giving the **false low results.**

If there is over- or undercharging, wash the chamber and coverslip with soap and water, dry them and recharge the chamber.

Focusing the Counting Grid

Examine the grid on each platform, without the coverslip, under low and high magnifications. Rack the condenser up and down, closing/adjusting the diaphragm at the same time. Find out the best combination of these two that shows the grid lines and squares clearly. When properly focused, the rulings (lines) appear as translucent darkish lines.
- First examine under low power (10x) one large square (1 mm × 1 mm) is visible in one field, i.e. a group of 16

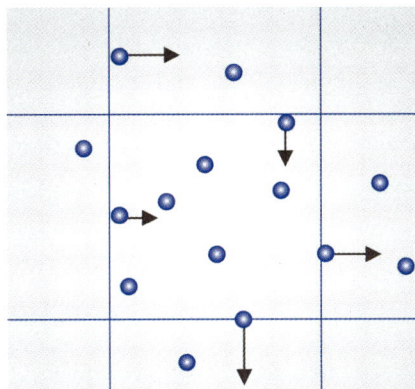

Fig. 1.4.6: Counting of cells. Arrows indicate the squares to which the cells belong.

medium squares (for WBC counting) or a group of 25 medium squares (for RBC counting).
- Then examine the squares under high power (40x).

Counting the Cells

Focus the appropriate squares under the required magnification and start counting as described below:

Rules of counting (Fig. 1.4.6)
1. Care should be taken not to count the same cells again.
2. The cells lying within a square and those lying on or touching the upper and left border is counted in that particular square.
3. The cells on the right and lower border are ignored as they will be counted in the adjacent squares. This is called **"inverted L pattern"**. Arrows indicate the squares to which the cells belong (Fig. 1.4.6).
4. In this way, you will avoid counting a cell twice.
5. In squares bound by triple lines, the middle line is considered the boundary of that square and the same rules of counting apply.
6. While counting the cells, continuously "rack", the fine adjustment up and down so that cells sticking to the underside of the coverslip are not missed.
7. Only one pattern should be followed for the entire counting.

SOURCES OF ERROR IN CELL COUNTING (REFER CHAPTER 1.5)

1. Pipette error
2. Dilution error
3. Chamber error
4. Statistical error
5. Field error
6. Charging error.

PRECAUTIONS

1. The pipette should be clean and dry and the bead should roll freely.
2. The pipette should not be lifted out of the blood drop while filling it with blood, otherwise air will enter into it.
3. The drawing up of diluent, after blood has been taken in the stem, should not be delayed, otherwise it will clot in it.
4. The pipette should be cleaned soon after the experiment is over.
5. Do not touch blood other than your own.
6. Ensure that the counting chamber and the coverslip are absolutely clean, grease-free and dry.
7. While charging the chamber ensures that it is neither under nor overcharged.
8. Never bring the objective lens down while looking into the microscope as the chamber is likely to be scratched or broken.

QUESTIONS

Q.1. What is the principle underlying the use of a counting chamber?

Q.2. What are the dimensions of WBC and RBC squares?

Q.3. What are the features of an ideally-charged chamber?

Q.4. How does the improved Neubauer's chamber differ from the older variety of Neubauer's chamber?

Q.5. How will you identify a red cell pipette and a white cell pipette?

Q.6. What is the function of the bead in the bulb?

Q.7. What are the units of markings on the pipettes?

There are no absolute units of volume marked on the pipette. They only denote relative volumes or parts in relation to each other.

Q.8. Why is it important to discard the first drop of diluted blood from the pipette before charging the counting chamber?

After the blood has been diluted in the pipette, the stem contains only the cell-free diluent. Therefore, this fluid has to be discarded before the chamber can be charged.

Q.9. How will you clean a pipette when blood has clotted in the stem?

The pipette is kept in strong nitric acid for 24 hours. A flexible suitably thick metal wire is used to clean the capillary bore after washing the pipette in running water.

Q.10. What are the other uses of these pipettes?

The RBC pipette can be used for counting platelets, WBCs (when their number is very high, as in some leukemias) or spermatozoa in the semen.

Q.11. How is the entry of air bubbles prevented while diluting the blood?

Q.12. If the blood is sucked above the 0.5 mark of the pipette how is it brought down?

STUDY NOTES

Teacher's Signature

Date ....

CHAPTER 1.5

Total Red Blood Cell Count

AIM
To determine the red blood cells (RBC) count.

INTRODUCTION
Red blood cells are the most abundant cells in the peripheral blood. The human RBC is normally a circular, non-nucleated, biconcave disc containing hemoglobin. The biconcave shape aids in exchange of oxygen and carbon dioxide maximally and also helps it to withstand osmotic lysis and to easily pass through narrow capillaries (diapedesis). The RBCs do not have mitochondria.

Red Cell Dimensions
- Shape: Biconcave disc
- Size: 7.4 (7–8) micron in diameter.

Sites of Formation
- Fetal life—spleen, liver, thymus and bone marrow
- Soon after birth—red bone marrow
- Adult life—long bone cavities and femur.

Normal Values
Adult
- Males: 5.4 (5.5–6.5) million/mm³ of blood.
- Females: 4.8 (4.5–5.5) million/mm³ of blood.
- Newborns: 6–8 million/mm³ of blood.

PRINCIPLE
The blood is diluted 200 times in a red cell pipette as the number of RBCs is very high. The cells are then counted in the Neubauer's counting chamber.

APPARATUS
1. **RBC pipette:** It should be clean and dry and the bead should roll freely (*Refer* Chapter 1.4) (Fig. 1.5.1).
2. **Improved Neubauer's chamber with coverslip:** These should be clean and dust free (Fig. 1.5.2).
3. Compound microscope.
4. Pricking apparatus.
5. **Hayem's fluid (RBC diluting fluid).**

Composition of Hayem's Fluid
- **Sodium chloride (NaCl):** 0.50 g—maintains **isotonicity** so that the red cells remain suspended in diluted blood without changing their shape and size.

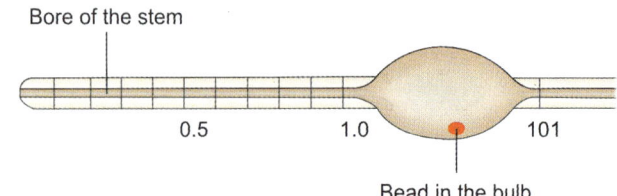

Fig. 1.5.1: The RBC pipette. It has three markings—0.5, 1.0 and 101.

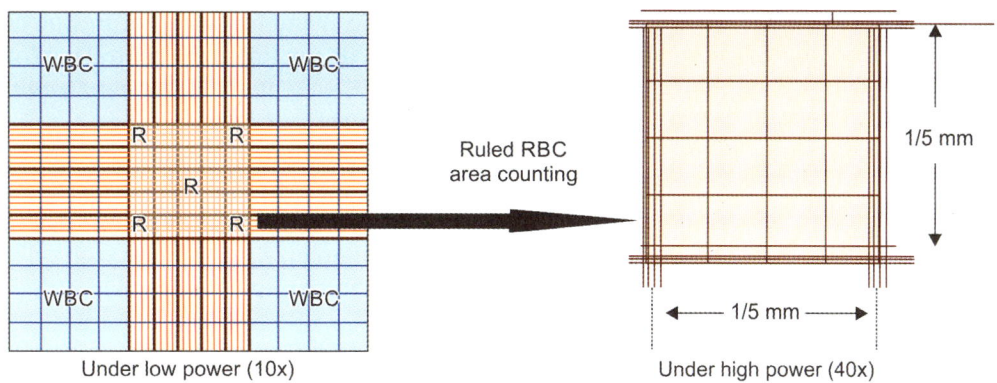

Fig. 1.5.2: Neubauer's chamber showing RBC squares (R) under low power. Also showing right lower medium-sized RBC square under high power.

- **Sodium sulfate (Na$_2$SO$_4$):** 2.50 g—acts as an **anticoagulant** and as a **fixative** to preserve their shape and to prevent rouleaux formation (piling together of red blood cells).
- **Mercuric chloride (HgCl$_2$):** 0.25 g—acts as an **antifungal** and **antimicrobial** agent, prevents contamination and growth of microorganisms.
- Distilled water—to make it 100 mL.

> **NOTE**
> **Alternatives to Hayem's fluid**
> **Dacie's solution:** It is simple to prepare and can be kept for a long time. It contains 3.13 g of trisodium citrate, 1 mL of 37% formalin (commercial formaldehyde) and distilled water to 100 mL.
> **Normal saline:** 0.9% sodium chloride solution can be used if Hayem's or Dacie's fluids are not available. However, the red cells have to be counted within an hour or so of filling the pipette. Also the RBCs are likely to form rouleaux. Further, a stock solution of normal saline cannot be kept for this purpose.

PROCEDURE

1. Place about 2 mL of Hayem's fluid in a watch glass.
2. Examine the Neubauer's chamber with the coverslip "centered" on it, under low magnification (10x). Adjust the illumination and focus the central 1 mm^2 (RBC square on the counting grid). The focus of the microscope should not be disturbed.
3. **Filling the pipette with blood and diluting it:** Taking all aseptic precautions prick the finger. Wipe the first drop of blood and fill the pipette from a fresh drop of blood up to the mark 0.5. Then suck Hayem's fluid to the mark 101 and mix the contents of the bulb by rotating the pipette between the palms of your hands by keeping the pipette horizontal for 3–4 minutes.
4. **Charging the chamber:** The first few drops of fluid from the pipette are discarded. They constitute the unmixed Hayem's fluid present in the stem of the pipette. A small drop of fluid is allowed to form at the tip of the pipette and this drop is gently brought in contact with the edge of the coverslip. The fluid is drawn into the chamber by capillary action. Both sides of Neubauer's chamber are charged (*Refer* Chapter 1.4 for details).
5. Move the chamber to the microscope and focus the grid once again to see the central 1 mm^2 with the red blood cells distributed all over. Wait for about 2 minutes for the cells to settle down.
6. **Counting the cells:** Switch over to high magnification (40x) and check the distribution of cells in the four corners and one central medium-sized RBC square, i.e. 16 × 5 = 80 small squares. If they are unevenly distributed, the chamber has to be washed, dried and recharged.
7. **Rules of counting (Fig. 1.5.3):** Count the cells lying within a square and those lying on or touching its upper horizontal and left vertical line (**inverted L pattern**) and those touching its lower horizontal and right vertical lines are to be omitted as they will be counted in the adjacent squares. Arrows indicate the squares to which the red blood cells belong.

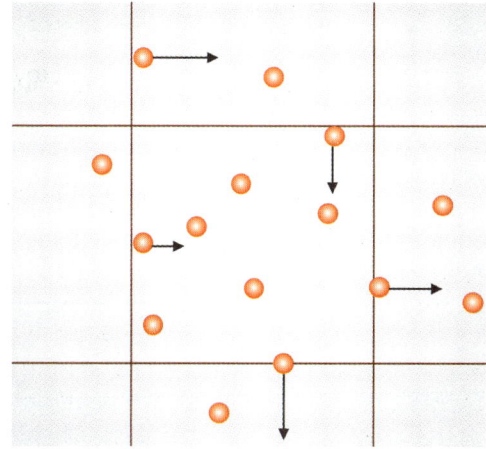

Fig. 1.5.3: Rules of counting.

8. **Calculations:**
   a. *Calculation of dilution obtained (dilution factor):*
      - As 0.5 part of blood mixes with 100.5 parts of RBC fluid in the pipette to make it 101. Blood mixes with the diluting fluid only in the bulb of the pipette. The fluid in the stem (1 part) is discarded as it does not take part in dilution.
      - Therefore, 0.5 part of blood mixes with 99.5 parts of the diluting fluid to form final volume of 100 parts (0.5 + 99.5).
      - Hence 0.5 part of blood is diluted in 100 parts. Thus, the dilution factor is

      $$= \frac{\text{Final volume attained (100 parts)}}{\text{Volume of blood taken (0.5 part)}}$$

      - Hence, the dilution factor is 200.
   b. *Calculation of volume of fluid examined:*
      - Area of 5 squares = $5 \times 1/5 \text{ mm} \times 1/5 \text{ mm} = 1/5 \text{ mm}^2$
      - Depth of the chamber = 1/10 mm
      - Hence, volume of fluid in 5 RBC squares = $1/5 \text{ mm}^2 \times 1/10 \text{ mm} = 1/50 \text{ mm}^3$ (μL)
   c. *Calculation of red cell count:*
      Let N be the total number of RBCs counted in 5 RBC squares (N_1 to N_5), i.e. cells in $1/50 \text{ mm}^3$ of diluted blood.
      Where, $N = N_1 + N_2 + N_3 + N_4 + N_5$
      Cells in 1 mm³ of diluted blood = N × 50
      Dilution employed was = 1 in 200
      Therefore, **number of cells in 1 mm³ (μL) of undiluted blood will be** = N × 50 × 200 = N × 10,000.

SOURCES OF ERROR

As mentioned in Chapter 1.4, despite all precautions in the procedures, the degree of error with this method is said to be about ± 15%. The following factors are responsible for the error:
1. **Pipette error:** It may be due to inaccuracy of graduations, inaccurate filling with blood and diluent or their mixing.
2. **Chamber error:** The counting grid and the depth of the chamber may not be accurate or the process of charging it may introduce an error.
3. **Field error:** The distribution of cells on the grid may not be uniform.
4. **Counting error:** Because of the high multiplication factor (i.e. 10,000), even an error in counting a single RBC will deviate the result by 10,000 cells per mm³ of blood.
5. **Charging error:** Overcharging and undercharging (*Refer* Chapter 1.4).

PRECAUTIONS

1. Observe all precautions described for getting a finger prick (*Refer* Chapter 1.2), filling the pipette with blood, diluent and charging the chamber (*Refer* Chapter 1.4).
2. Clean the chamber with a lint-free piece of cloth. Once cleaned, do not touch the central part of the chamber.
3. If there is overcharging or undercharging, wash, clean, dry and charge the chamber again.
4. Continuously rack the fine adjustment screw while counting the cells.
5. Do not draw diluents directly from the stock bottle as it may contaminate the solution with cells.
6. Discard the sample and recharge the chamber if the distribution of cells is not uniform.
7. Follow the rules of counting to avoid the counting the same cell twice.

PHYSIOCLINICAL SIGNIFICANCE

1. **Decrease in RBC count**
   a. *Physiological causes:*
      - Pregnancy
      - Females (**RBC count is higher in males because androgens stimulate erythropoiesis**)
   b. *Pathological causes:*
      - Anemia
      - Hemodilution, e.g. excess ADH secretion as in posterior pituitary tumors.
2. **Increase in RBC count**
   a. *Physiological causes:*
      - High altitude
      - Newborns
      - Hemoconcentration, e.g. excessive sweating.
   b. *Pathological causes:*
      - Hemoconcentration, e.g. diarrhea, vomiting
      - Chronic hypoxia, e.g. congenital heart disease, chronic obstructive pulmonary disease
      - Polycythemia vera.

Objective Structured Practical Examination–I

Aim: To dilute the given sample of blood 200 times using a pipette and diluent.
Procedural steps: See text above.
Checklist:
1. Select the correct pipette and check that it is clean, dry and patent. (Y/N)
2. Take enough diluents in a watch glass and suck blood to the exact 0.5 mark and see that there are no air bubbles. (Y/N)
3. Wipe off blood sticking to the outside of the tip of the pipette. (Y/N)
4. Suck diluting fluid exactly to the mark 101. (Y/N)
5. Hold the pipette horizontally between the palms and roll it gently to mix the contents of the bulb. (Y/N)

Chapter 1.5: Total Red Blood Cell Count

> **Objective Structured Practical Examination–II**
>
> **Aim:** To charge the Neubauer's chamber with diluted blood provided to you in a RBC pipette.
> **Procedural steps:** See text above.
> **Checklist:**
> 1. Ensure that the chamber and coverslip are clean and dry. (Y/N)
> 2. Mix the contents of the bulb between her palms. (Y/N)
> 3. Place the coverslip on the central plateau of the chamber to cover both the ruled areas. (Y/N)
> 4. Discard the first two drops from the pipette and allow a suitable-sized drop to form. (Y/N)
> 5. Place the tip of pipette on the chamber, touching the edge of the coverslip and allow the fluid to spread evenly over the counting grid without over- or undercharging. Charge the other side also. (Y/N)

QUESTIONS

Q.1. Why is blood diluted 200 times for RBC count?
Q.2. What is the function of the bead in the bulb?
Q.3. What are the units of markings on the pipette?
Q.4. If Hayem's solution is not available, can you use any other?
Q.5. Why should you discard the first few drops from the pipette before charging the chamber?
Q.6. What are the features of a properly charged chamber? How will over- or undercharging of the chamber affect the red cell count?
  Refer Chapter 1.4 for features of properly charged chamber. When the chamber is overcharged, diluted blood flows into the trenches where the red cells being heavier, sink down. This gives a false low count. Undercharging, due to less blood in the chamber will also give a low count.
Q.7. Why should both sides of the chamber be charged at the same time?
Q.8. How will you differentiate red cells from dust particles?
  Dust particles may be present on the objective, eyepiece or in the diluent. They are irregular and of different sizes (If they are on the eyepiece, they will rotate with the eyepiece). Red cells, on the other hand, are round discs, of uniform size and are light pink in color.
Q.9. Why is it necessary to follow the rules of counting?
Q.10. What are the sources of error in this experiment?
Q.11. What is the fate of leukocytes in this experiment? How does it affect the RBC count?
  An occasional leukocyte may be seen. It is larger than a red cell, appears refractile (shiny) and granular and it also contains a nucleus. Since the ratio of WBC to RBC is 1: 600–700. Therefore, hardly any WBCs are counted. So, WBCs do not affect the RBC count.
Q.12. What is the lifespan of red cells?
  The average lifespan of red cells is about 120 days (about 40 days in macrocytic anemia and spherocytosis).
Q.13. How is erythropoiesis regulated?
  Factors that regulate erythropoiesis:

1. *Erythropoietin (EPO):* Erythropoietin is a glycoprotein, about 95% of EPO is secreted by the peritubular interstitial cells of the kidneys and 15% from the perivenous hepatocytes of liver. Hypoxia is the most potent stimulator for EPO secretion. Cobalt salts and androgens also stimulate EPO secretion.
2. *Grade I proteins:* Proteins of animal origin, soyabeans, etc.
3. *Vitamins:* B_{12}, folic acid, pyridoxine, other B complex vitamins and vitamin C are needed for red cell formation.
4. *Trace metals:* Iron, copper, zinc and cobalt are required in trace amounts.
5. *Hormones:* Androgens, thyroxin, growth hormone and cortisol are required.

   Various other hormones or factors (hemopoietic growth factors) like colony-stimulating factors (CSFs), cytokines, interleukins (ILs), EPO, etc. also play a role.

Q.14. Which physiological condition causes a decrease in RBC count?
Q.15. What is anemia and what are its causes?
Q.16. What is polycythemia and what are its causes?
  Polycythemia: It refers to an increase in the number of red cells above the normal level. Erythrocytosis is a better term to describe an absolute increase in the total red cell mass.
  - **Polycythemia vera (erythremia or primary polycythemia):** A gene abnormality in the early red cells causes them to form more and more cells. Erythropoietin production is not raised, but may be decreased.
  - **Secondary polycythemia:**
    - Hypoxia due to lung diseases, congenital heart disease and cardiac failure increase the RBC count.
    - **Polycythemia due to hemoconcentration:** Fluid loss during severe vomiting and diarrhea and loss of plasma in burns. There is no increase in total red cell mass.

  Physiological polycythemia is seen during residence at high altitudes and in newborns. Emotional stress and severe exercise may cause a temporary increase in RBC count.

OBSERVATION

CALCULATION

RESULT

INTERPRETATION

STUDY NOTES

Teacher's Signature

Total Leukocyte Count

CHAPTER 1.6

Date ....

AIM

To determine the total leukocyte count (TLC).

INTRODUCTION

The white blood corpuscles (WBCs) or leukocytes constitute the major defense system of the body against invasion by bacteria, viruses, fungi, toxins and other foreign invaders. Their number is kept remarkably constant in health, but it increases or decreases in many diseases particularly acute and chronic infections.

Normal Count

- **Adults:** 4,000–11,000 cells/mm^3 of blood
- **Infants:** 18,000–20,000/mm^3 of blood

PRINCIPLE

A sample of blood is diluted with a diluting fluid which destroys the membrane of red blood cells and stains the nuclei of the leukocytes. The cells are then counted in a counting chamber using a microscope and their number in undiluted blood is reported as number of leukocytes/mm^3 of undiluted whole blood.

APPARATUS

1. Compound microscope
2. Counting chamber with a coverslip
3. Blood lancet or pricking needle
4. Sterile cotton or gauze swab
5. 70% alcohol
6. WBC pipette
7. WBC diluting fluid (Turk's fluid).

Composition of Turk's Fluid

- Glacial acetic acid: 3 mL—it destroys membrane of RBCs, WBCs and platelets; imparts refractility to the cells.
- Gentian violet (1% solution): 1 mL—it stains the nuclei of leukocytes.
- Distilled water: Make it to 100 mL.

PROCEDURE

1. Take 1 mL of WBC diluting fluid (Turk's fluid) in a watch glass.
2. Place the counting chamber on the microscope stage. Adjust the illumination and focus the WBC squares under low power (10x).
3. Taking all the aseptic precautions, prick the finger, discard the first drop of blood and let a good-sized drop to form.
4. **Filling the pipette:** Draw blood to the mark 0.5 of WBC pipette and then suck Turk's fluid up to the mark 11 (Fig. 1.6.1). Mix the contents of the bulb thoroughly for 3–4 minutes by rolling it between the palms.
5. **Charging the chamber:** Discard the first few drops of fluid from the pipette and charge the chamber on both sides. The chamber should neither be overcharged nor undercharged.
6. Allow the cells to settle for 2–3 minutes and then carefully transfer the chamber to the microscope.

> **NOTE**
> An ideally charged chamber preparation lasts for 90 minutes. After 40 minutes the charging starts to recede and WBC count becomes less.

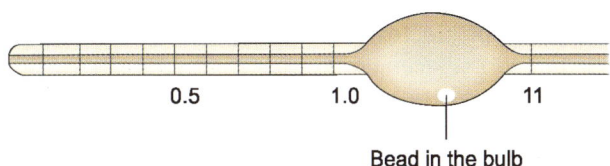

Fig. 1.6.1: The WBC pipette. It has three markings—0.5, 1.0, and 11.

7. **Identification of WBCs:** The leukocytes appear as round, shiny (refractile), darkish dots, with a halo around them. These "dots" represent the nuclei, which have been stained by gentian violet. The cytoplasm is not stained.

> **NOTE**
> Do not confuse with dust particles which have varying sizes and shapes, often irregular. They are usually opaque with no "halo" around them. They may be brown, black or yellow in color.

> **IMPORTANT**
> When examining cells or counting them, do not keep a fixed focus but continuously "rack" the microscope so that the cells and the lines come into and go out of focus. In this way, you will not miss cells sticking to the undersurface of the coverslip or confuse dust particles for WBCs.

8. **Counting the cells (Fig. 1.6.2):** The procedure for counting the WBCs is similar to that employed for red blood cells (*Refer* Fig. 1.5.3).
   - Count the cells under low power lens.
   - You may count the WBCs in 16 squares under low power (10x).
   - Count the cells in the 4 groups of 16 square each, i.e. in a total of 64 squares.
   - Draw appropriate squares in your workbook for entering the counts.

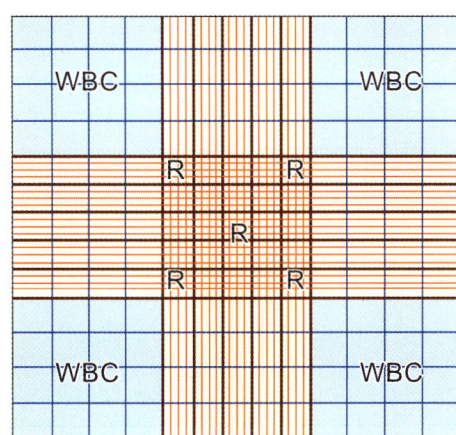

Fig. 1.6.2: Counting of WBC's in four corner squares..

9. **Calculations**
   a. *Calculation of dilution obtained (dilution factor):* As 0.5 part of blood mixes with 10.5 part of WBC fluid in the pipette. Blood mixes with the diluting fluid only in the bulb of the pipette. So the distal 0.5 is discarded as it does not take part in dilution.
   - Therefore 0.5 part of blood mixes with 9.5 parts of the diluting fluid to form final volume of 10 parts (0.5 + 9.5).
   - Hence 0.5 part of blood is diluted in 10 parts.

   $$\text{Dilution factor} = \frac{\text{Final volume achieved (10 parts)}}{\text{Original volume taken (0.5 parts)}} = 20$$

   - Hence dilution factor is 20.
   Volume of fluid:
   Area of 4 WBC squares = $4 \times 1 \times 1 = 4 \text{ mm}^2$
   Depth of the chamber = 1/10 mm
   Volume of fluid in the 4 WBC squares = $4 \times 0.1 = 0.4 \text{ mm}^3/\mu L$

   b. *Calculation of TLC:*
   Let N be the total number of WBCs in 4 WBC squares (N_1 to N_4)
   Where $N = N_1 + N_2 + N_3 + N_4$
   Total number of WBCs in 1 µL of undiluted blood
   = N × dilution factor (20)/0.4 = **N × 50**.

SOURCES OF ERROR

The sources of errors are the same as described for RBC counting (*Refer* Chapter 1.5) and include:
1. Pipette error
2. Chamber error
3. Field error
4. Experimental error
   The degree of error which may be 30% or more in RBC counting is much less in TLC (about 5–10%) because of the low dilution employed (1 in 20) in this case.

> **NOTE**
> In case when the leukocyte count is very high, as in leukemia, the dilution has to be increased. For this purpose the RBC pipette can be used in which the blood is sucked up to mark 1 and diluted 100 times. Further calculation is done accordingly.

PRECAUTIONS

1. Observe all precautions described for making a finger-prick, filling the pipette and charging the counting chamber as in RBC count.
2. When mixing the blood with the Turk's fluid, give sufficient time for complete hemolysis of red cells.
3. Continuously "rack" the microscope while identifying and counting the cells for reasons described earlier.

PHYSIOCLINICAL SIGNIFICANCE

Conditions that increase TLC: Leukocytosis (Above 11,000/mm³ of Blood)

1. **Physiological causes:**
   a. *Normal infants:* The count may be as high as 18,000–20,000/mm³ but it returns to normal level within 1–2 years.
   b. *Food intake:* There is a mild increase which returns to normal within an hour or so.
   c. *Physical exercise*
   d. *Mental stress*
   e. *Pregnancy:* The count may be quite high especially during the first pregnancy.
   f. *Parturition:* The high TLC is possibly due to tissue injury, pain, physical stress and hemorrhage.
   g. *Extremes of temperatures:* Exposure to sun or to very low temperature can increase the WBC count.

   > **NOTE**
   > **Redistribution within the blood:** The WBCs from the "marginal" pool are mobilized and poured into the circulating blood.
   > **Release from bone marrow reserve:** This is another process by which the number of WBCs can be raised in a short time.
   > These two processes raise the TLC without increasing their rate of production. There are no immature cells in the blood.

2. **Pathological causes:** A rise in TLC in disease is seen in:
   a. *Acute infection with pyogenic (pus forming) bacteria:* The infection due to cocci bacteria (*Streptococcus, Staphylococcus*) may be: (a) Localized, such as boils, abscess, tonsillitis, appendicitis, etc. and (b) Generalized, such as in septicemia and pyemia, bronchitis, pneumonia, peritonitis, meningitis, etc.
   b. *Myocardial infarction:* The rise in TLC is due to tissue injury. It is not seen immediately after a heart attack but only after 4–5 days.
   c. *Acute hemorrhage:* Maximum response occurs in 8–10 hours, the count returning to normal in 5–6 days.
   d. *Burns:* Maximum response occurs in 5–15 hours, the count returning to normal in 2–3 days.
   e. *Leukemia:* WBC more than 50,000/mm³ of blood along with presence of abnormal (blast) cells.
   f. *Surgical operations:* A postoperative rise in TLC is seen in all cases.

Conditions that Decrease TLC: Leukopenia (Below 4,000/mm³ of Blood)

1. **Physiological causes:** Exposure to extreme cold (even under arctic conditions and in spite of acclimatization) may reduce the count to only slightly below the 4,000/mm³.

2. **Pathological causes:**
   a. *Infection with nonpyogenic organisms:* Typhoid and paratyphoid fevers and sometimes in protozoal infection like malaria.
   b. *Viral infections:* Influenza, mumps, smallpox, acquired immunodeficiency syndrome (AIDS).
   c. *Drugs:* Chloramphenicol, sulfonamides, aspirin and cytotoxic drugs used in treating malignancies.
   d. Repeated exposures to X-rays.
   e. Chemical poisons that depress bone marrow: Arsenic, dinitrophenol, antimony and others.
   f. *Malnutrition:* Deficiency of vitamin B_{12} and folate, general malnutrition and starvation.
   g. *Hypoplasia and aplasia:* Partial or complete depression of bone marrow, i.e. failure of stem cells production.

> **Objective Structured Practical Examination–I**
>
> **Aim:** To dilute the given sample for total leukocyte count.
> **Procedural steps:** See text above.
> **Checklist:**
> 1. Check that the pipette is clean, dry and patent. (Y/N)
> 2. Take sufficient diluting fluid in a watch glass and suck blood exactly to the mark 0.5 and confirm that there is no air bubble. (Y/N)
> 3. Wipe off blood sticking to the outside of the pipette tip. (Y/N)
> 4. Suck diluting fluid to the mark 11. (Y/N)
> 5. Hold the pipette horizontally between the palms and rolls it gently. (Y/N)

> **Objective Structured Practical Examination–II**
>
> **Aim:** To charge the counting chamber for total leukocyte count with diluted blood provided in a pipette.
> **Procedural steps:** See text above.
> **Checklist:**
> 1. Check that the chamber and the pipette are clean and dry. (Y/N)
> 2. Place the coverslip on the floor piece and trenches. (Y/N)
> 3. Mix the contents of the pipette by rolling it between your palms and discard the first two drops. (Y/N)
> 4. Charge the chamber by slow and controlled release of diluted blood at the edge of the coverslip. (Y/N)
> 5. Allow the diluted blood to spread under the coverslip to cover the ruled area. Allow the cells to settle down. (Y/N)

QUESTIONS

Q.1. How will you differentiate a WBC pipette from a RBC pipette?
Q.2. What do the three markings on the pipette indicate?
Q.3. What is the volume of the bulb in the WBC pipette? Why is its bulb smaller than that of the RBC pipette?
   In WBC pipette the volume of the fluid in the bulb is 10 times the volume of fluid in the stem, which can give a dilution of

1 in 10 or 1 in 20. In RBC pipette, the volume of the bulb is 100 times the volume of the stem, which can give a dilution of 1 in 100 or 1 in 200. Since the count of leukocytes is in thousands/mm^3, the blood requires much less dilution as compared to red cell count which is in millions/mm^3.

Q.4. What is the function of the bead in the bulb?

Q.5. What are the other uses of WBC pipette?

The WBC pipette can be used for counting RBCs in cases of severe anemia or for counting platelets. It can also be used for doing sperm count.

Q.6. What is the composition of Turk's fluid? What is the function of each constituent?

Q.7. What is meant by the term "glacial"? Why should the acid in the Turk's fluid be glacial?

The term glacial means pure acetic acid. Only the glacial acid can give the typical "shine" (halo) or clear refractility around the WBCs due to swelling of nuclei. This differentiates them from dust particles which are opaque and of different shapes.

Q.8. Why are the red cells not seen when counting the leukocytes?

The red cells are not seen because they are hemolyzed by the acid. The remnants of red cell membranes are faintly visible—the so-called ghost cells.

Q.9. Can any other agent be used to hemolyze the red blood cells?

No. Any weak hemolytic agent would take blood a longer time to lyse the RBCs, whereas a strong agent, in addition to lysing the red cells membrane will also damage the nuclear membrane of WBCs.

Q.10. What are the sources of error in this practical?

Q.11. What is the normal total leukocyte count?

Q.12. What is meant by the terms leukocytosis? Name the physiological and pathological conditions which cause leukocytosis.

Q.13. What is the difference between leukocytosis, leukemoid reaction and leukemia?

Leukocytosis: It is an increase in TLC count above 11,000/mm^3, irrespective of the types of cells involved. It may be physiological or pathological. The pathological causes include infection and tissue injury. The count usually does not exceed 20,000–25,000/mm^3 and there are **no immature cells in the circulation**.

Leukemoid reaction: It is an extreme elevation of TLC above 50,000/mm^3 as a result of the presence of mature and/or immature neutrophils. The causes include: Severe chronic infections, especially in children, severe hemolysis, malignant growths (cancer of breast, lung and kidney).

Leukemia: Leukemia is a cancerous disease of hemopoietic cells (bone marrow or lymphatic tissues) characterized by uncontrolled and abnormal production of both immature (blast cells) and mature WBCs. The TLC is generally above 50,000/mm^3 or even a few lakhs which mainly consist of **immature blast cells**.

Q.14. What do you know about bone marrow transplantation?

Bone marrow transplantation is the intravenous transfusion of red bone marrow from a healthy donor (commonly taken from iliac crest) to a recipient.

OBSERVATION

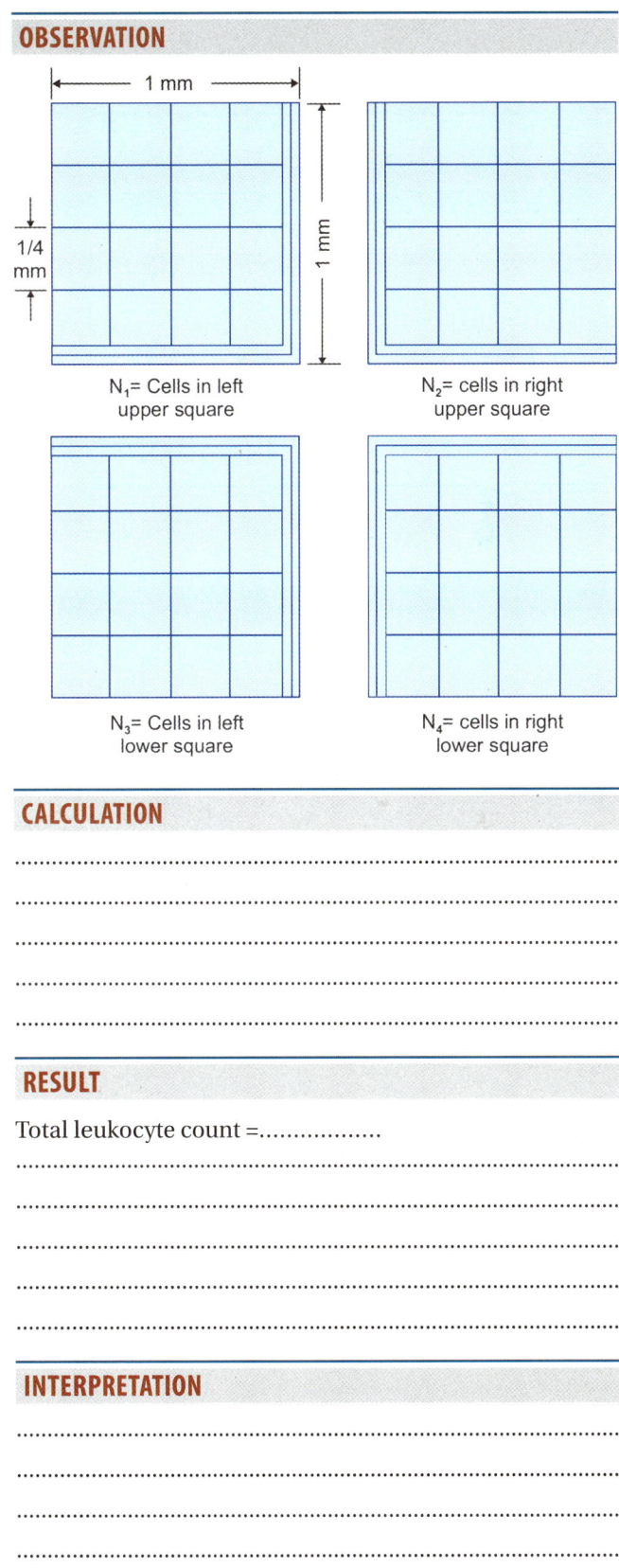

N_1 = Cells in left upper square

N_2 = cells in right upper square

N_3 = Cells in left lower square

N_4 = cells in right lower square

CALCULATION

....
....
....
....
....

RESULT

Total leukocyte count =..................
....
....
....
....
....

INTERPRETATION

....
....
....
....

STUDY NOTES

Date ....

CHAPTER 1.7
Preparation of a Peripheral Blood Smear and Determination of Differential Leukocyte Count

AIM
To prepare a peripheral blood smear (PBS) and determine differential leukocyte count (DLC).

INTRODUCTION
Many hematological and other disorders can be diagnosed by a careful examination of a stained blood film. The percentage distribution of leukocytes in the peripheral blood is known as DLC.

PRINCIPLE
A blood film is stained with Leishman stain and observed under oil immersion, from one end to the other. As each white blood cell (WBC) is encountered, it is identified until 100 leukocytes have been examined. The percentage distribution of each type of WBC is then calculated. Knowing the total leukocyte count (TLC) and the differential count, it is easy to determine the absolute number of each type of cell per cubic millimeter.

APPARATUS
1. Compound microscope
2. Four to five clean glass slides
3. Pricking apparatus
4. Glass dropper
5. Leishman stain
6. Distilled water (or buffered water, if available).

Leishman Stain
This stain is a simplification of the **Romanowsky** group of stains. It contains both an acidic and a basic dye. Its components are:
1. **Eosin:** It is an acidic dye (negatively charged) and stains basic (positive) particles—red blood cells (RBCs) and granules of eosinophils. It imparts a pink color.
2. **Methylene blue:** It is a basic dye (positively charged) and stains acidic (negatively charged) granules in the cytoplasm, nuclei of leukocytes, especially the granules of basophils. It imparts a blue-violet color.
3. **Acetone-free and water-free methyl alcohol:** The methyl alcohol is a **fixative** and must be free from acetone and water. It serves two functions:
   a. It fixes the blood smear to the glass slide. The alcohol precipitates the plasma proteins, which attaches (fixes) the blood cells to the slide so that they are not washed away during staining.
   b. The alcohol preserves the morphology and chemical state of the cells at the time of staining.

NOTE
- The alcohol must be free from acetone because acetone being a very strong lipid solvent, if present, will cause crenation, shrinkage or even destruction of cell membranes. This will make the identification of the cells difficult.
- The alcohol must be free from water since, if present, it may result in rouleaux formation and even hemolysis. The water may even wash away the blood film from the slide.

Section 1: Hematology

PROCEDURE

Preparation of a Blood Smear (Figs. 1.7.1A to C)

1. Place three or four clean, grease free glass slides on a white sheet of paper on your worktable, one of these is to be used as a *spreader*, the surface of which should be even and smooth.
2. Prick the finger under aseptic conditions.
3. Allow a medium-sized drop of blood to form on the fingertip.
4. Then touch the blood drop in the center line of the slide, about 1 cm from the one end of the slide.
5. Place the narrow edge of the spreader on the first slide, at an angle of 45°, just in front of the blood drop.
6. Pull the spreader backward till the blood runs along the full width of the spreader at the line of junction.
7. Slowly and smoothly move the spreader to the other end of the slide.
8. Dry the smear by waving the slide in the air (do not try to blot-dry the film).

Fixing of the Blood Smear

Fixation is the process that makes the blood smear and its cells adhere to the glass slide. It also preserves the shape and chemistry of blood cells as near living cells as possible.

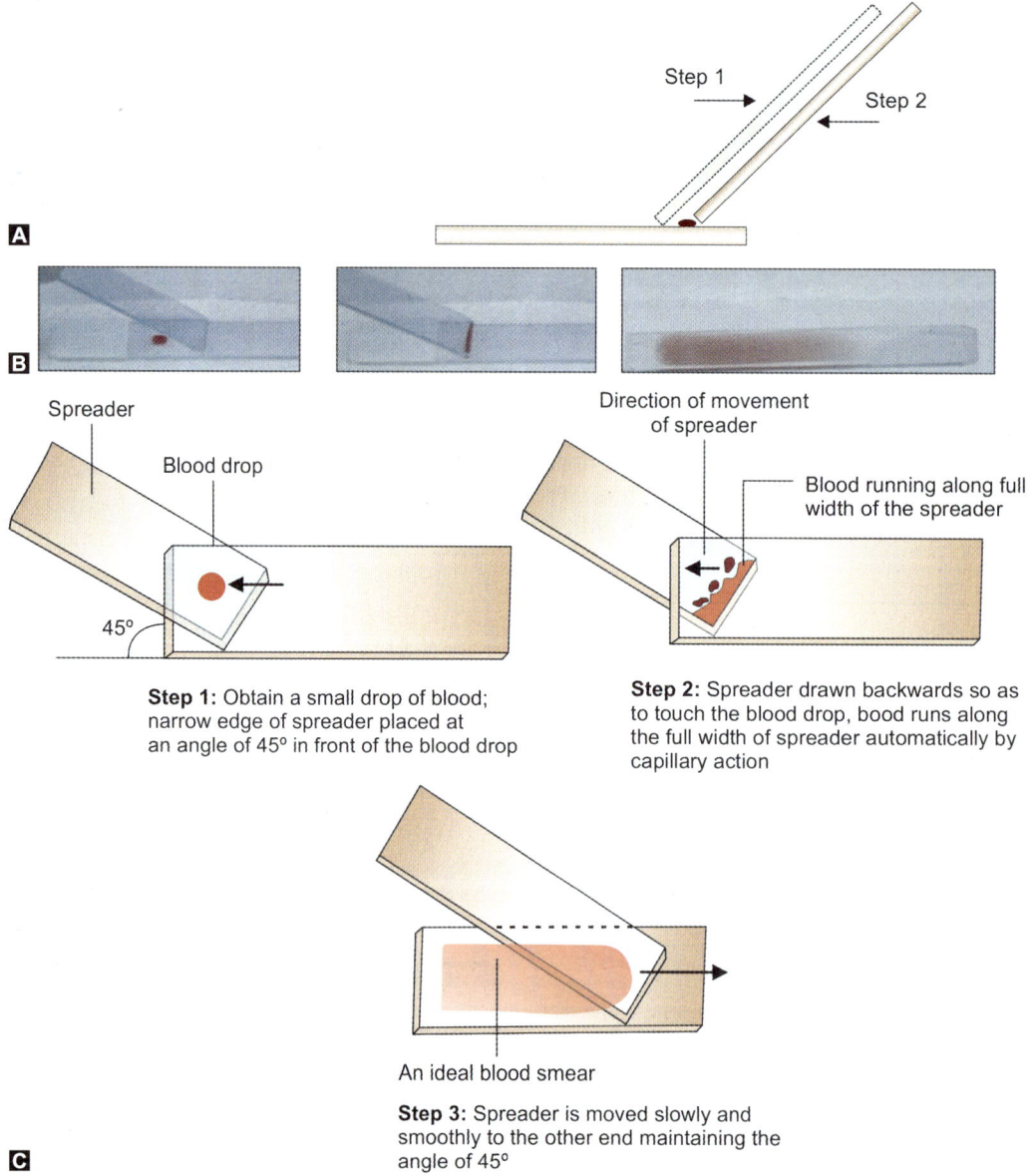

Step 1: Obtain a small drop of blood; narrow edge of spreader placed at an angle of 45° in front of the blood drop

Step 2: Spreader drawn backwards so as to touch the blood drop, bood runs along the full width of spreader automatically by capillary action

Step 3: Spreader is moved slowly and smoothly to the other end maintaining the angle of 45°

Figs. 1.7.1A to C: Method of making a blood film.

1. **Fixing the blood smear:** Place the slides, smear side up, on a "staining rack" assembled over a sink (two glass rods placed across the sink, with the ends fitted into short pieces of rubber tubing). Ensure that they are horizontal.
2. Pour 8–10 drops of the Leishman stain on each slide by using a dropper. This amount of stain usually covers the entire smear.
3. Allow the stain to remain undisturbed for 2 minutes. This time is known as **fixation time.** During this time, watch the stain carefully, especially during hot weather and see that it does not become thick due to evaporation of alcohol. If the stain dries, it will precipitate on the blood film and appear as round, blue granules. This can be prevented by pouring more stain on the slides as required.

Staining the Blood Smear

It is the process that stains (colors) the nuclei and cytoplasm of the cells. Both these purposes are achieved by the Leishman stain.
1. After the fixing time is over, add an equal number of drops of distilled water (or buffered water, if available) to the stain without spilling over.
2. Mix the stain and water by gently blowing at different places on the slides through a dropper. A glossy greenish layer (scum) soon appears on the surface of the diluted stain. Allow the diluted stain to remain on the slide for 8–10 minutes.
3. At the end of 10 minutes, pour off the stain.
4. Holding the slide in slanting position below the tap water, wash the slide with tap water gently and thoroughly, till the film gets a pink color. Wipe the back of the slide and allow it to air dry.

Examination of Peripheral Blood Smear

Examine the blood smear first under low power objective (10x) and then under high power objective (40x) to check the staining of the smear.

Features of an Ideal Blood Smear (Figs. 1.7.2 and 1.7.3)

1. The blood film should occupy the middle two-third of the slide, with a clear margin of about 2 mm on either side.
2. It should be tongue-shaped, i.e. broad at the head (starting point) and taper toward the other end, but without any "tail".
3. It should be translucent, uniformly thick throughout, with no vacant areas, striations (longitudinal or transverse) or "granular" areas.
4. It should be neither very thick nor very thin. The smear should be single cell thick with a uniform distribution of cells. A thin film looks faintly pink against a white surface, while a thick smear appears red. An ideal film appears light pink colored.

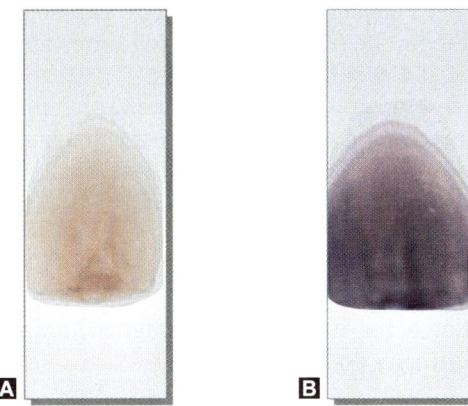

Figs. 1.7.2A and B: (A) Ideal blood film; (B) Ideal stained blood smear.

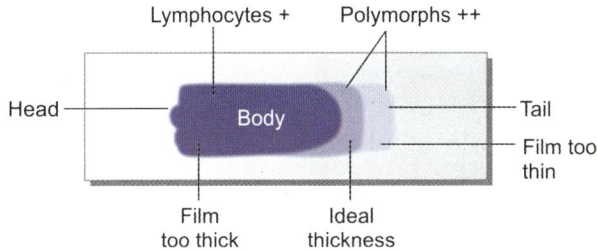

Fig. 1.7.3: Stained blood smear.

5. The red blood cells, as seen under the microscope, should lie separately from each other, without any crowding or rouleaux formation.

> **NOTE**
> A thick blood film results from taking too large a drop of blood, a faster movement and a smaller angle of the spreader.

Microscopic Appearance of an Ideal Stained Smear

1. **Under low magnification (10x):** The red blood cells appear as dots, uniformly spread out in a single layer. The WBCs cannot be differentiated.
2. **Under high magnification (45x):** The red cells are stained dull pink and show a central pallor (due to biconcavity). The WBCs, with their nuclei deep blue-violet, lie unevenly among the red cells. The platelets occur in small groups.
   At least one WBC is seen per high-power field.

Staining Defects

1. **Presence of stain granules:** They appear if the Leishman stain is old, if it has not been properly filtered or if it was allowed to dry up on the slide during fixing.
2. **Excessively blue appearance:** This appearance may be due to overstaining, overfixing, insufficient washing

or the use of alkaline stain or water. It can be corrected by reducing the fixing and staining times and proper washing under running water.

3. **Excessively reddish appearance:** This appearance may be due to understaining, overwashing or the use of more acidic stain or water. The defect may be rectified by restaining, if required.
4. **Faded appearance of blood cells:** This may result from the use of old stain, understaining or overwashing.

Examination of the Stained Smear Under Oil Immersion (100x) (Flowchart 1.7.1)

1. Place a drop of cedar wood oil in the center of the smear. Bring the oil immersion lens into position and focus the cells by keeping the condenser at the highest position and iris diaphragm fully opened.
2. Examine the slide all over for the distribution of different types of cells in different parts of smear.
3. The following cells can be identified:
   a. **Red cells:** Stained pink, the red cells appear as numerous, evenly spread out, non-nucleated, biconcave discs of uniform size of 7.2–7.8 μm. There may be some overcrowding and overlapping or even rouleaux formation in the **head end** of the blood film.
   b. **Leukocytes:** Five main types of WBCs are commonly seen in blood films. They are all larger than the red blood cells (RBCs), nucleated and unevenly distributed among the red blood cells. They include three types of granulocytes, i.e. neutrophils, eosinophils and basophils (neutrophils being the most numerous). Also present are two types of agranulocytes (monocytes and lymphocytes).

> **NOTE**
> There are fewer and poorly-stained WBCs in the head end and the extreme tail part of the PBS; and some of these may be distorted. There appear to be more monocytes in the tail end, probably dragged there by the spreader because of their larger size. Plenty of neutrophils are found along the edges, though they may be poorly stained and lymphocytes are seen in the middle of the blood smear.

   c. **Platelets:** They are membrane-bound round or oval bodies, with a diameter of 2–4 μm. They lie here and there in groups of 2–12. They stain pink-purple and being fragments of megakaryocytes, they do not possess nuclei.

Identification of Different Types of Leukocytes (Table 1.7.1 and Figs. 1.7.4)

A leukocyte is identified on the basis of following:
1. Size: The size of the leukocytes is compared with that of the surrounding RBCs.

Flowchart 1.7.1: Scheme of identification of cells in peripheral blood smear (PBS).

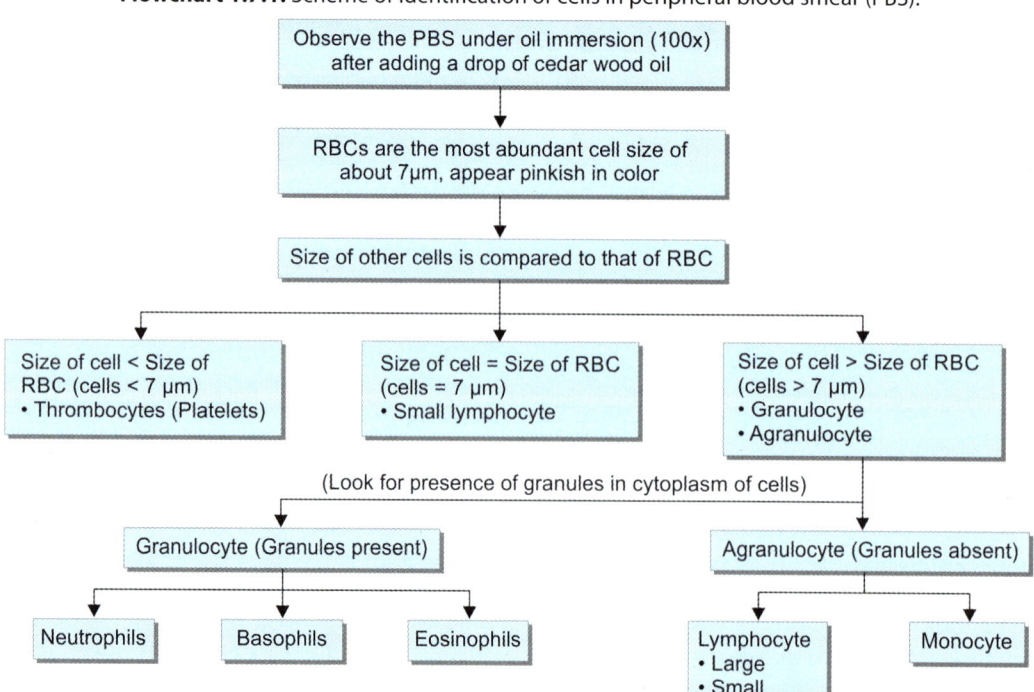

(RBC: red blood cell)

Chapter 1.7: Preparation of a Peripheral Blood Smear and Determination of Differential Leukocyte Count

Table 1.7.1: Characteristic features of white blood cells (WBCs) in a stained blood film.

Cell type	Diameter (μm)	Nucleus	Cytoplasm	Cytoplasmic granules	Functions
Granulocytes					
Neutrophils (40–70%)	10–14 μm (1.5–2 times the size of a RBC)	• Blue-violet • 1–6 lobes, connected by chromatin threads	• Slight blue in color	• Fine sand-like particles • Closely-packed violet pink in color • Do not cover nucleus	• First to arrive at the site of invasion by microbes. • Phagocytosis • Mediators of febrile response in our body (contain endogenous pyrogens)
Eosinophils (1–6%)	10–14 μm	• Blue-violet • Bilobed, lobes connected by thick or thin chromatin band (spectacle-shaped)	• Eosinophilic • Light pink-red • Granular	• Large, coarse • Brick red in color • Do not cover nucleus	• Antiallergic role: Release enzymes histaminase, leukotriene • Mild phagocytic function • Antiparasitic action
Basophils (0–1%)	10–14 μm	• Blue-violet • Bilobed • Not clearly seen because overlaid with granules	• Basophilic • Bluish • Granular	• Large, very coarse • Blue/purple in color • Completely fill the cell and cover the nucleus	• Liberate histamine, heparin and serotonin and eosinophil chemotactic factor of anaphylaxis (ECF-A) • Involved in immediate hypersensitivity reactions
Agranulocytes					
Monocytes (2–8%) **Largest Leukocyte**	12–20 μm (2–3 times the size of a RBC)	• Pale blue-violet • Large, single • May be indented horseshoe or kidney-shaped (can appear oval or round) • Peripheral in position	• Abundant • Slight blue in color • Nuclear/cytoplasmic ratio is 3:1 • Ground glass appearance	• Absent	• Second line of defense: Acute phagocytosis • They become tissue macrophages
Lymphocyte (20–40%)	Small lymphocytes (7–10 μm) (same as size of RBC)	• Deep blue-violet • Single, large, round, almost fills cell • Condensed, lumpy chromatin, gives "ink-spot" appearance	• Hardly visible • Thin crescent of clear, light blue cytoplasm	• Absent	• Role in immune responses of the body • Produce antibodies
	Large lymphocytes (10–14 μm) (1.5–2 times of a RBC)	• Deep blue-violet • Single, large, round or oval • May be central or eccentric	• Large crescent of clear light blue cytoplasm • Amount larger than in small lymphocyte	• Absent	

2. Nucleus.
3. Cytoplasm: Its color, whether granules are visible or not, their color and size, if visible.
4. Cytoplasm/Nucleus ratio.

Differential Counting of Leukocytes (Fig. 1.7.5)

Count a minimum of 100 WBCs and identify them. Enter these cells in the squares given below by using the

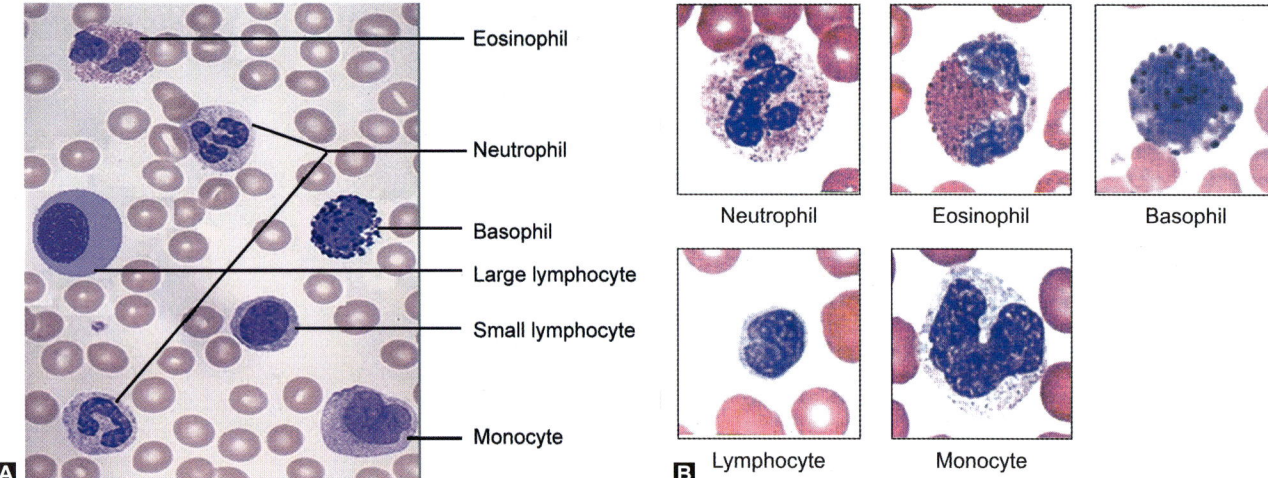

Figs. 1.7.4A and B: (A) Different types of blood cells in a blood film stained with Leishman stain. The size, shape of the nucleus and staining features of the cytoplasmic granules distinguish them from one another; (B) White blood cells under oil immersion.

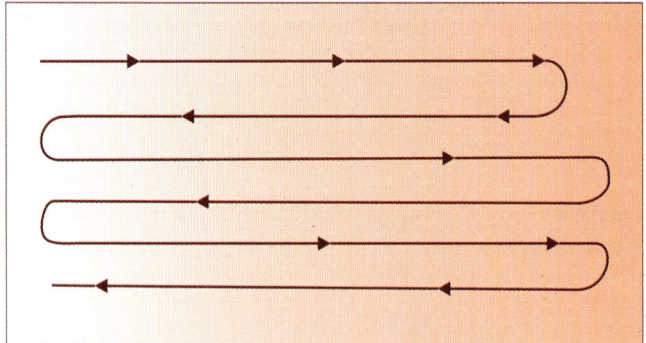

Fig. 1.7.5: Method of counting.

letters "N" for neutrophils, "M" for monocytes, "LL" for large lymphocytes, "SL" for small lymphocytes, "E" for eosinophils and "B" for basophils.

N	N	SL	N	L	L	N	N	N	L
LL	E	N	N	N	N	L	M	N	L

> **NOTE**
> **Alternative method (Tally bar method):** You can also indicate these cells in a column and as you identify a cell, put a short vertical stroke for each cell identified. In this way, you can place different types of cells in groups of five, a diagonal stroke representing the 5th cell (e.g. neutrophils = ||||).

- When counting has been done, calculate the percentage of each type of cell in your count of 100 white blood cells.
- **Absolute leukocyte count:** The absolute values are more significant than the DLC values alone. The reason is that the DLC may show only a relative increase or decrease of a particular type of cell with a corresponding change in the other cell types.

Absolute leukocyte count

$$= \frac{\text{Number of cells in DLC} \times \text{TLC count/mm}^3}{100}$$

Normal values: The normal values for differential and absolute counts are given in Table 1.7.2.

Table 1.7.2: Normal values for differential and absolute leukocyte counts.

Differential count	Percent (%)	Absolute count (per mm³)
Neutrophils	40–75	2,000–7,500
Lymphocytes (both)	20–45	1,300–3,500
Monocytes	2–10	500–800
Eosinophils	1–6	4–440
Basophils	0–1	0–100

PHYSIOCLINICAL SIGNIFICANCE

The suffix "-philia" means an increase in the number and the suffix "-penia" means a decrease in the number (of cells).

Neutrophils

Neutrophilia (Absolute Count ≥10,000/mm³)

1. **Physiological causes:**
   a. Muscular exercise, physical and mental stress after meals.
   b. During pregnancy and after parturition.
2. **Pathological causes (Absolute count):**
   a. Acute infections, especially localized due to pus-forming bacteria (streptococci and staphylococci).
   b. Surgery, trauma, burns, acute hemorrhage and hemolysis.
   c. Tissue necrosis (tissue death); myocardial infarction.
   d. *Drugs:* Adrenaline and glucocorticoids.

Neutropenia (Absolute Count ≤2,500/mm³)

1. **Physiological causes:** In children.
2. **Pathological causes:**
   a. Typhoid and paratyphoid infections, viral influenza, kala-azar.
   b. Acquired immunodeficiency syndrome (AIDS).
   c. Depression of bone marrow due to drugs, chemicals, radiation, etc.
   d. Autoimmune disease—diabetes mellitus, rheumatoid arthritis, purpura, etc.

Eosinophils

Eosinophilia (Absolute Count ≥500/mm³)

1. **Allergic conditions:** Bronchial asthma, skin diseases like urticaria, eczema and food sensitivity, etc.
2. **Parasitic infections:** Intestinal worms like hookworms, tapeworms, roundworms, especially those which invade tissues.

Eosinopenia (Absolute Count <50/mm³)

1. Adrenocorticotropic hormone (ACTH) and glucocorticoid treatment.
2. Cushing's syndrome (excess steroids).

Basophils

Basophilia (Absolute Count ≥100/mm³)

1. Viral infections
2. Allergic diseases
3. Smallpox and chickenpox.

Basopenia

1. Acute pyogenic infections
2. During glucocorticoid treatment.

Monocytes [Monocyte-Macrophage System/Reticuloendothelial System (RES)]

Monocytosis (Absolute Count ≥800/mm³)

1. Infectious mononucleosis (IM)
2. Malaria, kala-azar
3. Subacute bacterial endocarditis
4. Rheumatoid arthritis
5. Leukemias, collagen diseases and malignancies.

Monocytopenia

It may be seen in bone marrow depression.

Lymphocytes

Lymphocytosis (Absolute Count ≥5,000/mm³)

1. **Physiological:** Healthy infants and young children. DLC may be about 60%, though the TLC may be normal. This is sometimes called **"relative lymphocytosis"**.
2. **Pathological:**
   a. *Viral infections:* whooping cough, chickenpox, auto-immune disease, etc.
   b. Chronic infections like tuberculosis and hepatitis.
   c. Chronic lymphocytic leukemia.

Lymphocytopenia

1. Patients on steroid therapy.
2. Acquired immunodeficiency syndrome. The virus particularly attacks the helper/inducer (T4) cells.
3. Depression of bone marrow due to any cause.

OTHER USES OF PERIPHERAL BLOOD SMEAR

1. Diagnosis of malaria, from malarial parasite seen in the red blood cells.
2. Diagnosis of leukemia from the type and number of blast cells.
3. Various parasitic infections like filariasis, trypanosomiasis, etc.
4. Sex determination can be done from the presence of female sex chromatin which appears as a "drumstick" (Barr body) attached to a lobe of neutrophil nucleus.
5. Toxic granules can be seen within the neutrophils in bacterial infections.
6. Study of morphology of red blood cells in various types of anemias.
7. Estimation of platelet count by indirect method.

PRECAUTIONS

1. The slides should be absolutely free from dust and grease.
2. The edge of the spreader should be smooth, otherwise the slide would leave striations along or across the smear.
3. The blood film should be spread immediately after taking it on the slide. Any delay will cause clumping of cells due to partial coagulation.
4. The angle of the spreader should be 45°. The more the angle of the spreader approaches the vertical, the thinner the film and the lesser the angle, the thicker the film.
5. The pressure of the spreader on the slide should be slight and even and the pushing should be fairly quick while maintaining a uniform pressure throughout.
6. The film should be dried by waving it in the air immediately after spreading it. A delay can cause not only clumping, but also crenation and distortion of red cells in a damp atmosphere (if water is allowed to slowly evaporate from the blood plasma on the slide, crenation occurs due to gradual increase in the concentration of salts).

Objective Structured Practical Examination–I

Aim: To prepare a blood film from a sample of blood provided.
Procedural steps: See text above.
Checklist:
1. Select 3–4, clean, grease-free, dry slides and place these on a blotting paper. Mix the provided sample of blood thoroughly without frothing. (Y/N)
2. Using a dropper, she places a small drop of blood near the end of a slide about 1 cm from the end. (Y/N)
3. Supporting the left end of the slide between thumb and middle finger of left hand, she places the spreader in front of the blood drop at an angle of 40° and draws the spreader back and allows the blood to spread along its width. (Y/N)
4. Maintaining a light and even pressure and 40° angle, she moves the spreader forward, with a fairly fast and gliding motion, pulling the blood behind it in the form of a thin smear. (Y/N)
5. Make 3–4 more such smears. (Y/N)

Objective Structured Practical Examination–II

Aim: To stain the given blood film for differential count.
Procedural steps: See text above.
Checklist:
1. Place the blood film horizontally over the parallel glass rods assembled over the sink. (Y/N)
2. Pour 8–10 drops of Leishman stain from a drop bottle to cover the blood film. (Y/N)
3. After 1–2 minutes (or as advised), she adds equal amount of buffered water or double-distilled water, over the stain till the mixture stands from the edges of the slide. (Y/N)
4. Mix the stain by blowing on it through a glass dropper for 8–10 minutes. Watch that at no stage the stain is allowed to dry on the blood film. (Y/N)
5. Then drain off the stain under a gentle stream of distilled/tap water. Then put the slide against a support, stained side facing down. (Y/N)

Objective Structured Practical Examination–III

Aim: To examine the provided stained blood film under oil immersion lens and focus any leukocyte.
Procedural steps: See text above.
Checklist:
1. Check the stained slide to confirm the side on which the smear was made. Then examine it under low power and high power lenses by making suitable adjustments of light to check staining and cell distribution. (Y/N)
2. Raise the body tube, place a drop of cedar wood oil and swing the oil immersion lens into position. (Y/N)
3. Looking from the side, bring the oil immersion lens down slowly till it just enters the oil drop. (Y/N)
4. Raise the condenser and open the iris diaphragm. (Y/N)
5. Look into the microscope and scan the smear, "racking" the microscope all the time till she focuses a leukocyte. (Y/N)

QUESTIONS

Q.1. What precautions will you take while preparing blood films? Why are four or five (or more) slides prepared at a time?

Q.2. Why should the blood film be dried quickly soon after spreading it?

Q.3. What are the features of an ideal blood film?

Q.4. What is the composition of Leishman stain and what is the function of each component? Why should the stain be acetone free?

Q.5. What is buffered water? Why should it be preferred over distilled water?
Buffered water is a phosphate buffer in which the pH is adjusted at 6.8. At this pH, there is optimal ionization of the stain particles so that they can penetrate the cells better.

Q.6. Why is Leishman stain diluted after 2 minutes? What happens to the blood film during this period?

Q.7. Can tap water be used for diluting the stain after fixation?
Tap water should not be used because the methylene blue components may not stain the cells due to the unknown pH and salt content of this water. Also, tap water may contain impurities that may show up as artifact on the blood film.

Q.8. Can any other stain be used for blood films?
Yes. Giemsa stain, like Leishman stain, is a mixture of methylene blue, methylene azure and eosin.
Wright's blood stain is still another stain commonly used in some laboratories.

Q.9. What other information can be obtained from a blood film?

Q.10. Why is cedar wood oil used with oil immersion objective?
Q.11. Which part of the blood film should be avoided for counting the cells? Which is the best part?
Q.12. How are leukocytes classified and how can they be differentiated from each other?
Q.13. What is the clinical importance of doing differential leukocyte count?
Q.14. What is absolute leukocyte count and what is its importance?
Q.15. How does the differential leukocyte count of a child differ from that of an adult?
Q.16. Is it possible to know the sex of a person from the blood film?
Q.17. Draw a well-labeled diagram showing different cells in a peripheral blood smear.

RESULT

N : Neutrophil ....
L : Lymphocyte ....
E : Eosinophil ....
B : Basophil ....
M : Monocyte ....

....
....
....
....
....

OBSERVATION

INTERPRETATION

....
....
....
....
....

STUDY NOTES

Date ....

CHAPTER 1.8

Arneth Count (Cooke-Arneth Count)

AIM
To determine the Arneth count.

INTRODUCTION
Arneth count is the percentage distribution of neutrophils on the basis of number of lobes in the nucleus. It indicates the maturity (stage of development) of the neutrophils.

Young neutrophils have fewer lobes as compared to older cells which have 5 or 6 lobes (Table 1.8.1). The percentage of younger or older cells in a blood film can provide useful information about the functional status of the bone marrow (Fig. 1.8.1).

APPARATUS
Same as for differential leukocyte count (DLC) (*Refer* Chapter 1.7).

PROCEDURE
1. Prepare and stain a fresh blood film in the usual manner.
2. Stained smear is examined under the oil immersion objective (100x).
3. Examine 100 neutrophils, noting the number of lobes in each cell following the rule of counting as in DLC.
4. Enter your observations in your workbook.
5. Express your result as percentage of total neutrophils counted.

Table 1.8.1: Percentages of each stage with description.

Stage		Description	Percentage (%)
Stage I	(N_1)	Nucleus is C- or U-shaped, the two limbs being connected by a thick band of chromatin (**stab or Schaff cell**)–one lobed neutrophil	5–10
Stage II	(N_2)	The two lobes are connected by a narrow band of chromatin	20–30
Stage III	(N_3)	Three lobes connected by chromatin filaments. (Actively motile and functionally most effective)	40–50
Stage IV	(N_4)	Four lobes connected by chromatin filaments	10–15
Stage V	(N_5, N_6)	• Five lobes or more (N6 ≥6 lobes) • Outline may be irregular • Cytoplasmic granules poorly stained • Functionally less motile and less effective	3–5

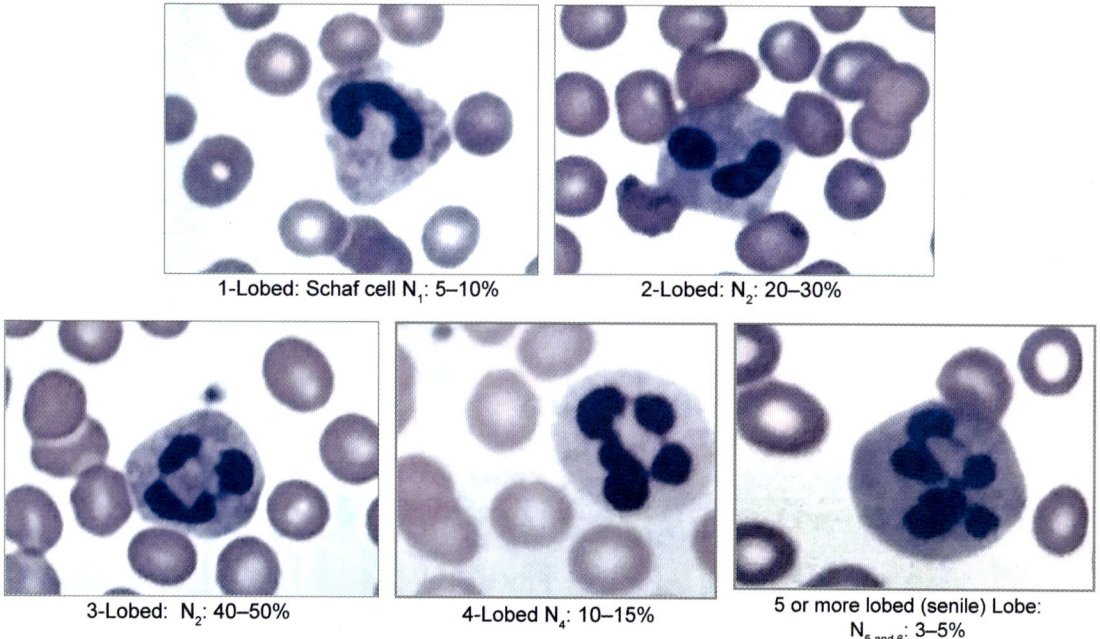

Fig. 1.8.1: Cooke-Arneth count. The percent distribution of neutrophils in the circulation based on the number of their lobes is shown.

> **NOTE**
> - When two lobes of the nucleus are connected only by a band of chromatin they are called as separate lobes of the nucleus. There should be no nucleoplasmic connection between them.
> - The neutrophil size decreases with aging.
> - The older neutrophil contain fewer granules.

PHYSIOCLINICAL SIGNIFICANCE

Left Shift (Regenerative Shift) (Fig. 1.8.2)

$(N_1 + N_2 + N_3) \geq 80\%$. This indicates a **hyperactive bone marrow**.

A shift to the left indicates that the bone marrow is actively forming and releasing neutrophils into the circulation. Shift to left occurs in:
1. Acute pus-producing infections.
2. Tuberculosis: Though there is lymphocytosis, a shift to the left may be due to removal of older neutrophils from the blood.
3. Hemorrhage.
4. Low-dosage irradiation is said to stimulate bone marrow while heavy doses cause a shift to the right.

Right Shift (Degenerative Shift) (Fig. 1.8.2)

$(N_4 + N_5 + N_6) \geq 20\%$. This indicates a **hypoactive bone marrow**.

A shift to the right indicates decreased production and release of neutrophils. Shift to right occurs in:

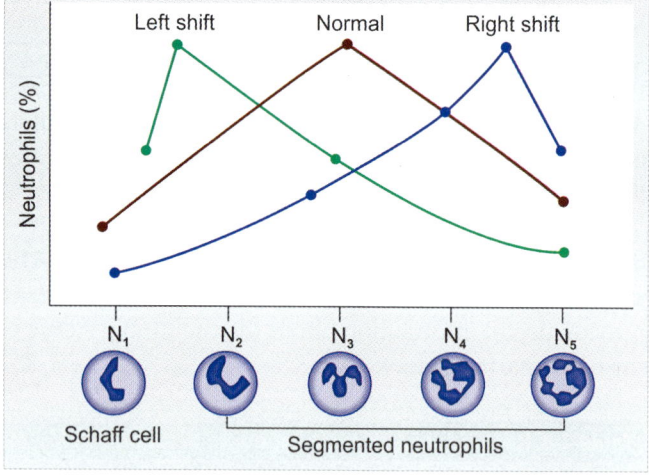

Fig. 1.8.2: Arneth curve showing right and left shift.

1. Bone marrow depression (hypoplasia and aplasia) due to any factor.
2. Drugs, toxins and chemical poisons.
3. Megaloblastic anemia, septicemia, uremia, etc.

PRECAUTIONS

1. Choose a stained slide that shows neutrophils to best advantage.
2. If the lobes cannot be seen, consider the size of the cell and the number of granules in the cytoplasm.

Chapter 1.8: Arneth Count (Cooke-Arneth Count)

Objective Structured Practical Examination

Aim: To focus a stage 3 neutrophil in a blood smear.
Procedural steps: See text above.
Checklist:
1. Make an ideal stained smear. (Y/N)
2. Check the stained slide to confirm the side on which the smear was made. Then examine it under low power and high power lenses by making suitable adjustments of light to check staining and neutrophil distribution. (Y/N)
3. Raise the body tube, place a drop of cedar wood oil and swing the oil-immersion lens into position. (Y/N)
4. Looking from the side, bring the oil-immersion lens down slowly till it just enters the oil drop. (Y/N)
5. Raise the condenser and open the iris diaphragm. (Y/N)
6. Look into the microscope and scan the smear, "racking" the microscope all the time till she focuses a stage 3 neutrophil. (Y/N)

QUESTIONS

- **Q.1.** What is the relation between the number of lobes of the nucleus and the age of a neutrophil?
- **Q.2.** What is meant by the terms left shift and right shift? Is the Cooke-Arneth count of any clinical value?
- **Q.3.** If a person has a slight rise in total leukocyte count (TLC) (about 10,500/mm^3), how can the possibility of an early leukocytosis be ruled out?
  In this case on doing the Arneth count if there is no increase in number of young neutrophils (stage 1 and stage 2) the possibility of an early leukocytosis is ruled out.
- **Q.4.** If Cooke-Arneth count can provide such useful information about the functioning of bone marrow, why it is not used as a routine test?
  The reason for this test not being used as a routine: Some physiological conditions can cause shifting of neutrophils from various pools into the circulating blood. This leads to confusion about left or right shift. Therefore, better methods, e.g. bone marrow biopsy, are now available for assessing bone marrow function.
- **Q.5.** Plot a graph of your own values with the neutrophil stages on the X-axis and their percentage on the Y-axis. Draw another graph with the values given in your book and compare the two graphs.
  The student should be able to do this exercise easily and be able to explain the differences, if any.
- **Q.6.** What are the typical features of senile neutrophils?

OBSERVATION

RESULT

Express the results as percentage of the total neutrophils counted.
N_1: Single lobed.....................%
N_2: Two lobed........................%
N_3: Three lobed.....................%
N_4: Four lobed......................%
N_5 and N_6: Five or more lobed....................%

INTERPRETATION

Section 1: Hematology

STUDY NOTES

Teacher's Signature

CHAPTER 1.9

Determination of Blood Groups (A, B, O and Rh System)

AIM
Determination of blood groups ABO and Rh.

INTRODUCTION
Blood groups are based on the presence or absence of antigens on the surface of red blood cells and antibodies in the plasma.

PRINCIPLE
The surfaces of human red cells contain a variety of genetically determined glycolipids and glycoproteins that act as **antigens (agglutinogen)**. The plasma contains **antibodies (agglutinins)** that can react with these antigens when the two are mixed. Since the red cell antigens cause **agglutination** of RBCs in the presence of suitable antibodies, they are also called *agglutinogens*; the antibodies in the plasma are called *agglutinins*.

The Landsteiner law (1900), which has two major components, states that:
1. If an agglutinogen is present on the red cells of an individual, the corresponding agglutinins must be absent in the plasma.
2. If an agglutinogen is absent in the red cells, the corresponding agglutinins must be present in the plasma.

The exception to the second component of the law is that absence of Rh agglutinogen from the red cells in Rh –ve persons is not accompanied by the presence of anti-Rh agglutinins.

BLOOD GROUP SYSTEMS
There are 30 commonly occurring antigens and hundreds of rare antigens that have been found on the surfaces of human red cell membranes. Of different blood group systems, only two are of great clinical importance—the ABO system and the Rh system.

ABO Blood Group (Classical)

Blood group	Antigens	Antibodies
AB	A and B	None
A	A	B
B	B	A
O	None	A and B

Rh Blood Group

- In addition to antigens of ABO system, the red cells of 80–85% of humans also contain an additional antigen, called Rh antigen (or Rh factor) (Table 1.9.1). The Rh factor is so named because this antigen was discovered in the rhesus monkey by Landsteiner and Wiener in 1940. They injected red blood cells of rhesus monkey into rabbits. The rabbit's immune system reacted by forming antibodies against rhesus red cells and when the rabbit's plasma was tested against human red cells, agglutination occurred in 80–85% of individuals.

Section 1: Hematology

Table 1.9.1: Differences between ABO and Rh antibodies.

ABO system antibodies	Rh antibodies
The antibodies anti-A and anti-B are of the larger IgM type. They cannot cross the placenta.	Rh antibodies are of the IgG type. They can easily cross the placenta.
These antibodies react best with the antigens at low temperatures of 5–20°C. They are, therefore, called "cold" antibodies.	The antigen-antibody reactions occur best at body temperature. Hence, they are called "warm" antibodies.
ABO incompatibility between a mother and her fetus rarely causes any problems.	Rh incompatibility between a mother and her fetus may cause serious complications.

- Persons whose red cells contain this additional antigen are called **"Rh positive" (Rh+)** while those who lack this antigen are called **"Rh negative" (Rh−)**. There are several varieties of Rh antigens—C, D, E, c, d and e—but the D antigen is the most common and antigenically, the most potent.

In addition to the ABO and Rh antigens, many other antigens are expressed on the surface of RBC membrane, e.g. M and N antigen, Kell antigen and the Lewis system.

APPARATUS

1. Pricking apparatus
2. Microscope
3. Clean, dry blood group slides with well
4. 0.9% normal saline
5. Applicator sticks, dropper, glass marking pencil
6. Anti-A serum, anti-B serum, anti-D serum (Fig. 1.9.1).

PROCEDURE

Preparation of Red Cell Suspension (Fig. 1.9.2)

1. Place 2 mL of saline in a small (5 mL) test tube.
2. Then using aseptic precautions give a bold finger prick and allow a blood drop to form.
3. Now place the pricked fingertip on top of the test tube and invert it. Mix the blood and saline by inverting the tube two or three times.
4. A suspension of red cells is now ready.

Determination of Blood Groups

1. Mark the wells in blood group slides as A, B and D separately.
2. Put one drop of anti-A serum, anti-B serum and anti-D serum separately in the three wells marked as A, B and D on the blood group slide.
3. In addition also take 1 drop of normal saline as control in a separate well.
4. Add a drop of red cell suspension drawn from the bottom of the test tube by a dropper on each of anti-A, anti-B and anti-D sera and one drop on the normal saline taken on the "control" side (The nozzle of the dropper should not touch any of the antisera) (Figs. 1.9.3A and B).

    In this way, the red cells–saline mixture on the "control" side will act as a control to confirm agglutination or no agglutination on the corresponding test side (Fig. 1.9.4).
5. Gently mix the antisera and red cells suspension, using three separate applicator sticks.
6. Wait for 8–10 minutes then inspect the three antisera—red cell mixtures and the "control" mixture, first with the

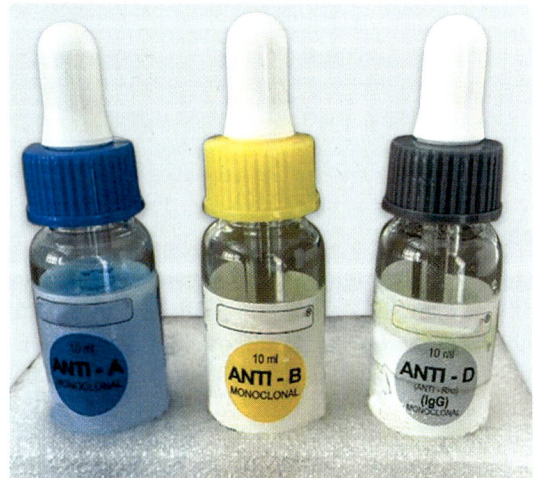

Fig. 1.9.1: Commercially available anti-A, anti-B, and anti-D serum.

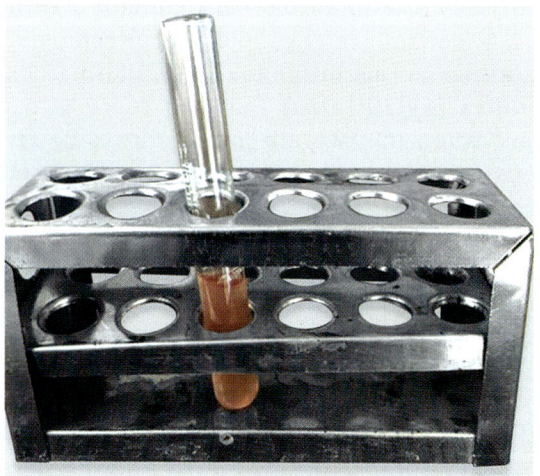

Fig. 1.9.2: Preparation of red cell suspension.

Chapter 1.9: Determination of Blood Groups (A, B, O and Rh System)

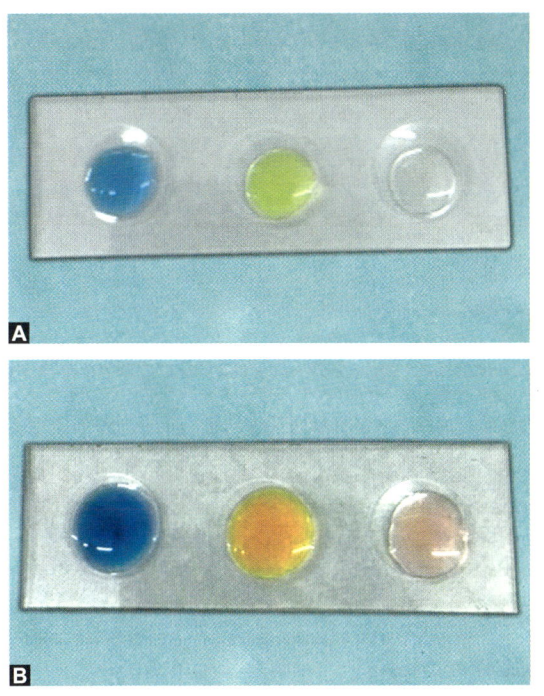

Figs. 1.9.3A and B: Marking of serum anti-A, anti-B and anti-D.

naked eye to see whether agglutination (clumping of red cells) has taken place or not.

7. Then confirm under low magnification microscope, comparing each "test mixture" with the "control mixture".
   - If there is no agglutination, the RBCs remain evenly distributed and separated from each other.
   - If there is agglutination, the RBCs are clumped together and lose their outline.
8. Reaction of different blood groups with different antibodies is given in Table 1.9.2.

> **NOTE**
> **False positive reaction:** This can occur when the antisera are contaminated with bacterial growth.
> **False negative reaction:** It may occur due to improper storage of antisera leading to loss of its potency.

PHYSIOCLINICAL SIGNIFICANCE OF BLOOD GROUPING

Blood grouping/typing is important in:
1. Blood transfusion.
2. Determination of Rh incompatibility between the mother and child.
3. Paternity disputes: The ABO, Rh and MNS blood grouping is used to settle cases of disputed paternity. It is possible to prove that a person is not the father. But not possible to prove that he is the father.
4. Organ transplantation.

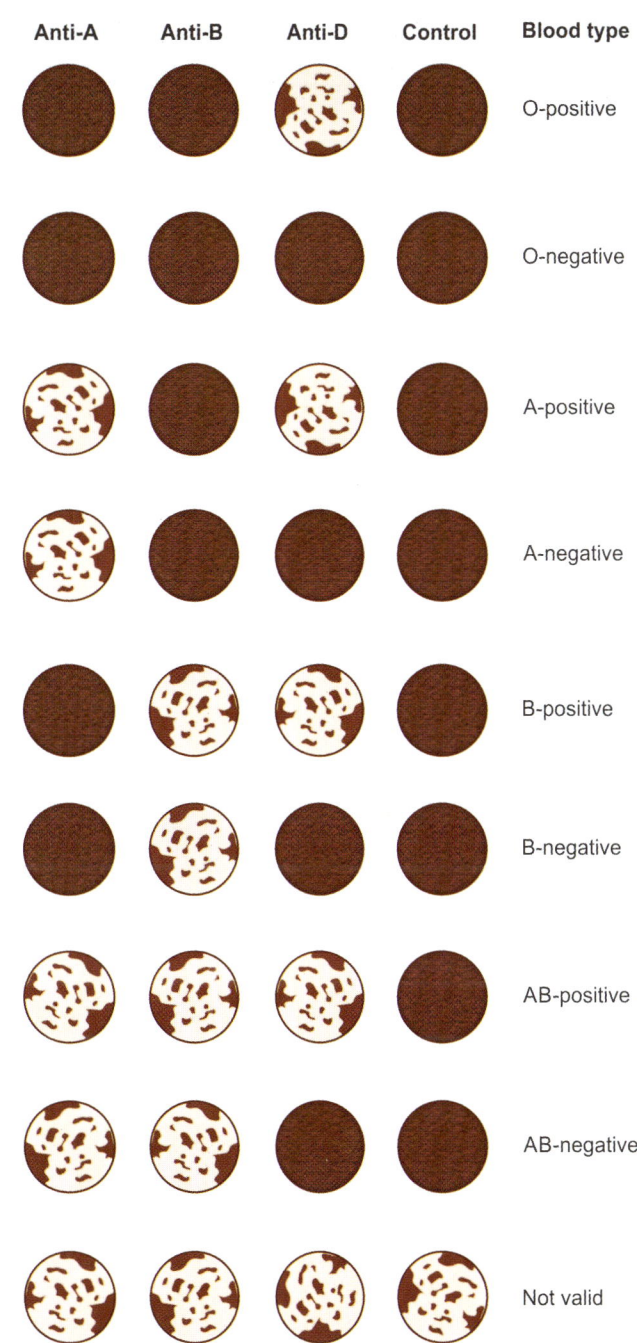

Fig. 1.9.4: Determination of blood groups showing agglutination (hemolysis and clumping of red cells) and no agglutination (cells remain uniformly distributed).

5. Genetic studies
6. Medicolegal use
7. Susceptibility to disease: The people of blood type O are more susceptible to peptic ulcer. Blood type A is more commonly prone to carcinoma of stomach and to some extent in diabetes mellitus.

Table 1.9.2: Reaction of different blood groups with different antibodies

Blood group	Antigen on cell membrane	Antibodies in serum	Reaction with		
			Anti-serum A	Anti-serum B	Anti-serum Rh
A	A	B	–	+	
B	B	A	+	–	
O	No antigen	A, B	+	+	
AB	A, B	No antibodies	–	–	
Rh+	Rh	No antibodies			+
Rh–	No Rh antigen	No antibodies			–

"+": **Agglutination present**—RBCs are massed together in clumps and lose their outline.
"–": **No agglutination**—RBCs remain separate and evenly distributed.

PHYSIOCLINICAL SIGNIFICANCE OF Rh FACTOR

Although there are no natural anti-Rh antibodies and they never develop spontaneously, they can be produced when a Rh –ve person is given Rh +ve blood or when a Rh –ve mother carries a Rh +ve fetus.

1. **In transfusions:** When a Rh –ve person receives Rh +ve blood, there is no immediate reaction since there are no antibodies. But during the next few weeks/months, he/she may produce anti-Rh antibodies that will remain in the blood. However, if later, there is another exposure to Rh +ve blood, there will be agglutination and hemolysis, thus resulting in a serious transfusion reaction.
2. **In pregnancy:** The most common problem due to Rh incompatibility may arise when a Rh –ve mother carries a Rh +ve fetus. At the time of delivery small amount of fetal blood leaks into the mother as the placenta separates from the uterine wall, resulting in high concentration of anti-Rh antibodies in the mother.

   During the first pregnancy, however, the anti-Rh antibody levels do not reach high enough levels to cause complications. However, during the second and subsequent pregnancies, the mother's anti-Rh antibodies cross the placental membrane into the fetus where they cause agglutination and hemolysis. The clinical condition that develops in the fetus is called **"hemolytic disease of the newborn (HDN)" or "erythroblastosis fetalis."**

Chief clinical forms of HDN:
- Hydrops fetalis
- Icterus gravis neonatorum (Grave jaundice of the newborn)
- Kernicterus.

PRECAUTIONS

1. The slides should be dry, dust-free and grease-free.
2. Mark all the slides beforehand.
3. There should not be intermixing of different antisera placed on the slide.
4. Separate applicator should be used to mix each of the antisera with the red cell suspension.
5. Examine the slides with the naked eye and then under the microscope after 8–10 minutes but before the sera–blood mixture dry up.
6. Do not add undiluted blood from the fingerprick directly on to the antisera for two reasons, one, the sera may get intermixed and two, false-positive reaction may develop. Sometimes, it is not possible to say with certainty whether agglutination has occurred or not. In such cases, the grouping must be repeated with diluted blood.
7. A control should always be used to exclude false-positive result.

QUESTIONS

Q.1. What is a blood group system?

Q.2. How can antibodies be present in a person when the corresponding antigens are absent?

The specific blood group antibodies are absent at birth. However, they are produced in the next few weeks/months, reaching a maximum by the age of 10 years. These antibodies are produced in response to A and/or B antigens (or antigens very similar to these), which are present in intestinal bacteria or are taken in foods, such as seeds, plants and in house dust. These antigens are absorbed into blood and stimulate the formation of antibodies against **antigens not present in the infants' red cells,** i.e. those antigens that are recognized as "non-self" by the body's immune system.

Q.3. What is Landsteiner law? How does it apply to all blood groups?

Q.4. What are cold and warm antibodies?

Q.5. How are antisera A and antisera B obtained?

The antisera can be obtained from the humans or from animals:
1. Antisera A, B and Rh are obtained by injecting their antigen into rabbit and collecting antibodies from their serum.

2. Antisera can be obtained from the serum of individuals of blood group A (anti-B serum) and of blood group B (anti-A serum).
3. **Monoclonal antibodies:** Also, since the titer (concentration) of antibodies is variable, monoclonal antibodies are used. If a single plasma cell could be isolated, it could be made to proliferate in a tissue culture and produce large quantities of identical antibodies.

Q.6. What is the importance of using a control on each of the three test slides? What are false-positive and false-negative results?

The control in each case is only a suspension of red cells in saline. Its purpose is to avoid "false-positive" (formation of large rouleaux and contamination) and "false-negative" results.

Q.7. What is the difference between agglutination and rouleaux formation? How will you confirm that agglutination has occurred on the microscope slide?

Q.8. What is zone phenomenon?

For agglutination to occur, the concentration of agglutinogens and agglutinins has to be about the same. This is the reason for making a red cell suspension in isotonic saline solution.

Q.9. Why should you wait for 8–10 minutes before checking for agglutination?

This much time is required for antigen-antibody reaction to occur.

Q.10. What is cross-matching?

The red cells and the plasma of the donor and recipient blood are separated by centrifugation.

1. **Direct (major) cross-matching:** The donor red cells are then tested with the recipient plasma. Since the reaction between donor red cells and recipient plasma is of prime importance, it is called "major cross-matching".
2. **Indirect (minor) cross-matching:** The donor plasma is tested against the red cells of the recipient. The whole process is called "cross-matching". This reaction is not very important and usually does not occur even in a mismatch, because the agglutinins are greatly diluted in the recipient plasma. Thus, the donor agglutinins can usually be ignored, if their potency is not too high. It is for these two reasons that this reaction is called "minor cross-match".

If there is no agglutination in either case, the donor blood can safely be given to the recipient.

> **NOTE**
> Cross-matching must always be done before every blood transfusion.

Q.11. What is meant by the terms universal donor and universal recipient?

Since type O persons do not have either A or B antigens on their red cells, they are called "universal donors" because their blood can, theoretically, be given to all four blood types. Type AB persons are called "universal recipients" because they do not have circulating agglutinins in their plasma and can, therefore, receive blood of any type.

> **NOTE**
> Though it is a rule never to give blood without cross-matching, an exception could be made in a most extreme emergency, where group O Rh –ve blood may be given immediately as O –ve blood group is considered as **universal donor.**

Q.12. What is Rh factor and what is its clinical significance?

Q.13. If an Rh –ve mother carries Rh +ve fetus, what are the complications that are likely to occur?

Q.14. How can hemolytic disease of the newborn be prevented?

The hemolysis of red cells (HDN) is due to the crossing over of anti-Rh antibodies from the Rh –ve mother (through the placenta) into the Rh +ve fetus. The condition can be prevented by desensitizing all Rh –ve mothers by giving them injections of massive doses of **anti-Rh antibodies called anti-Rh gamma globulin** after childbirth. This is to prevent active antibodies formation in the mother.

Q.15. Why does the ABO incompatibility rarely produce hemolytic disease of the newborn?

The ABO incompatibility between the mother and fetus rarely causes HDN. The reason is that the anti-A and anti-B (anti-ABO) antibodies belong to IgM type of gamma globulins (cold antibodies) that do not cross the placenta.

Q.16. What is the most common blood types in Indian populations?

Blood group B +ve.

Q.17. What is the importance of blood grouping?

Q.18. What are the indications for blood transfusion?

1. Acute hemorrhage
2. Chronic anemias that cannot be treated with diet and drugs.
3. Exchange transfusion: It is employed in hemolytic disease of the newborn.
4. Bleeding disorders: Fresh blood or platelet concentrates are given in purpura. Fresh frozen plasma or cryoprecipitate is given in hemophilia and other clotting factor deficiencies.
5. Bone marrow depression.
6. Autologous transfusion: In addition to receiving blood from a donor, an individual may also receive one's own stored blood, (i.e. during elective surgery), a procedure called predonation.

Q.19. What is blood doping?

Blood doping is the procedure in which some athletes get a unit or two of their own blood (or red cells) removed and stored for a few weeks. It is then reinjected in 2–3 sessions a few days before an event.

Q.20. What are the hazards (dangers) of blood transfusion?

1. **Transmission of diseases such as** human immunodeficiency virus (HIV)/AIDS, hepatitis B, hepatitis C, syphilis and malarial parasite.
2. **Mismatched transfusion reactions**: This is the most serious and potentially fatal complication. Whether the transfusion reactions are immediate or delayed, as well as their severity is determined by the speed and extent of hemolysis of donated red cells.

- Body aches and pains: These symptoms are due to blockage of capillaries by clumps of agglutinated cells. Chills and fever generally accompany pains.
- Renal failure

3. **Allergic reactions:** Reactions such as skin rashes and asthma may occur.
4. **Pyrogenic reactions:** Reactions such as chills and fever are probably due to the presence of antibodies to leukocytes and platelets.
5. **Tetany:** With massive transfusions, the normal conversion of citrate to bicarbonate in the tissues may be delayed. This will result in a fall in plasma ionic calcium and hence tetany.
6. **Iron overload.**

Q.21. How is donated blood stored? What is the fate of transfused citrate in the body?

Storage of blood: After a donor has been screened for donation, one unit of blood (450 mL) is collected, under aseptic conditions, from the antecubital vein directly into a special plastic bag containing 63 mL of CPDA (citrate–phosphate–dextrose–adenine) mixture. The blood bag is suitably sealed, labeled and stored at 4°C, where it can be kept for about 20 days.

The *citrate* prevents clotting of blood, *sodium diphosphate* acts as a buffer to control decrease in pH, *dextrose* supports adenosine triphosphate (ATP) generation via glycolytic pathway and also provides energy for Na^+–K^+ pump that maintains the size and shape of red cells and increases their survival time and *adenine* provides substrate for the synthesis of ATP, thus improving postdonation viability of red cells.

Blood is stored at low temperatures for two reasons: one, it decreases bacterial growth and two, it decreases the rate of glycolysis and thus prevents a quick fall in pH.

Changes in red cells during storage: Changes occur due to decreased metabolism and include increase in their Na^+ and decrease in K^+ concentration due to reduced Na^+–K^+ pump activity, the result being a net increase in total base and water content of the cells that swell and become more spherocytic. The ATP content decreases and inorganic phosphate content increases.

Q.22. What is Bombay blood group?

This blood type is a rare phenomenon in which the H antigen is absent. Since there is no H antigen, there is no antigen A or antigen B on the red cells. However, the plasma contains anti-A, anti-B and anti-H antibodies. As a result, such a person can receive blood only from a person having Bombay blood type.

OBSERVATION

Control	Anti-serum A	Anti-serum B	Anti-serum D	Blood group

RESULT

....
....
....
....
....

INTERPRETATION

....
....
....
....
....

STUDY NOTES

CHAPTER 1.10

Bleeding Time and Clotting Time

AIM

To determine bleeding time (BT) and clotting time (CT).

INTRODUCTION

The term hemostasis (Greek: hema = blood; stasis = halt) refers to the process of stoppage of bleeding after blood vessels are punctured. It involves the following four interrelated steps:
1. Vasoconstriction (contraction of injured blood vessels)
2. Platelet plug formation
3. Formation of a blood clot
4. Fibrinolysis (dissolution of the clot).

TESTS FOR HEMOSTASIS

1. Bleeding time
2. Clotting time
3. Capillary fragility test of Hess (tourniquet test)
4. Platelet count
5. Clot retraction time (CRT)
6. Clot lysis time (CLT)
7. Prothrombin time (PT).

Bleeding Time

Bleeding time is the time interval between the skin puncture and spontaneous stoppage of bleeding. The BT test is an in vitro test of platelet function. However, a peripheral blood film is always examined for the number of platelets and their morphology.

It is determined by two methods:
1. **Duke's method**
2. **Ivy's method.**

Duke's Method

This method is more commonly used as it is easy to perform.

Apparatus
1. Pricking apparatus.
2. Clean filter papers.
3. Stopwatch.

Procedure
1. Give a deep fingerprick under aseptic conditions to get free-flowing blood. Start the stopwatch and note the time. The time of puncture of the finger is known as **Zero time**.
2. Blot the blood drops every 30 seconds by touching the puncture site with the filter paper along its edges, without pressing or squeezing the wound.
3. Note the time when bleeding stops, i.e. when there is no trace of blood spot on the filter paper. Encircle this spot and number it as well. This is the end point (Fig. 1.10.1). (Do not keep the filter paper on the table and then press your wound on it).
4. You can also count the number of blood spots on the filter paper and multiply it by ½ to get the bleeding time in minutes.

Normal BT is 2–6 minutes.

Precautions
1. The skin should be dry and the puncture should be 3–4 mm deep to give free-flowing blood. Do not squeeze.

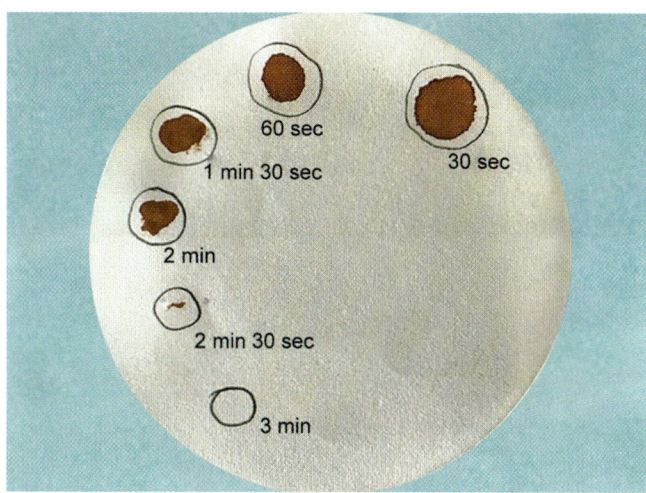

Fig. 1.10.1: Bleeding time.

2. Do not press the filter paper on the puncture site.
3. If bleeding continues for more than 10–12 minutes, stop the test and press a sterile gauze on the wound. Inform your teacher about the bleeding.

Ivy's Method

This method is more reliable than the Duke's method. However, it requires some practice to apply the blood pressure (BP) cuff and maintain the pressure. Ivy's method is more painful and requires experience, hence Duke's method is commonly used in the laboratories.

Procedure

1. Clean the skin over the anterior surface of the forearm with spirit.
2. Apply a BP cuff on the upper arm, raise the pressure to 40 mm Hg and maintain it there till the end of the experiment.
3. Clean the skin area once again. Make a 1–3 mm deep skin puncture, about 5–6 cm below the cubital fossa on the anterior surface of the arm. Note the time.
4. Remove the blood every 30 seconds by absorbing it along the edges of a clean filter paper by gently touching the wound with it till the bleeding stops. This is the end point.

Normal BT with **this method is up to 9 minutes**.

Physioclinical Significance of Bleeding Time

1. Although a BT of over 10 minutes has a slightly increased risk of bleeding, the risk becomes greater when the BT exceeds 15 or 20 minutes.
2. Prolonged BT with normal CT is seen in the following conditions:
   a. **Low platelet count (thrombocytopenia):** It may be due to:
      ♦ Decreased production of platelets
      ♦ Increased destruction of platelets.
   b. **Functional platelet defects:** Prolonged BT with normal platelet count suggests the following defects:
      ♦ **Drugs:** Aspirin, large doses of penicillin, other drugs
      ♦ **Von Willebrand disease**
      ♦ Other diseases: Uremia, cirrhosis, leukemia, etc.
   c. **Vessel wall defects:** These defects are generally acquired, but may be inherited.
      ♦ Prolonged treatment with corticosteroids
      ♦ Allergic purpura
      ♦ Infections
      ♦ Deficiency of vitamin C
      ♦ Senile purpura
      ♦ Connective tissue diseases.

> **NOTE**
> BT and CT are two simple tests that are used as a routine before every minor and major surgery (e.g. tooth extraction), biopsy procedures and before and during anticoagulant therapy, whether or not there is a history of bleeding.

Clotting Time

Clotting time is the time taken from the onset of bleeding to the formation of a fibrin thread. It is determined by two methods:
1. **Wright's capillary glass tube method.**
2. **Lee and White method.**

Wright's Capillary Glass Tube Method

Apparatus
1. Pricking apparatus.
2. Clean 10–12 cm long, glass capillary tubes with a uniform bore diameter of 1–2 mm.
3. Stopwatch.

Procedure
1. Give a fingerprick under aseptic precautions. Note the time of prick. This is called **Zero time**.
2. Now dip one end of the capillary tube in the blood; the blood rises into the tube by capillary action (Fig. 1.10.2). This can be enhanced by keeping its open end at a lower level.
3. Hold the capillary tube between the palms of your hands to maintain the blood near body temperature.

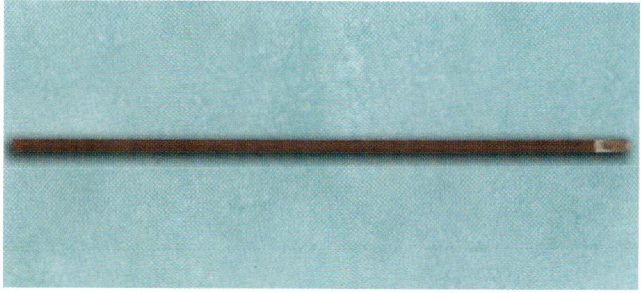

Fig. 1.10.2: Glass capillary tube filled with blood.

4. At the end of 1 minute (from zero time) break off 1 cm of the tube from one end.
5. Then gently break off 1 cm bits of glass tube from one end at intervals of 30 seconds and look for the formation of fibrin thread between the broken ends. The endpoint is reached when fibrin thread spans a gap of at least 5 mm between the broken ends (**fibrin thread formation**). Note the time (Fig. 1.10.3).
6. The CT is taken as total time from the time of puncture (zero time) till there is formation of fibrin thread.

Normal CT is 3–8 minutes (at 37°C).

> **NOTE**
> In capillary tube method clotting method involved is the **intrinsic pathway.** This is brought by exposure of the blood to electronegatively charged surface (glass tube).

Lee and White Test Tube Method

Single Test Tube Method

This method needs more arrangements than the capillary tube method but is more sensitive and reliable method for the determination of CT.
1. Draw 2 mL venous blood by a clean, nontraumatic venepuncture. Note the time when blood starts to enter the syringe. This is the zero time. Transfer the blood to a clean and dry test tube.
2. Holding the test tube in a water bath at 37°C, take it out at 30 second intervals and tilt it. The end point is when the tube can be tilted without spilling the blood.

Normal CT with this method is 5–10 minutes.

> **NOTE**
> If a siliconized test tube is used at the same time, a delayed CT (40–70 minutes) can be shown. The CT depends on the condition of the glass itself and even on the size of the test tube. Therefore, a high degree of standardization is needed.

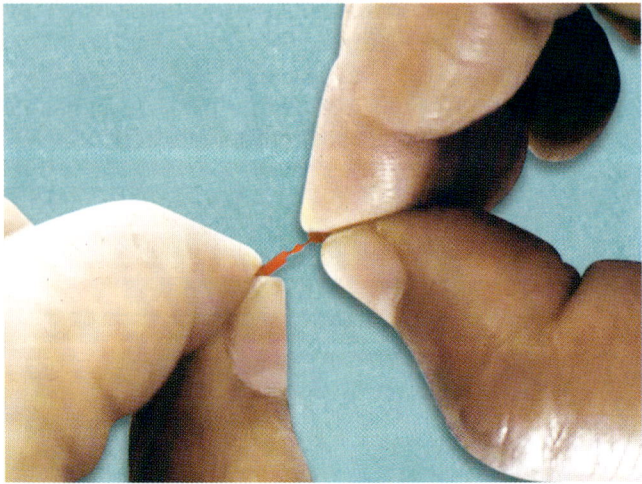

Fig. 1.10.3: Formation of fibrin thread.

Physioclinical Significance of Clotting Time

1. **The coagulation time is increased in the following conditions:**
   a. *Hereditary coagulation disorders:*
      - Hemophilias—A, B, C, D.
      - Von Willebrand disease
      - Afibrinogenemia and dysfibrinogenemia.
   b. *Acquired coagulation disorders:* These may develop in a variety of diseases as mentioned here.
      - Vitamin K deficiency
      - Liver diseases
      - Intravascular clotting
      - Anticoagulant therapy.
   c. *Newborns:* Newborns especially premature babies sometimes have a tendency to bleed because the plasma levels of certain factors are low, especially prothrombin. Usually, these levels reach normal by the 2nd or 3rd week after birth. Vitamin K is given if bleeding persists.
2. **The CT is decreased in:**
   - *Physiological conditions:* Malnutrition, parturition.
   - *Pathological conditions:* There is no pathological condition in which the CT is decreased.

QUESTIONS

Q.1. What is the clinical importance of doing BT and CT?
Bleeding time and CT are important in the following situations:
- History of frequent and persistent bleeding from minor injuries or spontaneous bleeding into tissues.
- Before every minor and major surgery (tooth extraction, etc.).
- Before taking biopsy especially from bone marrow, liver, kidney, etc.
- Before and during anticoagulant therapy.
- Family history of bleeding disorders.

Q.2. How does BT differ from CT? What is the interrelation between them and which aspects of hemostasis are tested by them?
Both BT and CT are done together in all disorders of hemostasis. They are interrelated in the sense that platelets are involved in both tests. **The BT tests the platelet plug formation and the condition of the microvessels (arterioles, capillaries, venules), while CT tests the formation of the clot.** Increase in BT (e.g. in purpura) or CT (e.g. in hemophilia) usually occurs independently of each other.

Q.3. What are the factors on which BT and CT depend?
Bleeding time depends on:
- Breadth and depth of the wound.
- Degree of hyperemia of the skin puncture site.
- Number of platelets and their functional status.
- Functional status of the blood vessels.
- Temperature: In cold weather, low temperature promotes vasoconstriction and thus shortens BT.

Clotting time depends on:
- Nature of contact surface (glass in this case; siliconized surface would prolong the CT).
- Presence or absence of clotting factors.
- Temperature: Low temperature may prolong the CT.

Q.4. What happens to BT and CT in purpura and hemophilia?
In purpura, BT increases while CT is normal.
In hemophilia, CT increases markedly while BT is normal.

Q.5. What is the relation between the platelet count and the severity of bleeding?
Broadly speaking, the relation between the platelet count and the severity of bleeding is as follows:

Platelet count	Severity of bleeding
• Above 100,000/mm³	No clinical symptoms, bleeding is rare.
• 50,000–100,000/mm³	Bleeding may occur after major surgery.
• 20,000–50,000/mm³	Bleeding occurs with minor trauma of everyday life or gentle sports.
• Below 20,000 mm³	Spontaneous hemorrhages in urinary and GI tract, nose bleeds, etc.
• At very low counts	Fatal hemorrhages may occur in the brain.

Q.6. What is the mechanism of clotting of blood?
Mechanism of coagulation of blood: The intrinsic and extrinsic pathways for blood clotting are shown below:

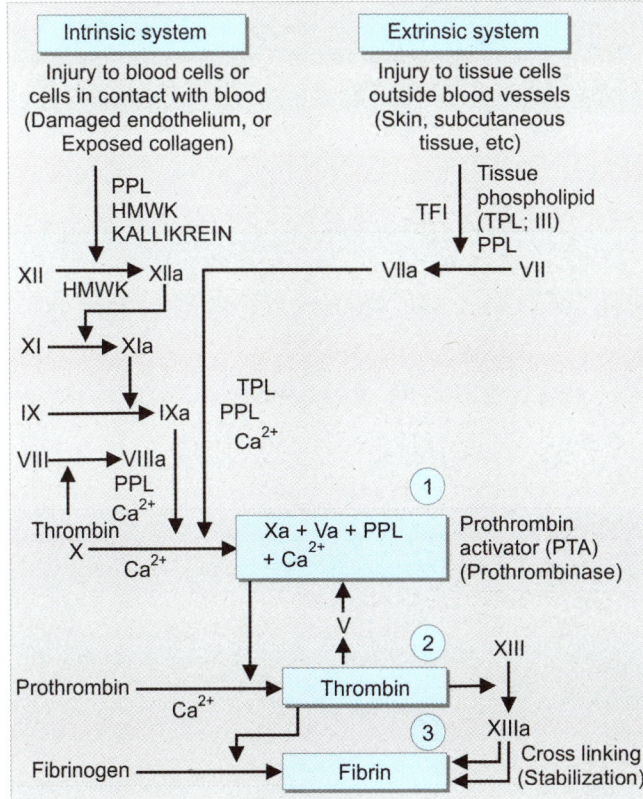

Stage 1: generation of prothrombin activator (PTA); Stage 2: formation of thrombin from prothrombin; Stage 3: formation of fibrin from fibrinogen; HMWK: high molecular weight kininogen; TFI: tissue factor pathway inhibitor; PPL: platelet phospholipid.

Q.7. How does clotting occur in the glass capillary tube in your experiment?

Q.8. What is purpura?
Purpura is a condition characterized by red or purple discolored spots on the skin which is the result of capillary abnormality leading to hemorrhages into the skin, mucous membranes and internal organs.
Types of purpura are:
- **Idiopathic thrombocytopenic purpura:** Decrease in platelet count.
- **Athrombocytopenic purpura:** Purpura with normal platelet count.
- **Thromboasthenic purpura:** Abnormal platelets with normal platelet count.
- **Drug-induced purpura**.

Q.9. What is hemophilia?
Hemophilia is a group of bleeding disorders that result from deficiency of factors VIII, IX, X or XII. These four types have been called as hemophilia A, B, C and D.
Hemophilia A which is also called *classical hemophilia* due to clotting factor VIII deficiency.
Hemophilia B called as **Christmas disease** is due to clotting factor IX deficiency.

Q.10. Why does calcium deficiency not cause a bleeding disorder though it is essential for many steps of blood coagulation?
The reason is that only minute amounts of ionic calcium are required for clotting. A very severe calcium deficiency will lead to life-threatening symptoms like tetany before clotting disorders occur.

> **NOTE**
> Except for the first two stages in the intrinsic system of coagulation, calcium ions are required for the promotion of all blood clotting reactions.

Q.11. How is blood maintained in a fluid state within the body?
A balance between clotting and anticlotting mechanisms is required to prevent hemorrhage and at the same time, to prevent intravascular clotting. **Hemofluidity within the body** is maintained by the following factors:
1. Continuous motion (circulation) of blood does not allow clotting factors to accumulate at one point.
2. Endothelial surface factors
3. Antithrombin action of antithrombin III-heparin complex and fibrin
4. Fibrinolytic system (the plasmin system)

Q.12. Which test can be used to monitor oral anticoagulant therapy?
Prothrombin time.

OBSERVATION

....
....
....
....
....

Section 1: Hematology

RESULT	INTERPRETATION
Bleeding Time by Duke's Method	....
Clotting Time by Capillary Glass Tube Method	....

STUDY NOTES

Teacher's Signature

CHAPTER 1.11

Erythrocyte Sedimentation Rate and Packed Cell Volume

AIM

To determine erythrocyte sedimentation rate (ESR) and packed cell volume (PCV).

ESTIMATION OF ESR

Principle

The rate at which the red blood cells (RBCs) sediment when a sample of blood, to which an anticoagulant has been added, is allowed to stand in a narrow vertical tube for **1 hour** is called erythrocyte sedimentation rate. It is expressed in millimeter of clear plasma at the end of the 1st hour.

Sedimentation of Red Cells

The settling or sedimentation of red blood cells in a sample of anticoagulated blood occurs in three stages:
1. In the **first stage**, the RBCs pile up (like a stack of coins) and form rouleaux during the first 10–15 minutes.
2. During the **second stage**, the rouleau being heavier sinks to the bottom. This stage lasts for 40–45 minutes.
3. In the **third stage**, there is packing of massed bunches of red cells at the bottom of the blood column. This stage lasts for about 10–15 minutes.

Thus, most of the settling of the red blood cells occurs in the 1st hour or so.

> **NOTE**
> A longer tube will make the second stage last longer and greater will be the ESR.

Determination of ESR

Two methods are commonly used:
1. Wintrobe method
2. Westergren method.

Wintrobe Method

Apparatus

1. Pricking apparatus, penicillin bottles and powdered mixture of double oxalate mixture (6 mg ammonium oxalate and 4 mg potassium oxalate).
2. **Wintrobe tube with stand (Figs. 1.11.1A and B)**:
   a. It is 11 cm long, thick-walled, cylindrical glass tube, with a uniform bore diameter of 2.5 mm. Its lower end is closed and flat.
   b. The tube is calibrated in centimeter and millimeter from 0 to 10 cm from above downward on one side of the scale (for ESR) and 10–0 cm on the other side (for PCV). Each centimeter is further divided into millimeter (mm).
3. **Pasteur pipette:** It is a glass tubing drawn to a long thin nozzle about 14 cm long. It is used for filling the Wintrobe tube (Fig. 1.11.2).

Procedure

1. Draw 5 mL of venous blood from antecubital vein and transfer it to penicillin bottle having double oxalate mixture (anticoagulant). Mix the contents gently. Do not shake, as it will cause frothing.
2. Using the Pasteur pipette, fill the Wintrobe tube from below upward with anticoagulant mixed blood. Ensure that there are no air bubbles.

Chapter 1.11: Erythrocyte Sedimentation Rate and Packed Cell Volume

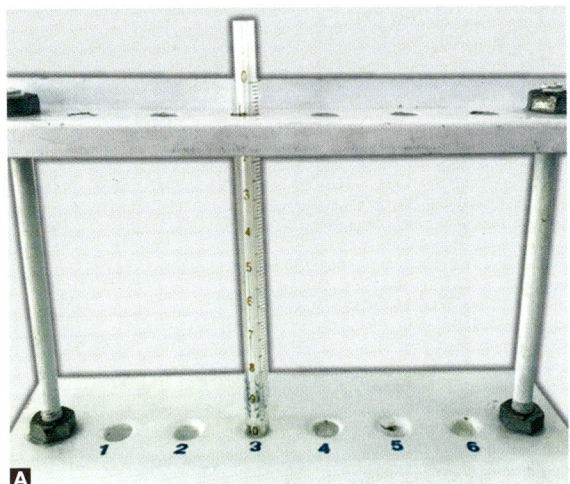

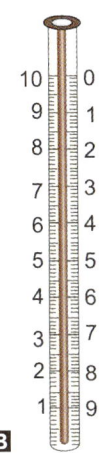

Figs. 1.11.1A and B: (A) Wintrobe tube with stand; (B) Wintrobe tube.

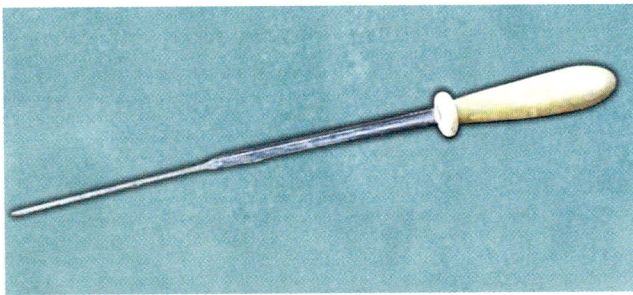

Fig. 1.11.2: Pasteur pipette.

3. Fill the tube up to the zero mark.
4. Transfer the tube to its stand. Leave the tube undisturbed in vertical position for 1 hour. At the end of which read the millimeter of clear plasma above the red cells.
5. Express your result as............mm at the end of 1st hour.

Normal values
Males: 0–9 mm at the end of one hour
Females: 0–20 mm at the end of one hour.

Westergren's Method

Apparatus
1. Pricking apparatus and penicillin bottle.
2. 3.8% sodium citrate as the anticoagulant.
3. **Westergren pipette** (Figs. 1.11.3A and B)
   a. It is 300 mm long glass pipette, open from both the sides with an internal bore diameter of 2.5 mm.
   b. It is calibrated in centimeter and millimeter from 0 to 200, from above downward in its lower two-thirds.
   c. The Westergren stand can accommodate up to four tubes at a time. For each pipette, there is a screw cap that slips over its top and at its lower end, the pipette presses into a rubber pad or cushion.

Procedure
1. Draw 2.0 mL of venous blood and transfer it into penicillin bottle containing 0.5 mL of 3.8% sodium citrate solution. This will give a blood:citrate ratio of 4:1. Mix the contents gently. Do not shake, as it will cause frothing.
2. Fill the Westergren pipette with blood–citrate mixture by sucking up to the "0" mark, immediately close the upper opening with a thumb to prevent blood from flowing out.
3. Keeping your finger over the pipette, transfer it to the Westergren stand by firmly pressing its lower end into the rubber cushion. Now slip the upper end of the pipette under the screw cap. Fix the tube in an exact vertical position with leveling screws.
4. Leave the pipette undisturbed for 1 hour at the end of which read the millimeter of clear plasma above the red cells.
5. Express your result as: ....mm at the end of 1st hour.

Normal values
Males: 3–5 mm at the end of one hour
Females: 4–7 mm at the end of one hour.

> **NOTE**
> ESR estimation by Westergen method is more sensitive than the Wintrobe method.

Sources of error
1. Tilting of the tube and high temperature can lead to high values.
2. Low temperature gives false low values.
3. Hemolyzed blood may obscure the sharp line separating red cells and the plasma.

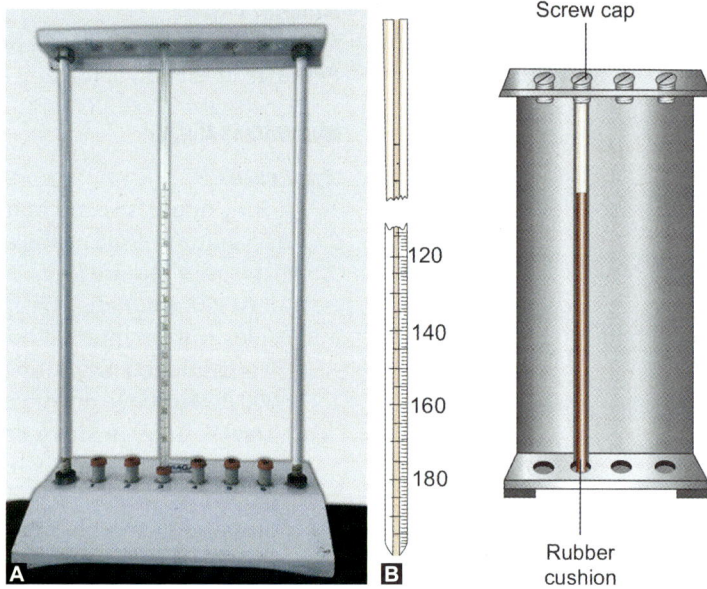

Figs. 1.11.3A and B: (A) Westergren pipette and stand; (B) Westergren stand with the Westergren pipette in position.

Precautions

1. All glass apparatus like tubes and pipettes should be absolutely dry.
2. To prevent hemolysis, detach the needle after venepuncture and then gently transfer the blood into the penicillin bottle.
3. Proper anticoagulant should be used for each method. It should be taken in a specific amount for a given method.
4. The blood should be collected in the fasting state.
5. There should be no air bubble while filling the Wintrobe tube or the Westergren pipette with blood.
6. The test should preferably be done within 2–3 hours of collecting the blood sample at room temperature.
7. The hematocrit (Hct) should be checked and correction factor should be applied in cases of anemia (nomograms are available for this purpose).
8. Clotted or hemolyzed blood must be discarded.
9. The Wintrobe tube or Westergren pipette should not be disturbed from the vertical position during the test.

MEASUREMENT OF PACKED CELL VOLUME

Packed cell volume is the volume of the cellular components per unit volume of whole blood expressed as a percentage.

Apparatus

1. **Wintrobe tube**
2. **Pasteur pipette**
3. **Centrifuge machine:** It packs the RBCs in the Hct tube by centrifugal force.

Procedure

1. Draw 5 mL of venous blood and transfer it to a penicillin bottle containing double oxalate. Rotate the bulb between your palms.
2. Fill the Pasteur pipette with blood and take its nozzle to the bottom of the **Wintrobe tube**. Expel the blood gently by pressing the rubber teat. Fill the tube from below upward while withdrawing the pipette, always keeping its tip below the level of blood. Ensure that there is no air bubble trapped in the blood.
3. Bring the blood column exactly to the mark 10 (or the mark 0 on the other side of the scale) at the top.
4. Close the mouth of the tube with its rubber cap and centrifuge it at 3,000 rpm for 30 minutes.
5. At the end of 30 minutes, take the reading of upper level of packed red cells on the side of the scale where zero is at the bottom.

Observations and Results

Note that the blood has been separated into three layers (Fig. 1.11.4):

1. A tall upper layer of clear plasma (amber- or straw-colored). A pink or red color indicates hemolysis of red cells in the sample. If there is hemolysis, the test must be repeated on a fresh sample.
2. A grayish-white, thin layer (about 1 mm thick) is called the **"buffy layer"** and consists of platelets above and leukocytes below it.
3. A tall bottom layer of red blood cells, closely packed together. A grayish red line separates red cell layer from the layer of leukocytes above it. The line marks the upper limit of the red cell layer.

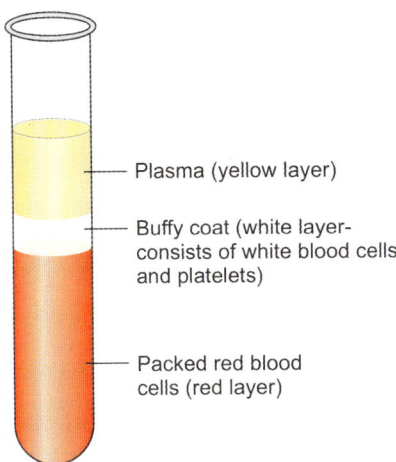

Fig. 1.11.4: Formation of three layers after centrifugation of blood.

> **NOTE**
> Do not include the buffy coat while reading the height of the red cell column.

Take out the tube and read the PCV directly off the graduation given on the tube. The height of the column of cellular component is taken as PCV.

Express the value as the percentage of the blood.

4. **Normal values:** The average value of PCV is 42% when the RBC count is 5 million/mm^3 and their size and shape are normal.
Adult males: 44% (38–50%)
Adult females: 42% (36–45%)
PCV for newborns is about 50%.
"True" Hct [true cell volume (TCV)]: Even under optimum conditions, it is impossible to completely pack the red cells together as about 2% plasma remains trapped in between the red cells. To compensate for the trapped plasma, the "true" cell volume (true Hct) can be obtained by multiplying the observed Hct value with 0.98.
Venous blood Hct: The Hct of venous blood is 3% higher than that of arterial blood, due to the chloride shift.

Precautions

1. The test should be done within 6–8 hours of collection of the sample.
2. The Wintrobe tube should be filled carefully using Pasteur pipette, placing the tip of the pipette at the bottom of the tube.
3. The pipette should be gradually withdrawn as the blood fills in the Wintrobe tube from below upward, so that no air bubble is trapped in the tube.
4. The Hct should be checked and correction factor should be applied in cases of anemia (nomograms are available for this purpose).

Physioclinical Significance

Erythrocyte Sedimentation Rate

1. **Physiological variations in ESR**
   a. *Age:* ESR is low in infants (0.5 mm in 1st hour by Westergren) because of polycythemia. It gradually increases to adult levels in the next few years.
   b. *Sex:* The ESR is somewhat higher in females, probably due to lower Hct (PCV).
   c. *High altitude:* People living at high altitudes have relatively higher ESR.
   d. *Pregnancy:* The ESR is higher during pregnancy due to increased fibrinogen: albumin ratio.
   e. *Body temperature:* Within limits, ESR varies with body temperature, which tends to affect the viscosity.
   f. After a meal.

2. **Pathological variations in ESR**
   Pathological increase: The ESR is increased in any condition that is associated with inflammation and tissue damage. It is seen in—
   a. All acute and chronic infections (localized or generalized), e.g. pneumonia and tuberculosis.
   b. All anemias, except spherocytosis, sickle cell anemia and pernicious anemia.
   c. Bone diseases: osteomyelitis.
   d. Connective tissue diseases: Systemic lupus erythematosus and rheumatoid arthritis.
   e. All malignant diseases (cancers), e.g. carcinoma of breast and leukemia
   f. Acute noninfective inflammation, e.g. gout, rheumatoid arthritis.
   g. Trauma and surgery.

   Pathological decrease:
   a. Polycythemia
   b. Anemias: Spherocytosis, pernicious anemia and sickle cell anemia.
   c. Afibrinogenemia
   d. Shock, e.g. burns and dehydration.

Clinical significance of ESR

1. **Value of ESR as a prognostic tool:** ESR is a valuable prognostic test in following the course of the disease, such as tuberculosis, rheumatoid arthritis, etc. while a patient is on treatment.
2. As an indicator of bodily reaction to tissue injury and inflammation:
   ESR increases with age, the upper limit of normal can be calculated as:
   Males = Age ÷ 2
   Females = (Age + 10) ÷ 2.

Section 1: Hematology

Hematocrit/PCV

- It is a very good indicator of RBC population and Hb content of the blood.
- Hct is an important factor that determines viscosity of blood.

Increased PCV is seen in:
1. Excessive sweating due to hemoconcentration.
2. All cases of polycythemia, hypoxia due to lung and heart diseases, etc.
3. Congestive heart failure, burns (loss of plasma), dehydration, after severe exercise and emotional stress.

Decreased PCV is seen in:
1. Pregnancy (hemodilution) and ingestion of large amounts of water.
2. All types of anemia.
3. Bone marrow depression.

Objective Structured Practical Examination–I

Aim: To fill the Wintrobe tube with the anticoagulated blood for measuring ESR.
Procedural steps: See text above.
Checklist:
1. Select the tube and see that it is clean and dry. (Y/N)
2. Mix the blood sample and draw blood into a Pasteur pipette or a dropper with a long nozzle. (Y/N)
3. Fill the tube with blood, starting from its bottom and withdrawing the pipette till blood column reaches the zero mark. (Y/N)
4. Check that there are no bubbles; if there are, it is removed with a filter paper strip. (Y/N)
5. Place the tube vertically in the Wintrobe stand and note the time. (Y/N)

Objective Structured Practical Examination–II

Aim: To fill the Westergren pipette with the anticoagulated blood for measuring ESR.
Procedural steps: See text above.
Checklist:
1. Select the Westergren pipette and check that it is dry and clean. (Y/N)
2. Mix the blood sample. (Y/N)
3. Suck blood into the pipette and take it to the zero mark, taking care to avoid any bubbles. (Y/N)
4. Press the lower end of the pipette into the rubber cushion of the stand and the upper end under the screw cap. (Y/N)
5. Place the pipette vertically and note the time. (Y/N)

Objective Structured Practical Examination–III

Aim: To fill the Wintrobe tube with the anticoagulated blood for measuring hematocrit.
Procedural steps: See text above.
Checklist:
1. Select the Wintrobe tube. (Y/N)
2. Mix the blood sample. (Y/N)
3. Fill blood in the Wintrobe tube properly using the Pasteur pipette till the 0 mark. (Y/N)
4. Place the Wintrobe tube in the centrifuge machine. (Y/N)
5. Note the final reading after adequate time. (Y/N)

QUESTIONS

Q.1. Why do the red cells settle down in a sample of anticoagulated blood?
The red blood cells settle down because they are heavier (specific gravity = 1.095) than the plasma (specific gravity = 1.032) in which they are suspended.

Q.2. Can you use oxalate mixture in Westergren method and citrate in Wintrobe method?
No, the anticoagulants employed for each method cannot be interchanged because both methods have been standardized and employed in clinical practice for the last many years (Sodium citrate cannot be used in Wintrobe method because the blood will be too much diluted as compared to the height of the tube; and this will give high false values for ESR).

Q.3. What is the advantage of using Wintrobe method?
The **advantage** of this method is that the same sample of oxalated blood can first be used for ESR and then, after 1 hour, for Hct (PCV) by centrifuging it.

Q.4. What is the advantage of Westergren method?
The **advantage** of this method is that it is more sensitive since the tube is sufficiently long and its diameter is also larger. The higher sensitivity and the longer tube are particularly important in cases where ESR is high (>80 mm).

Also, as the pipette is kept closed from both ends, the effect of atmospheric pressure is neutralized.

Q.5. Why is ESR reading taken after 1 hour?
The reason for this is that more than 95–98% red cells settle down by the end of this time. After 1 hour, the rate of sedimentation does not significantly affect the ESR. Further, the method has been standardized for 1 hour and in clinical practice for long.

Q.6. What are the factors on which the rate of sedimentation of red cells depends?
The factors that affect the ESR include the following:
1. **Technical and mechanical factors:** Factors like the length of the tube, diameter of the bore (if less than 2 mm) and **the anticoagulant used** affect the values of ESR obtained, e.g. sodium citrate in Westergren method changes red **cell–plasma ratio**, which increases the ESR.

2. **Physiological factors:** The red cell count, their size, shape and their tendency to **rouleaux formation**.
   - *Number of red cells:* A decrease in RBC count promotes rouleaux formation, while an increase in count (e.g. polycythemia) decreases ESR.
   - *Size and shape of red cells:* Biconcave shape of red cells favors rouleaux formation, while an increase in MCV, hereditary spherocytosis and in sickle cell disease, ESR is decreased.
3. Rate of settling of red cells depends on:
   - A downward gravitational force acting on the red cells due to their weight (mass).
   - An upward force due to **viscosity of plasma**. Increased viscosity of blood, whether due to increase in RBC count or plasma protein concentration, decreases ESR, while a decrease in viscosity increases ESR (Viscosity of water:plasma:blood = 1:3:5).

   Thus, the rate of settling of red cells will depend on the balance between these two opposing forces.

Q.7. What is rouleaux formation? What are the factors that increase the rate of rouleaux formation and hence the ESR?

Rouleaux formation: The pilling up of the RBCs like stack of coins is called a Rouleaux.

Factors affecting rouleaux formation:
1. Concentration of large, asymmetric molecules of fibrinogen and globulins.
2. Bacterial proteins and toxins and products of inflammation and tissue destruction such as acute-phase reactants (e.g. C-reactive proteins of acute rheumatic fever).

Q.8. Name the physiological and pathological variations in ESR.
Q.9. What is the clinical significance of ESR?
Q.10. What is the importance of determining hematocrit?
Q.11. Which cells make up the buffy layer?
Q.12. How thick is the buffy layer and when can it increase in thickness?

The buffy layer is about 1 mm thick but the thickness increases in cases of severe leukocytosis, leukemia and thrombocytosis.

Q.13. What is the difference between the PCV of arterial and venous blood?
Q.14. Name the conditions where the PCV is increased and those where it is decreased?

OBSERVATION

ESR		PCV
Wintrobe's method	Westergren's method	

RESULT

....
....
....
....
....

INTERPRETATION

....
....
....
....
....

STUDY NOTES

CHAPTER 1.12

Red Blood Cell Indices

AIM

Determination of red blood cell indices.

PRINCIPLE

The basic values of hemoglobin (Hb), red blood cell (RBC) count and packed cell volume (PCV) [hematocrit (Hct)] do not give any information about the condition of an average red cell, such as its volume, Hb content or its percentage saturation with Hb. However, this information, in the form of RBC indices (absolute values of blood indices), can be calculated from three basic values of Hb, RBC count and PCV.

PHYSIOCLINICAL SIGNIFICANCE

It is helpful in morphological classification of anemias (based on its size and hemoglobin concentration).

APPARATUS

The apparatus and materials required are those used for Hb, RBC count and PCV.

PROCEDURE

Use the values of Hb, RBC count and PCV obtained during the previous experiment to calculate the RBC indices.

The various blood indices are:

Mean Corpuscular Volume (MCV)

The MCV is the average or mean volume of a single RBC expressed in cubic micrometers (μm^3 or femtoliters). It is calculated using the formula:

$$\frac{PCV \times 10}{RBC \text{ count in million/mm}^3} \text{ or } \frac{PCV \text{ per liter}}{RBC \, (10^3/mm)}$$

For example:
PCV = 45%, RBC count = 5.0 million/mm^3

$$MCV = \frac{45 \times 10}{5} = 90 \, \mu m^3$$

(Normal range = 74–95 μm^3)

On the basis of MCV, the RBC can be:
1. Normocytic: RBC with normal MCV
2. Macrocytic: RBC with MCV above the normal range
3. Microcytic: RBC with MCV below the normal range.

Mean Corpuscular Hemoglobin (MCH)

The MCH, which is also determined indirectly, is the average Hb content (weight of Hb) in a single RBC expressed in picograms (pg = 10^{-12} g). It is calculated by using formula:

$$\frac{Hb \text{ in g\% } \times 10}{RBC \text{ count in million/mm}^3}$$

For example:
Hb = 15 g%
RBC count = 5 million/mm^3

$$MCH = \frac{15 \times 10}{5} = 30 \, pg$$

(Normal range = 27–32 pg)

Mean Corpuscular Hemoglobin Concentration (MCHC)

It is amount of hemoglobin expressed as a percentage of the volume of a RBC. It is the Hb concentration in a RBC.

This represents the relationship between the red cell volume and its degree or percentage saturation with Hb, that is, how many parts or volumes of a red cell are occupied by Hb. The MCHC does not take into consideration the RBC count, but represents the actual Hb concentration in red cells only, (i.e. not in whole blood) expressed as saturation of these cells with Hb. **So, it is a more reliable index as compared to other indices.**

> **NOTE**
> The Hb synthesizing machinery of red cells does not have the Hb concentrating capacity beyond a certain limit, i.e. RBCs cannot be, say 70% "filled" with Hb; this upper limit is only 38%. If the MCHC is within the normal range, the cell is normochromic, if it is below the range, the cell is hypochromic. However, it can never be hyperchromic. A large cell may contain more Hb, but its percentage saturation will not be more than 38%.

MCHC is calculated from the following formula:
For example:
Hb = 15 g%, PCV = 45%

$$MCHC = \frac{Hb \text{ in g per 100 mL blood}}{PCV \text{ per 100 mL blood}} \times 100$$

$$= \left[\frac{Hb\ g\%}{PCV\%} \times 100\right]$$

$$MCHC = \frac{15}{45} \times 100 = 33.3\%$$

(Normal range = 30–38%)

Color Index

It is the ratio of Hb percentage to the RBC percentage. It is calculated using the formula:

$$\text{Color index} = \frac{Hb \text{ concentration (percentage of normal)}}{RBC \text{ count (percentage of normal)}}$$

$$= \frac{100}{100} = 1.0$$

(Normal range = 0.85–1.15)

The normal 100% RBC count is fixed at 5 million/mm³ and the normal Hb at 15 g%, irrespective of age and sex.

> **NOTE**
> The color index is low in iron-deficiency anemia and high in macrocytic anemias. But since both RBC count and Hb may decrease simultaneously in a way that the CI remains normal, the CI does not have much clinical value.

PHYSIOCLINICAL SIGNIFICANCE

These blood indices form the basis of morphological classification of anemia is depicted in Table 1.12.1.

Table 1.12.1: Morphological classification of anemias.

	Normochromic	Hypochromic
Normocytic	• After acute hemorrhage • Hemolytic anemias, except thalassemias • Renal disease • Aplastic anemia, chronic infection	After chronic blood loss — — —
Microcytic	Inflammation — —	• Iron deficiency anemia • Thalassemias (due to globin deficiency) • Hypoproteinemia
Macrocytic	Deficiency of vitamins B_{12} and folic acid	• Secondary to liver disease

QUESTIONS

Q.1. Which absolute corpuscular value is most useful?
MCHC is the most reliable and useful value for the following two reasons:
1. It does not take RBC count into consideration for its calculation. MCH and MCV, on the other hand, both depend on the RBC count, which has a high degree of error of ±15%.
2. MCHC tells us the actual Hb concentration in red cells only and not in whole blood.

Q.2. Why cannot the MCHC exceed the saturation limit of 38?

Q.3. How will you classify anemias according to their causes?

Q.4. How will you classify anemias on the basis of MCV and MCHC?
Anemias can be classified on this basis as given in Table 1.12.1.

Q.5. Calculate all blood indices from the given data: PCV = 40%; RBC count and hemoglobin concentration of your blood.

CALCULATION

....
....
....
....

RESULT

....
....
....
....

INTERPRETATION

....
....
....
....

STUDY NOTES

Date ....

CHAPTER 1.13

Platelet Count

AIM

To determine the platelet count.

INTRODUCTION

Platelets play an important role in hemostasis. They are small in size (2–4 μm) and are non-nucleated. There are two methods for platelet counting:
1. Direct method
2. Indirect method.

DIRECT METHOD

Ammonium Oxalate Method

Apparatus

- Microscope
- Red blood cell (RBC) pipette
- Improved Neubauer's counting chamber with coverslip
- Equipment for finger-pick, and
- Freshly prepared 1% ammonium oxalate solution.

> **NOTE**
> **Note: Platelet diluting fluid** (1% ammonium oxalate) acts an anticoagulant, preserves the platelets and destroys the RBC.

Principle

Blood is diluted with 1% ammonium oxalate, which lyses the RBCs. Platelets are counted microscopically using an improved Neubauer's counting chamber. The total platelet count of the undiluted sample is then calculated.

Procedure

1. Get a fingerprick and draw blood up to the mark 0.5. Suck the diluting fluid to the mark 101.
2. Mix the contents thoroughly and wait for 20 minutes. The red cells will be hemolyzed, leaving only the platelets. Mix the contents once again and discard the first two drops and charge the chamber on both sides. Place the charged chamber on wet filter paper and cover it with a petri dish to avoid evaporation. Wait for 20–30 minutes to allow the platelets to settle down.
3. Focus the RBC squares under HP 40x; adjust the diaphragm and position of condenser till you see the platelets—which appear as small, round or oval structures lying separately, highly refractile bodies with a silvery appearance (Fig. 1.13.1).

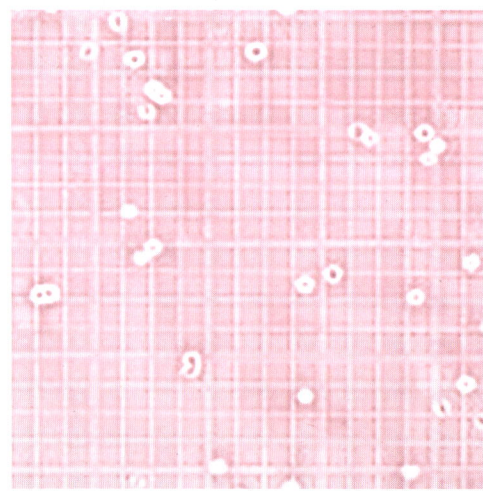

Fig. 1.13.1: Platelets in 25 RBC squares.

4. Rack the microscope continuously and count the platelets in all the 25 RBC squares, as done for red cell count. Record the observation in Figure 1.13.2.

   Knowing the dilution (1 in 200) (*Refer* Chapter 1.5) employed and the dimensions of the squares, calculate the number of platelets in 1 mm³ of undiluted blood.

Calculations

Dilution factor = 200
Volume of fluid = $1 \times 1 \times 0.1 = 0.1$ mm³ or 0.1 μL
Let N be the total number of platelets in 25 RBC squares
= 0.1 mm³ of diluted blood
Therefore, number of platelets in 1 μL of undiluted blood

$$= \frac{N \times \text{dilution factor (200)}}{0.1}$$

$N \times 10 \times 200 = N \times 2{,}000$.

Precautions

1. The chamber and the pipette must be cleaned with absolute alcohol to remove any dust particles, etc. to which platelets could adhere. Use a lint-free piece of cloth for final cleaning.
2. Same as that in RBC count.

Rees-Ecker Method

When blood is diluted with a solution of brilliant cresyl blue which stains the platelets light blue. Platelets are then counted by hemocytometry.

Disadvantage of this method is that the RBCs are not lysed.

The Rees-Ecker fluid contains the following:
- Brilliant cresyl blue 0.1 g—the dye stains the platelets
- Sodium citrate 3.8 g—prevents clotting and makes the fluid isotonic
- Formalin (40% formaldehyde)—0.2 mL—prevents fungal growth and lyses red cells
- Distilled water—100 mL.

INDIRECT METHOD

1. Place a drop of 14% magnesium sulfate solution on your fingertip and get a prick through this drop.
2. Spread a blood film with the diluted blood, dry it and stain it with Leishman's stain.
3. Examine the stained film under oil-immersion lens. Count the platelets and red cells in every 5th field until 1,000 red cells have been counted. Determine the "platelet RBC ratio", i.e. the ratio of platelets to red cells (usually, there is 1 platelet to 16–18 red cells).

Calculation

With the knowledge of platelet count and the RBC count, the actual number of platelets per mm³ blood can now be calculated.

Normal platelet count is 250,000–500,000/mm³.

AUTOMATED METHOD

It is a very accurate method. It is carried out on an electronic cell counter. The red cells and platelets in the diluted blood sample pass through an aperture.

QUESTIONS

Q.1. **What is the normal platelet count? Write the lifespan and site of destruction of platelets.**
Normal platelet count is 250,000–500,000/mm³.

About 60–70% of platelets formed in the bone marrow are in the circulating blood, while the rest are in the spleen. Their lifespan is 8–12 days, about 20% being consumed each day in the repair of microvessels. The aged and dead platelets are removed by the tissue macrophages [reticuloendothelial system (RES)] mainly in spleen, but also in the liver.

Q.2. **What is capillary fragility test of Hess?**
Capillary fragility test of Hess (also called "tourniquet" test): This is an important test to assess the mechanical fragility of the capillaries (and formation of a platelet plug) by raising the pressure within them. It may reveal latent purpura.
1. Mark a 1 inch diameter circle on the front of the forearm and using blue ink, mark any pink, purple or yellow spots within the circle.
2. Apply a blood pressure cuff on the upper arm and note the systolic and diastolic pressures. Then, after a pause of about 2 minutes or so, raise the pressure to midway between systolic and diastolic levels and maintain it there for 15 minutes. Appearance of more than 10 new petechiae (pink or red spots in the skin) is a positive test, which may be seen in various types of purpura and vessel wall abnormalities.

Q.3. **How does aspirin act as an antiplatelet agent and what is its clinical value?**
Prostacyclin produced by endothelial and smooth muscle cells in the walls of blood vessels and **thromboxane A2** formed in the platelets before they enter the circulation are both prostaglandins and synthesized from arachidonic acid (an essential fatty acid) via the enzyme cyclooxygenase.

Small doses of aspirin irreversibly inhibit cyclooxygenase so that both prostacyclin and thromboxane A2 are reduced. The balance shifts in favor of prostacyclin for many hours so that platelets are prevented from aggregating at the sites of endothelial damage—a process which precedes the formation of clots.

Aspirin is widely used on a long-term basis to prevent formation of clots in the coronary and cerebral vessels.

Q.4. Enumerate the functions of platelets.
The functions of platelets are:
1. **Hemostatic plug formation.**
2. **Role in blood coagulation**
3. **Clot retraction**
4. **Phagocytosis:** The platelets can ingest carbon particles, immune complexes and viral particles.
5. **Transport:** They synthesize, store and transport a number of substances. They can take up 5-HT against a concentration gradient and transport large amounts from the argentaffin cells of the intestinal glands.
6. **Role in local blood flow regulation:** Products of platelet aggregation (and many other stimuli) also cause the release of nitric oxide (NO), a powerful vasodilator from the intact endothelial cells. Thus, platelets may have a role in dilating the vessels in the vicinity of vasoconstriction and plug formation in microvessels as described above.

Q.5. What are the physiological variations in the platelet count?
Increased counts may be seen after severe exercise and sometimes at high altitudes.

Decreased counts near the lower side of the normal may be seen in the newborns and in females, during menstruation.

Q.6. What is meant by the terms thrombocytopenia and thrombocytosis? Enumerate the pathological variations in platelet count.

Thrombocytopenia: The term refers to a decreased count of platelets. It may be due to decreased production or increased destruction.
1. **Decreased production:**
   a. *Bone marrow injury/depression/failure*
   b. *Bone marrow invasion*
   c. *Periodic thrombocytopenic purpura (purpura hemorrhagica):* Cause not known.
2. **Increased destruction (i.e. decreased survival time):**
   a. *Drugs:* Thiazides, quinine, ethanol, estrogens, methyldopa, quinidine.
   b. *Immune thrombocytopenic purpura (ITP):* Autoimmune destruction of platelets. May be idiopathic.
   c. *Sequestration in spleen:* There is increased trapping and/or destruction by enlarged spleen.
   d. *Disseminated intravascular coagulation (DIC)*
   e. *Hemorrhage with extensive transfusion.*

Thrombocytosis refers to increase in platelet count.
1. *Primary thrombocytosis:* Platelet count more than 800,000/mm^3—it is a myeloproliferative disease involving megakaryocytes. Bleeding and thrombosis may occur.
2. *Secondary (or reactive) thrombocytosis:* Platelet count more than 500,000/mm^3—this condition occurs after removal of spleen or after severe hemorrhage.

Q.7. What is purpura and what are its causes?
The term purpura is derived from the purple-colored petechial hemorrhages and bruises in the skin. The blood that leaks out from the capillaries, etc. changes color from red to purple to dark blue to green over a period of time. These colors are due to changes in the pigments derived from hemoglobin.

Causes of purpura: These include:
1. Thrombocytopenia
2. Functional platelet defects
3. Vessel wall defects (Thrombasthenic purpura)
4. Allergy and old age.

Purpura may be primary or secondary.
- **Primary purpura** (idiopathic; cause not known): In many cases, antibodies develop against platelets (ITP), causing their excessive destruction.
- **Secondary purpura:** It is much more common than the primary form. The causes include: Drugs (aspirin) and chemicals, bone marrow depression/destruction, hypersplenism, etc.

Q.8. What do the platelets look like in a blood film stained with Leishman's stain?

Q.9. Which other diluting fluid may be used for counting platelets?

OBSERVATION

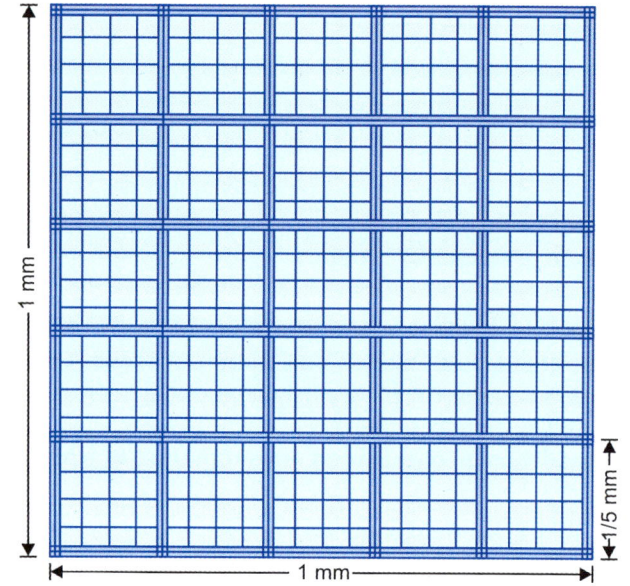

Fig. 1.13.2: Enter the observations in the corresponding squares.

RESULT

....
....
....
....
....

INTERPRETATION

....
....
....
....
....

STUDY NOTES

Teacher's Signature

CHAPTER 1.14

Absolute Eosinophil Count

AIM
To determine the absolute eosinophil count (AEC).

INTRODUCTION
Absolute eosinophil count is required when the differential leukocyte count shows a high percentage of these cells. This is especially true in cases of bronchial allergy, asthma, urticaria, intestinal parasites, pulmonary eosinophilia, etc.

COUNTING METHODS
The absolute count of eosinophils can be done by two methods:
1. **Direct method:** The cells are counted directly by employing hemocytometry.
2. **Indirect method:** The percentage of eosinophils is determined from differential leukocyte count (DLC). If total leukocyte count (TLC) is done simultaneously, the absolute count can be calculated.

$$AEC = \frac{\text{Differential count of eosinophil}}{100} \times TLC$$

> **NOTE**
> The direct method will be used in this experiment.

Direct Method of Counting Eosinophils

Principle
Blood is diluted 10 times in a white blood cell (WBC) pipette using Pilot's diluting fluid. The stained cells are then counted in a counting chamber.

Apparatus
1. Microscope, counting chamber, WBC pipette, coverslips.
2. Pricking apparatus.
3. **Pilot's diluting fluid.**

Composition of Pilot's Fluid
- Propylene glycol (50 mL) lyses red blood cells and is a solvent for the stain.
- Phloxine (10 mL): Stains only eosinophil granules
- Sodium carbonate (1 mL): Lyses all leukocytes except eosinophils and enhances the staining of eosinophilic granules.
- Heparin: 100 units (anticoagulant).
- Distilled water to make 100 mL.

Procedure
1. Give a fingerprick under aseptic conditions, discard the first drop and then fill the WBC pipette with blood to the mark 0.5.
2. Suck the Pilot's fluid to the mark 11 in the pipette. Mix the contents for 2 minutes by rolling the pipette between palms.
3. Place the pipette on moistened filter papers and cover it with a petridish. Allow it to stand for 15 minutes for proper lysis and staining (The purpose of moist filter paper is to prevent evaporation of water from the pipette).
4. Take out the pipette and mix the contents once again for 30 seconds. Discard the fluid in the stem and charge each side of the chamber.
5. Using HP objective 40x count the eosinophils seen as pink cells with nuclei in the four corner WBC squares (Fig. 1.14.1).
6. Determine the absolute eosinophil count per µL of blood (N × 50) (*Refer* Chapter 1.6).

Normal absolute eosinophil count is 10–400/mm^3 (eosinophil count of capillary blood is usually 10–15% higher).

Chapter 1.14: Absolute Eosinophil Count

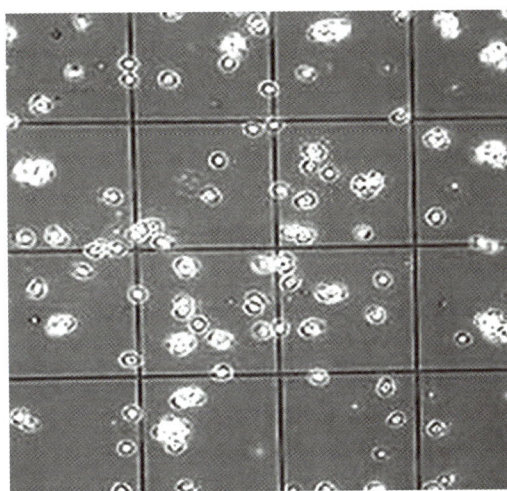

Fig. 1.14.1: Eosinophil as seen under high power (40x).

PHYSIOCLINICAL SIGNIFICANCE

Formerly, eosinophil count was considered as an index of adrenocorticotropic hormone (ACTH) activity in the blood. However, the absolute count helps in diagnosing various allergic and parasitic conditions.

> **NOTE**
> When ACTH is injected into a person with normal adrenocortical function, there is a drastic reduction in the absolute eosinophil count. This test called **"Thorn's test"** used to be employed to assess adrenocortical function. However, with better hormone assay tests, this test is no longer employed.

Eosinophilia is seen in:
1. Allergic conditions
2. Parasitic infestations
3. Pulmonary eosinophilia.

Eosinopenia is seen in:
1. Cushing's syndrome
2. Acute pyogenic infections
3. Aplastic anemia.

PRECAUTIONS

1. Observe all precautions same as for TLC (*Refer* Chapter 1.6).
2. Do the cell counting within 20–30 minutes of charging the chamber because the cells begin to disintegrate in the diluting fluid.
3. The pipette should be placed on moist filter paper.
4. If possible, use the indirect method to check on your results.

QUESTIONS

Q.1. What is the clinical significance of absolute eosinophil count?
Q.2. Can any other diluting fluid be used for the count?
Yes. In *Dunger's diluting fluid,* eosin replaces phloxine and acetone replaces propylene glycol.

In *Randolph's diluting fluid* which is similar to Pilot's solution, methylene blue is added to stain other leukocytes blue compared to red-orange eosinophils.
Q.3. Name the conditions in which absolute eosinophil count increases and decreases.
Q.4. What is the advantage of determining absolute eosinophil count over the indirect method?

OBSERVATION

Enter your observations in appropriate squares.

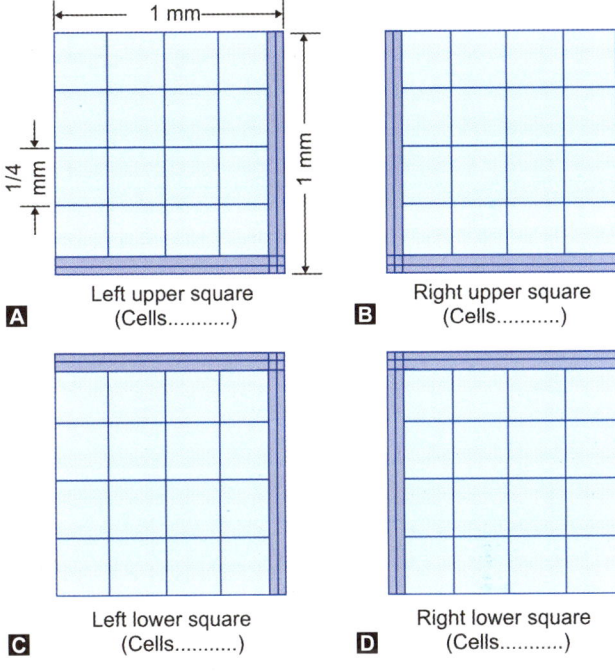

A Left upper square (Cells...........)
B Right upper square (Cells...........)
C Left lower square (Cells...........)
D Right lower square (Cells...........)

CALCULATION

....
....
....
....
....

RESULT

....
....
....
....
....

INTERPRETATION

....
....
....
....

STUDY NOTES

CHAPTER 1.15

Reticulocyte Count

AIM

To determine the reticulocyte count.

INTRODUCTION

Reticulocytes are the non-nucleated immediate precursors of red blood cells that develop in the red bone marrow from the pluripotent hematopoietic stem cell (HSC). They contain large amounts of **remnants of RNA and ribosomes.** They are slightly larger (diameter = 9.0 μm) than red blood cells (RBCs) and are present in large numbers in bone marrow and in small numbers in blood (1% of RBCs).

PRINCIPLE

A mixture of blood and a dye (stain) is spread in the form of a thick smear on a glass slide. The reticulocytes are then counted per 1,000 red cells under oil immersion and their percentage is calculated.

Reticulocyte Staining: The reticulocyte can only be stained with certain dyes such as brilliant cresyl blue. The dye enters the cells and stains the basophilic material to form bluish precipitates of dots, short strands and filaments. This reaction can occur only in **supravitally (or vitally)** stained cells, i.e. in "unfixed" and "living" cells.

Vital staining means that a dye is capable of penetrating living cells or tissues and does not induce any immediate degenerative changes.

> **NOTE**
> More the immature cells, greater is the amount of precipitable ribosomal material present in them.

The reticulocyte count which is 1–2% of the total circulating red blood cells is an indicator of erythropoietic activity of red bone marrow.

APPARATUS

1. Microscope, glass slides, pricking apparatus, petri dish, blotting paper.
2. Reticulocyte stains (**supravital stains**): These stains are used for staining unfixed, "living" cells and tissues in vitro (outside the body).
   a. **Brilliant cresyl blue:** 1 g of this dye dissolved in 100 mL of citrated saline (one volume of 3.8% sodium citrate and 4 volumes of normal saline). The dye stains the RNA of reticulocytes, citrate prevents clotting of blood and normal saline provides tonicity (1% solution of the dye in methyl alcohol can also be used).
   b. **New methylene blue:** While methylene blue does not stain the reticulum, new methylene blue (**which is chemically different from methylene blue**) stains this material more deeply and uniformly. 1 g of the dye is dissolved in 100 mL of citrate saline.

PROCEDURE

1. Take 1 mL of anticoagulated blood in a small test tube; add an equal amount of the supravital stain.
2. Mix gently and incubate at 37°C for 15–20 minutes. The test tube is incubated at body temperature to simulate the living conditions so that the stain may penetrate the reticulocytes.
3. Mix it gently to re-suspend the blood cells and prepare moderately thick 4–5 smears from this mixture. Choose the best smear for reticulocyte counting under oil immersion.

Alternate Method

1. Take 2–3 clean glass slides and place a drop of reticulocyte stain in the center of each slide about 1 cm from its end.
2. Give a fingerprick under aseptic precautions and add an equal-sized drop of blood to each drop of stain. Stir with a pin and put the slides on moist filter paper and cover with a petri dish. Allow the mixture to remain on the slides for 1 minute.
3. Spread a smear of the blood-dye mixture on each slide, then counterstain with Leishman's stain in the usual manner (This will stain all cells).

IDENTIFICATION OF RETICULOCYTES

1. Place a piece of paper with a hole in the center below the eye piece lens. This restricts the microscopic field.
2. Using oil-immersion objective, bring the blood cells into focus and identify the reticulocytes (Fig. 1.15.1). They stain lighter than the red cells and also contain dots, strands and filaments, etc. of bluish-stained material. Reticulocytes are non-nucleated cells and are slightly larger (diameter about 9 μm) than the red cells (average diameter = 7.5 μm).
3. Count the RBCs in different microscopic fields. Count 1,000 RBCs and record the number of reticulocytes encountered in each field (Table 1.15.1).

Express the reticulocyte percentage as:

$$\text{Reticulocyte \%} = \frac{\text{Number of reticulocytes counted}}{\text{Total RBCs counted}} \times 100$$

NORMAL VALUES

1. Newborns: 30–40%. Their number decreases to 1–2% during the first week of life.
2. Infants: 2–6%
3. Children and adults:
   a. 0.2–2.0% (average 1%)
   b. Absolute count: 20,000–90,000/mm^3.

ABSOLUTE RETICULOCYTE COUNT

A direct reticulocyte counting by Neubaeur's chamber is not possible. An indirect absolute count can be obtained from the relative percentage of reticulocytes by doing a total red blood cell count.

Absolute reticulocyte count

$$= \frac{\text{Reticulocyte (\%)} \times \text{RBC count}/\mu\text{L of blood}}{100}$$

Normal value = 25,000–100,000/μL.

PHYSIOCLINICAL SIGNIFICANCE

1. **Reticulocytosis:** The term indicates an increase in the number of reticulocytes in the blood.
   a. *Physiological causes:*
      - Newborn infants
      - High altitude
      - Menstruation.
   b. *Pathological causes:*
      - Reticulocyte response: Increase in reticulocyte count following treatment of deficiency anemias
      - After hemorrhage
      - Chronic hemolytic anemias, hereditary spherocytosis, sickle cell anemia, thalassemia
      - Bone marrow proliferation.
2. **Reticulocytopenia:** Decrease in reticulocyte count may be seen in:
   a. Aplastic anemia.
   b. Hypopituitarism, myxedema.

PRECAUTIONS

1. Observe all the precautions as for differential leukocyte count.

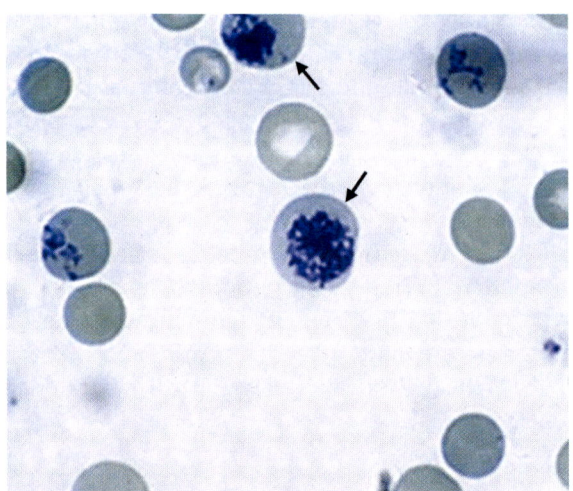

Fig. 1.15.1: Peripheral blood smear showing reticulocytes.

2. The blood film should be thick so that the red cells lie separately from each other without any crowding or overlapping.
3. There should be no rouleaux formation on the slide.

QUESTIONS

Q.1. What are the indications for doing reticulocyte count?
Indications are:
1. Hemolytic anemia
2. To see response after treatment of anemia.

Q.2. What are reticulocytes? Are they normally present in blood? Do you see these cells in the Leishman-stained blood films?

Q.3. What is the chemical nature of reticular material in the reticulocyte?
It is the remnant of RNA and ribosomes.

Q.4. What is meant by the term "vital" staining? How does it differ from Leishman's staining you employ for blood films?
Vital staining is a special method of staining employed for unfixed, "living cells" (or as nearly living as possible) including tissue cultures. There are two types of vital staining:
1. **Supravital staining:** It is an in vitro method where the living cells are stained by immersing them in a dye solution.
2. **Intravital staining:** It is an in vivo method where a dye is injected into a living organism for selective staining.

Q.5. How does a reticulocyte differ from a red cell?

Q.6. What are the normal reticulocyte counts in newborns, infants, children and adults?

Q.7. What is a reticulocyte response? Is it of any practical value?
Reticulocyte response is an increase in the number of reticulocytes in the circulating blood in response to the administration of a hematinic agent. It indicates a high rate of erythropoiesis. Its practical importance is as follows:
1. It is useful in assessing the erythroid activity of the red marrow.
2. It can be employed to check if the diagnosis and treatment of an anemic patient is proceeding on correct lines.
3. The potency of a particular hematinic drug can also be assessed. The response starts 2–8 days after the therapy is started and reaches a peak in the next 8–10 days. After that, there is a gradual fall in the response, while the RBC count continues to rise steadily.

Q.8. What is meant by the term reticulocytosis? Name the physiological and pathological conditions that cause an increase and decrease in the number of reticulocytes.

Q.9. Is there any automated (electronic) method for counting reticulocytes?
Yes, there is a method in which the cells are stained with a fluorochrome dye that specifically stains RNA. The reticulocytes fluoresce when exposed to ultraviolet light and the cells can then be counted.

Q.10. Why is it necessary to restrict the microscopic field to count the cells?
It is necessary as this will allow the easy counting of the cells and avoid the recounting of the RBCs.

OBSERVATION

Table 1.15.1: Count the number of reticulocytes and the number of RBCs in different microscopic fields.

Field No.	Number of reticulocytes	Number of RBCs
1.		
2.		
3.		
4.		
5.		
6.		
7.		
8.		
9.		
10.		

CALCULATION

RESULT

INTERPRETATION

STUDY NOTES

CHAPTER 1.16

Osmotic Fragility of Red Blood Cells

AIM

To determine the osmotic fragility of red blood cells (RBCs).

INTRODUCTION

Osmotic fragility of red blood cells is defined as the RBC resistance to hemolysis while being exposed to varying levels of dilution of a saline solution. Osmotic fragility tests the ability of RBCs to withstand hypotonic saline without bursting. It is employed as a screening test for hemolytic anemias.

It is expressed as the concentration of the hypotonic solution in which the red blood cells are hemolyzed.

PRINCIPLE

1. The normal red blood cells can remain suspended in isotonic solution, e.g. normal saline 0.9% NaCl; 5% glucose; 10% mannitol and 20% urea solution for hours without rupturing or any change in their size or shape. But when they are placed in decreasing strengths of hypotonic solutions (<0.9% NaCl), they imbibe water (due to osmosis) and finally burst.
2. The ability of RBCs to resist this type of hemolysis can be determined quantitatively.
3. When RBCs are placed in isotonic solution, there is no change in the shape because fluid neither goes out of cells nor enters into it.
4. In hypertonic solution (>0.9% NaCl), they shrink because the fluid goes out of the cells.

APPARATUS

1. Test tube rack with 12 clean, dry, 7.5 cm × 1.0 cm glass test tubes.
2. Glass marking pencil.
3. Glass dropper with a rubber teat.
4. Sterile swabs moist with alcohol.
5. 2 mL syringe with needle.
6. Freshly prepared 1% sodium chloride solution.
7. Distilled water.

PROCEDURE

1. Number the test tubes from 1 to 12 with the glass marking pencil and put them in the rack.
2. Prepare the saline solutions of increasing hypotonicity as shown in Table 1.16.1.
3. Using the glass dropper, place the varying number of drops of 1% saline in each of the 12 test tubes. Then, after thorough rinsing of the same dropper with distilled water, add the number of drops of distilled water to each of the 12 tubes (Table 1.16.1).
4. Mix the contents of each test tube by placing a thumb over it and inverting it a few times. Mark the tonicity of saline on each of the test tubes. Note that tube no. 1 contains normal saline which is isotonic with plasma, while tube no. 12 contains only distilled water which has no tonicity.
5. Draw 2 mL of blood from a suitable vein and gently eject one drop of blood into each of the 12 tubes. (The blood may be put into a container of anticoagulant

Section 1: Hematology

Table 1.16.1: Preparation of saline solutions for testing the osmotic fragility of red cells.

Test tube number	1	2	3	4	5	6	7	8	9	10	11	12
No. of drops of 1% NaCl	22	16	15	14	13	12	11	10	9	8	7	0
No. of drops of distilled water	3	9	10	11	12	13	14	15	16	17	18	25
Tonicity strength of NaCl (in %)	0.88	0.64	0.60	0.56	0.52	0.48	0.44	0.40	0.36	0.32	0.28	0

Note: Use the same dropper, after thorough rinsing each time, for measuring saline and distilled water. This will ensure that the volume of all drops is equal for all test tubes.

and a drop can be put into each tube with a pipette). Mix the contents gently by placing a thumb over it and inverting the tube only once.

6. Leave the test tubes undisturbed for 1 hour in order that unhemolyzed RBCs settle to the bottom of the tube. Then observe the extent of hemolysis in each tube by holding the rack at an eye level with a white paper sheet behind it (Fig. 1.16.1).
7. While judging the degree or extent of hemolysis from the depth of the red color of supernatant saline, tube no. 1 (normal saline) and tube no. 12 (distilled water) will act as controls, i.e. no hemolysis in normal saline (no. 1) and complete hemolysis in distilled water (no. 12).
   a. The test tubes in which **no hemolysis** has occurred, the RBCs will settle down and form a red dot (mass) at the bottom of the tube, leaving the saline above clear.
   b. If there is **some hemolysis**, the saline will be tinged red with Hb with the unruptured RBCs forming a red dot at the bottom. **This marks the onset of fragility. Normally, this is seen in 0.48% NaCl solution.** The color of the saline will be seen to be increasingly deeper with decreasing tonicity of saline.
   c. The test tubes in which there is **complete hemolysis**, the saline will be uniformly deep red with no RBCs at the bottom of these tubes. **This marks the end of fragility. This usually occurs in 0.36% NaCl solution.**

Normal Range of Osmotic Fragility

Normally, hemolysis begins in about 0.48% saline (tube no. 6 in this case).

Hemolysis is complete at about 0.36% saline (tube no. 9).

PRECAUTIONS

1. Use the same dropper, after thorough rinsing each time, for measuring saline and distilled water.
2. The test tubes should not be shaken vigorously after adding blood, because this is likely to cause mechanical hemolysis.
3. The test tubes should be left undisturbed for exactly 1 hour before taking the observations.

QUESTIONS

Q.1. What is meant by the terms fragility and hemolysis?
Fragility: This term refers to the susceptibility of red cells to being broken down by osmotic or mechanical stresses.
Hemolysis: This term refers to the breaking down (bursting) of red cells resulting in release of Hb into the surrounding fluid.

Q.2. Define osmosis and osmotic pressure. How much osmotic pressure is exerted by the blood and what is its importance?
Osmosis: It is the process of net movement of water from a weaker solution (of a solute and solvent) to a stronger

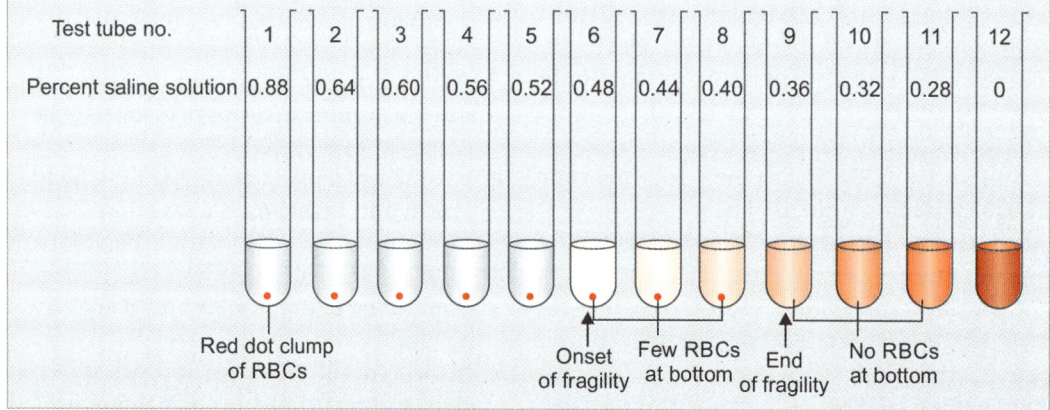

Fig. 1.16.1: Osmotic fragility test showing RBC suspension after 1 hour in increasing hypotonicity of NaCl solution and distilled water.

solution through a selectively permeable membrane, that is permeable only to water but not to solute.

Osmotic pressure: It is the pressure required to be applied to the stronger solution to prevent the movement of solute (water) from the weaker to the stronger solution.

Osmotic pressure of blood: The total osmotic pressure of blood (or plasma) due to all crystalloids and colloids is about 5,000 mm Hg (6–7 atmospheres).

Q.3. What will be the effect of vigorous shaking of the test tubes after adding blood to each of them?
Vigorous shaking in an attempt to mix the contents of the test tubes is likely to cause mechanical rupture of RBCs with release of Hb into the saline.

Q.4. How do red cells behave in hypotonic and hypertonic saline solutions? How do they resist hemolysis in hypotonic saline?
The red cell membrane is selectively permeable membrane which allows water to pass through easily while the movement of various solutes is restricted to varying degrees.
Red cells in hypertonic saline: In hypertonic solutions, the RBCs, like other body cells, shrink (crenate) due to movement of water out of the cells **(exosmosis)**.
Red cells in hypotonic saline: In hypotonic saline, water moves into the red cells **(endosmosis)**. They swell up and lose their biconcave shape becoming smaller and thicker. When they swell and become completely spherical, further increase in volume is not possible without an increase in their surface area.

Osmotic fragility of RBCs also indicates the shape of the cells. The more fragile the cells, the greater is their degree of spherocytosis. Also, fragility of red cells is greater in venous blood.

> **NOTE**
> The red cell membrane has protein pumps and ion channels. Its structural proteins, including spectrin, actin, tropomyosin, adducin, etc. are attached to the transmembrane skeletal protein meshwork by the protein ankyrin (The Hb molecules are not present free within the cells but absorbed onto the protein meshwork). The structural proteins give the red cells the remarkable property of "deformability".

Q.5. Give the normal range of fragility of red cells.

Q.6. What will be the effect of waiting for 5–6 hours before observations are made on the test tubes?
If observations are made after, say, 5–6 hours, hemolysis is likely to occur in all hypotonic solutions. The reason is that without energy supply, various membrane pumps (especially Na^+-K^+ pump) will fail to function. Sodium chloride will enter the cells, they will swell up and finally rupture.

Q.7. What is the clinical significance of doing osmotic fragility test?
Though the fragility test is not done as a routine test, it is employed as a screening test in hereditary spherocytosis.

Q.8. Name the conditions where red cell fragility increases and those where it decreases?
1. **Increased red cell fragility:**
   a. *Hereditary spherocytosis*
   b. *Autoimmune hemolytic anemia*
   c. *Toxic chemicals, poisons, infections and some drugs (aspirin)*
   d. *Deficiency of glucose-6-phosphate dehydrogenase (G6PD)*
   e. *Venom of cobra and some insects contains* lecithinase which dissolves lecithin from red cell membranes, thus making them more fragile.
2. **Decreased red cell fragility:**
   a. *Acholuric jaundice.*
   b. *Pernicious anemia.*

Q.9. What are the complications of hemolysis occurring in the circulating blood?
The Hb released from red cells will increase the osmotic pressure of blood thereby affecting tissue fluid exchanges. Further, if the tubular fluid is acidic, acid hematin crystals may be precipitated in the renal tubules and cause renal damage.

Q.10. Name some hemolytic agents.
Some of the hemolytic agents are:
- Hypotonic saline
- Incompatible blood transfusion
- Snake venom
- Severe infection
- Reaction to certain drugs. Aspirin is a common drug that may cause hemolysis at any time.

Q.11. What is the effect of 5% glucose, 10% glucose, urea solution of any strength and urine on red cells?
- **5% glucose:** It is isotonic with blood (and plasma). The RBCs do not show any change in size or shape.
- **10% glucose:** Since it is hypertonic, the red cells will shrink due to exosmosis (water moving out). However, in the intact body, when 10% or even 20% glucose is given intravenously, the RBCs will shrink in the beginning. But later on, after some time, glucose gets metabolized and there are no harmful effects.
- **Urea solution:** As urea tends to move into the red cells, this is followed by water. The final result is hemolysis.
- **Urine:** Since urine is hypotonic, the red cells imbibe some water and swell up. In a highly concentrated urine sample, the red cells shrink to some extent.

Q.12. How does hemolysis occur in the body?
Hemolysis of red cells within bloodstream may occur in many different ways. It may be due to structural abnormalities (hereditary spherocytosis, sickle cell anemia), mismatched blood transfusion, bacterial toxins, chemicals, adverse drug reactions, venom of snake and insects.

Q.13. Name some isotonic solutions for mammals.
Isotonic solutions of medical interest are:
- Sodium bromide: 1.5%
- Magnesium sulfate: 3.3%
- Sodium chloride: 0.9%
- Sodium nitrate: 2.5%
- Dextrose: 5%
- Sucrose: 10%
- Sodium bicarbonate: 0.9%.

Q.14. Enumerate the factors affecting osmotic fragility test.
The factors affecting are:
1. Final pH of blood in saline. The fragility of RBCs increased by a fall in pH. A shift of 0.1 of a pH unit is equivalent to altering saline concentration by 0.01 g%.

2. The relative volume of blood in saline.
3. Temperature: A rise in temperature decreases the fragility, a rise of 0.5°C is equivalent to an increase in saline concentration of 0.01 g/dL.

Q.15. Do all the normal RBCs in a person or in a sample of blood have similar osmotic fragility?

The red cells in a person or in a sample of blood vary in their osmotic fragility because they belong to many generations of RBCs. Younger cells are more resistant, while older cells are more osmotically and mechanically fragile (The old and worn out cells fragment in the circulation and are taken up by the Reticulo-endothelial system). After removal of spleen, the cells become flat which decreases the volume to surface ratio, thereby decreasing osmotic fragility.

OBSERVATION

Express your result in % saline.
- Hemolysis begins in .... % saline.
- Hemolysis is complete in .... % saline.

Osmotic fragility of RBC in given sample of blood ranges from .... % to .... % saline.

RESULT

....
....
....
....
....

INTERPRETATION

....
....
....
....
....

STUDY NOTES

CHAPTER 1.17

Specific Gravity of Blood

AIM

To determine the specific gravity (SG) of blood.

INTRODUCTION

Specific gravity is the ratio of the weight of a given volume of a fluid to the weight of the same volume of distilled water, measured at 25°C. The specific gravity of serum, plasma, blood and red cells is as mentioned in the Table 1.17.1.

Table 1.17.1: Specific gravity of serum, plasma, blood and red cells.

	Specific gravity
Serum	1.22–1.024
Plasma	1.028–1.032
Blood	1.058–1.062
Red cells	1.092–1.095

The following methods are used for this experiment, which are as follows:

1. **Direct method:** Equal volumes of blood and water taken in capillary tubes called pycnometers and weighed. The ratio of their weights determines the specific gravity of blood.
2. **Indirect method:** There are two methods:
   a. *Hammerschlag's method:* In this method, the densities of the two miscible liquids (for example, chloroform—specific gravity 1.470 and benzene—specific gravity 0.88) are equalized to match that of blood to determine the specific gravity.
   b. *Philips and Van Slyke's $CuSO_4$ method:* The procedure essentially involves comparing the specific gravity of blood, plasma or serum against the specific gravity of a series of $CuSO_4$ solutions. After the specific gravity has been determined, line charts (or tables) are consulted to read the concentration values.

Indirect Method

Philips' and Van Slyke's $CuSO_4$ Method

This is the most commonly used method.

Principle: The specific gravity of blood is compared with the solutions of $CuSO_4$ with known specific gravity.

Apparatus

1. Well-stoppered bottles of 150 mL capacity—20 in number.
2. **Stock solution of copper sulfate** (specific gravity = 1.100).
3. Syringe and needle, Pasteur pipette, sterile swabs moist with alcohol.

Procedure

1. Mix distilled water with stock solution of $CuSO_4$ (Table 1.17.2), to prepare 10 mL of $CuSO_4$ solutions of specific gravity (SG) ranging from 1.050 to 1.066.
2. Mix each solution properly.

Chapter 1.17: Specific Gravity of Blood

Table 1.17.2: Preparation of standard copper sulfate solutions for the determination of specific gravity of blood.

Bottle number	1	2	3	4	5	6	7	8	9
Stock solution (mL)	4.9	5.1	5.3	5.5	5.7	5.9	6.1	6.3	6.5
Distilled water (mL)	5.1	4.9	4.7	4.5	4.3	4.1	3.9	3.7	3.5
Specific gravity	1.050	1.052	1.054	1.056	1.058	1.060	1.062	1.064	1.066

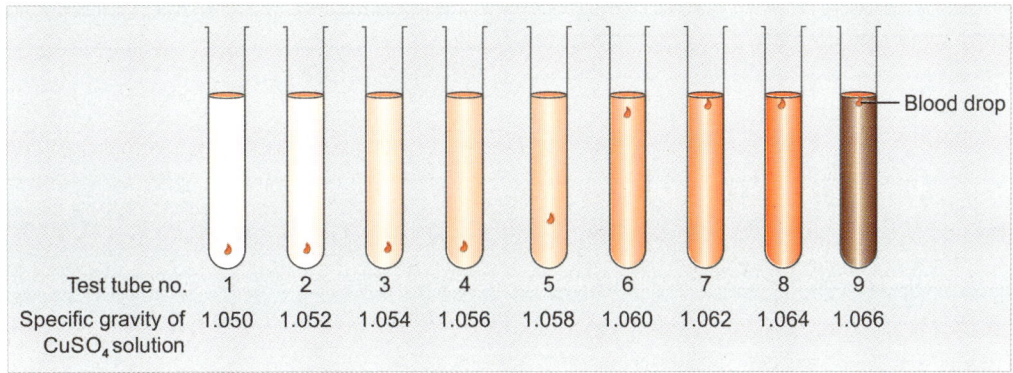

Fig. 1.17.1: Position of blood drop in $CuSO_4$ solutions ranging from SG 1.050 to 1.066.

3. Allow a drop of blood to fall from a Pasteur pipette from a height of about 1 cm into each solution.
4. Observe the behavior of blood drop in the solution.
5. The blood drop will travel for some distance due to momentum (Fig. 1.17.1):
   a. If the drop continues to sink, move to the next higher specific gravity solution.
   b. If it begins to rise, move to the lower specific gravity solution till you come to a solution where the drop remains stationary for about 15 seconds.
6. Note the SG of the solution in which blood drop remains suspended for 15–20 sec. This gives the SG of the blood sample.

NOTE

When the blood drop falls into the $CuSO_4$ solution, it becomes encased in a layer of copper proteinate and there is no change in its specific gravity for the next 15–20 seconds. This is the reason why the behavior of the drop is to be observed during this period. Within a short time, however, the drop becomes heavier and sinks to the bottom as a precipitate. In fact, the drops which initially float on the surface ultimately become heavier and settle down as shown in the Figure 1.17.1.

QUESTIONS

Q.1. Define specific gravity. What is the specific gravity of serum, plasma, blood and red blood corpuscles?

Q.2. Why is copper sulfate method preferred over the other method?

This method is chosen because the chemical is cheap and it is not hygroscopic. Also, its temperature coefficient of expansion is about the same as that of blood. No correction factor for temperature is, therefore, required.

Q.3. What is the clinical significance of determining the specific gravity of blood?

It is used to measure the hemoglobin content, PCV, blood proteins and degree of dehydration. It also gives an idea of hemoconcentration.

The test is employed in the screening of blood donors, mass surveys for anemia and in handling emergency cases of burns requiring repeated transfusions of plasma, plasma expanders or blood.

Q.4. What are the physiological and pathological conditions in which the specific gravity of blood is increased and decreased?

The specific gravity of blood is affected by:
1. Red cell count
2. Hemoglobin concentration
3. Plasma (or serum) protein concentration
4. Water content of blood.

Physiological conditions:

It is **increased** in:
1. Newborns
2. At high altitude due to polycythemia.

It is **decreased** in:
1. Pregnancy (due to hemodilution)
2. After excess water intake.

Pathological conditions:

The specific gravity is **increased** in:
1. Polycythemia due to any disease (e.g. congenital heart disease, cardiac failure)
2. Polycythemia vera

3. Severe dehydration (diarrhea, vomiting)
4. Hemoconcentration (loss of plasma due to burns).

The specific gravity **decreased** in:
1. Anemias
2. Hemodilution (excessive secretion or prolonged treatment with glucocorticoids)
3. Kidney disease (loss of albumin and water retention).

OBSERVATION

RESULT

INTERPRETATION

STUDY NOTES

Section 2

Amphibian (Frog) Experiments

CHAPTERS

- 2.1 Introduction to Amphibian Experiments
- 2.2 Study of Apparatus
- 2.3 Dissection of Gastrocnemius Muscle-Sciatic Nerve Preparation of Frog
- 2.4 Simple Muscle Twitch
- 2.5 Effect of Temperature on Simple Muscle Twitch
- 2.6 Conduction Velocity of Sciatic Nerve of Frog
- 2.7 Effect of two Successive Stimuli (of Same Strength) on Skeletal Muscle Contraction
- 2.8 Effect of Increasing Strength of Stimulus on Skeletal Muscle Contraction
- 2.9 Genesis of Tetanus
- 2.10 Genesis of Fatigue
- 2.11 Effect of Load on Skeletal Muscle Contraction (Freeload and Afterload)
- 2.12 Recording of a Normal Cardiogram of Frog's Heart and Effect of Temperature on it
- 2.13 Properties of Cardiac Muscle
- 2.14 Effect of Stimulation of Vagosympathetic Trunk and White Crescentic Line on Frog's Cardiogram
- 2.15 Effect of Variables on Intact Frog's Heart
- 2.16 Perfusion of Isolated Frog's Heart

Date ....

CHAPTER 2.1

Introduction to Amphibian Experiments

To study the response of a living tissue to a stimulus, three things are required:
1. Living tissue
2. Stimulus
3. Recording device.

LIVING TISSUE

The student usually begins the experimental work on the amphibian nerve and muscle tissues after removing them from the frog's body. The living tissue of frog is preferred because:
- They can function as isolated preparations for many hours when handled carefully and kept moist with a suitable solution.
- The tissues get their oxygen from the atmospheric air and therefore, no separate oxygenation is required.
- Frogs are cold-blooded animals, so no temperature control is required.
- Frogs are easily available.

STIMULUS

A stimulus is a change in the environment of an excitable tissue, which causes the tissue to respond in its own particular fashion.

Out of the various (mechanical, chemical and electrical) types of stimuli, electrical stimuli are usually preferred because:
- Their strength (in volts), duration (in ms), timing and site can be easily controlled.
- Since their duration of use is very short, they do not cause any damage to the tissues. Thus, they can be applied repeatedly, if required, without producing any harmful effects.
- They resemble the natural mode of excitation of the tissues, i.e. the phenomena of resting potentials and action potentials are electrical in nature.

Types of Current

1. Faradic (induced) current
2. Galvanic current.

The living tissue is stimulated by an **induced** or **faradic current**. This current is produced or obtained by feeding a **galvanic current** [direct current (DC)] into an induction coil known as Du Bois–Reymond induction coil, which converts low voltage, high ampere and DC (galvanic) into a high voltage, low ampere and phasic current (faradic). This induced current is of short duration and therefore, stimulates the tissue without causing any injury. Its intensity can be adjusted as required. Since, the usual household electric supply, alternating current (AC), 220 volts, 50 Hz is lethal and is never employed without modifying it. It can be used by converting it to DC-low volts (6 volts) by means of step-down transformer having a rectifier. This 6 volts DC supply is fed to 2-pin plug point to form low-voltage mains.

Strength of Stimuli

1. A **threshold** (minimal or liminal) stimulus is the minimum strength of stimulus that is just sufficient to produce a response.

Section 2: Amphibian (Frog) Experiments

2. A **subthreshold** (subminimal or subliminal) stimulus is weaker than a threshold stimulus and is unable to produce a response.
3. A **maximal** stimulus produces a maximum response.
4. **Submaximal** stimuli are weaker than a maximal stimulus.
5. **Supramaximal** stimuli are stronger than a maximal stimulus.

Recording Device

The recording of the responses is done by using a writing lever and kymograph with drum.

QUESTIONS

Q.1. Why the frogs are preferred for amphibian experiment?
Q.2. Name the various types of stimuli?
Q.3. What are the different types of currents used in amphibian experiments?

STUDY NOTES

Teacher's Signature

Date ....

CHAPTER 2.2

Study of Apparatus

The different apparatus the students will be using include the following:
1. **Source of current:**
   a. **Two-pin plug point (low-voltage mains):** It is supplied by 6 voltage DC from a step-down transformer having a rectifier plugged to the 220 V high voltage mains.
   b. **Three-pin plug point (high voltage mains):** It is supplied with 220 V AC mains and it is used exclusively for running the kymograph.
   Caution: The **high-voltage mains** is potentially lethal. Handle the electric kymograph with utmost caution.

2. **The keys:** A key is used as a switch to complete ("make") or interrupt ("break") an electrical circuit. The different types of keys are:
   a. **Simple key/primary key (Figs. 2.2.1):** It is used to open or close the primary circuit.
   b. **Short-circuiting key/secondary key (Fig. 2.2.2):** It is connected in parallel in the secondary circuit.
      - It is kept closed to prevent accidental passage of current into the tissues.
      - In the open position, the current passes to stimulate the tissue.
   c. **Reversing key (Fig. 2.2.3):** It is employed for shunting current from one electrode to the

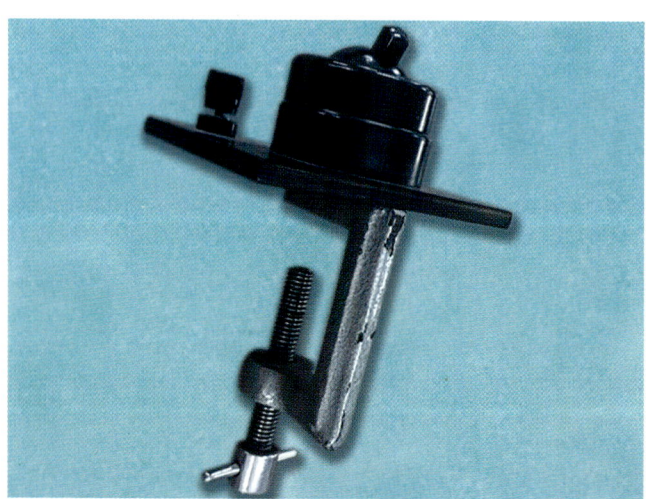

Fig. 2.2.1: Simple key.

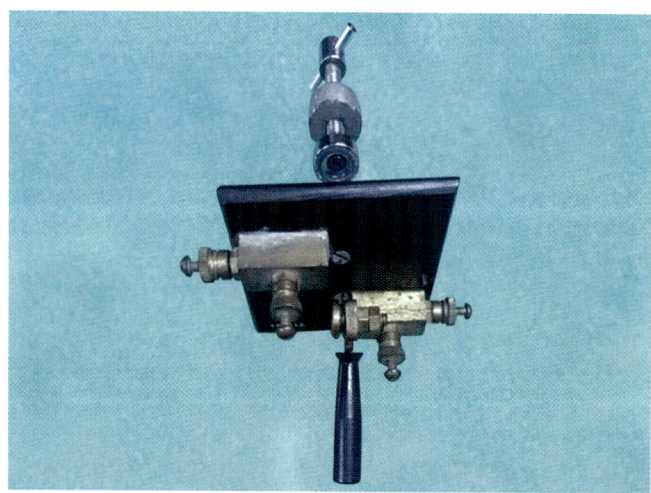

Fig. 2.2.2: Secondary key.

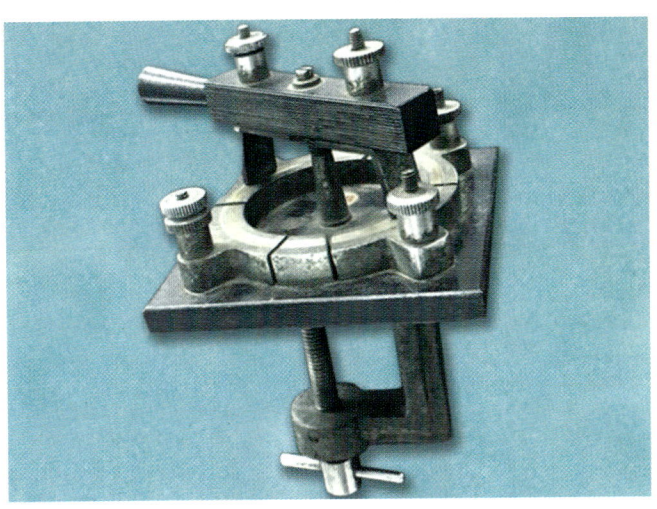

Fig. 2.2.3: Reversing key.

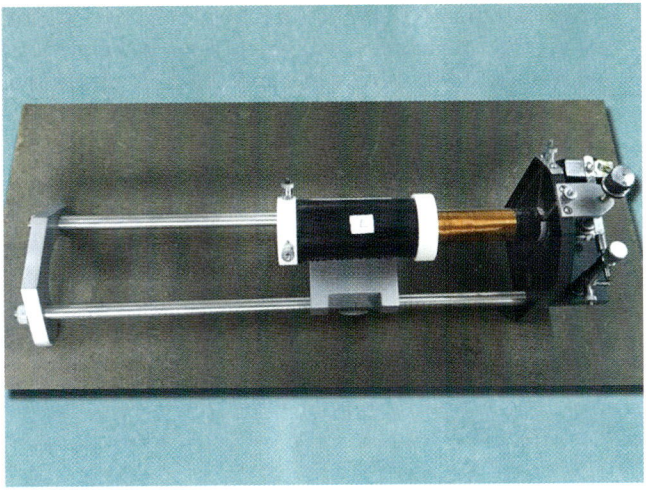

Fig. 2.2.5: Du Bois–Reymond induction coil.

other in experiments where two electrodes are used.

d. **Tapping key (Fig. 2.2.4):**
   - It is used to make or break the circuit for a limited time as and when required by gently tapping the key and releasing it suddenly.
   - It is connected in series with the low-voltage mains in the primary circuit.
   - It is used in experiments for determining the auditory and visual reaction time.

3. **Du Bois–Reymond induction coil (Fig. 2.2.5):**
   - It is a simple device to convert galvanic (low voltage, direct) current into the faradic (induced, high voltage phasic) current.
   - **Principle:** A flow of current in a wire (or a coil) produces a magnetic field in the space around it, which, in turn, can induce a current in another wire or coil placed nearby. In other words, a change in the magnetic field around a wire or a coil induces an electric current in it.
   - **It consists of two coils: Primary** and **secondary** coil which are made up of well insulated copper wire wrapped around a soft iron core. The secondary coil has a much larger number of turns than the primary coil.
   - The primary coil terminals are connected to the DC source (2-pin plug point) and the secondary coil is connected to the stimulating electrodes.
   - **"Break-induced" current versus "make-induced" current:** When the primary circuit is closed, the magnetic flux within the secondary coil increases from zero to maximum and an induced electromagnetic flux (EMF) is developed in the secondary circuit. While when the primary circuit is broken, the magnetic flux within the secondary coil drops **very rapidly** to zero and an induced EMF develops. As a result, the change in the magnetic field is greater at "break" than at "make". Therefore, *the "break-induced" current is stronger than the "make-induced" current.*

   Factors affecting strength of induced current:
   The following factors are involved:
   - The number of turns of wire in the two coils.
   - The strength of DC fed into the primary coil.
   - The distance between the primary coil and secondary coil—greater the distance and weaker the induced current.
   - The angle between the two coils—when the secondary coil is at right angle to the primary, there is no induced current; as the angle is decreased, the strength increases.

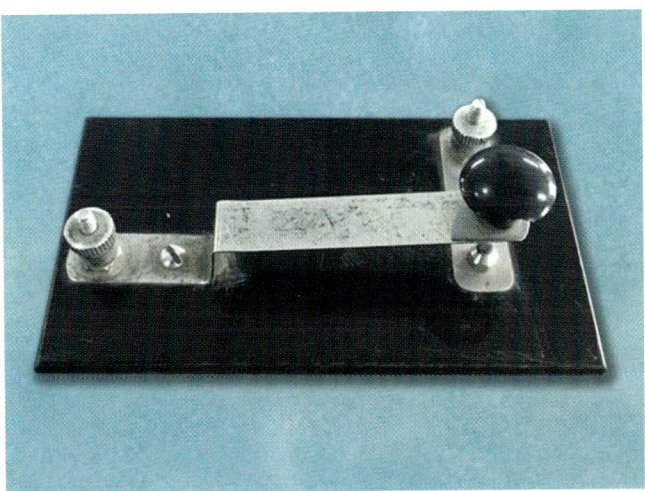

Fig. 2.2.4: Tapping key.

Neef's hammer: It is fitted on the side of the induction coil (Fig. 2.2.6) and is included in series in the primary circuit when multiple, repeated stimuli are required. It works on the principle of an electric bell. It consists of an electromagnet and a horizontally mounted T-shaped iron bar with a spring. When the current is switched on, the iron bar vibrates up and down, thus repeatedly "making" and "breaking" the primary circuit at a rate of 30–40/second.

4. **Kymograph (Fig. 2.2.7):** It is a machine for recording graphically the time course of events in tissues manifesting movement (i.e. muscle contractions).
   a. *Electric motor:* It runs on the mains 220 volts AC current.
   b. *Shaft:*
      - Two switches operate as ON/OFF switches—the **mains switch** labeled ON/OFF—this should always be put "ON".
      - It is connected to the motor and can be rotated at different speed. The speed is selected by means of a calibrated **speed setting lever.**
      - It has a groove on one side and a screw at the top. A small rectangular plug mounted on the screw inside the shaft butts out through the groove. It can be raised or lowered along the groove by rotating the screw at the top. It supports the weight of the drum and prevents it from sliding down. The level of the drum can therefore be adjusted by the top screw.
   c. *Gear:* A **variable speed lever** permits speed between 2.5 mm/s (slowest) and 640 mm/s (fastest). It is used to change the speed of the shaft.
   d. *Clutch lever:* Which engages or disengages the gears. This is used as ON/OFF switch to prevent damage to the gears. The cylinder may be rotated easily by hand when the clutch lever is in the horizontal (OFF) position. There is one slot marked "N" (neutral) where the gears get disengaged from the motor.
   e. *Dual electric contact arms* (also called the **"striker"**): They are fitted, one over the other, at the base of the vertical shaft and rotates along with it. The two arms of the striker can be drawn apart, as and when two stimuli, one after the other is required.

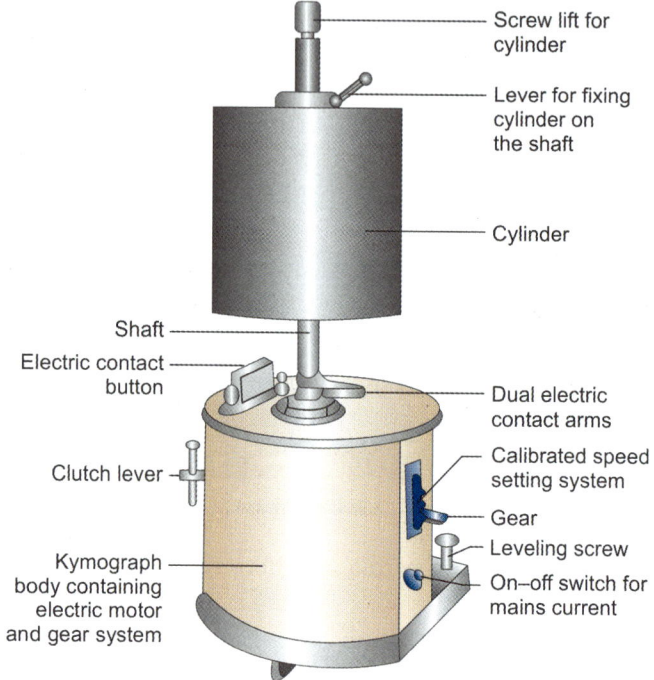

Fig. 2.2.7: Electric kymograph.

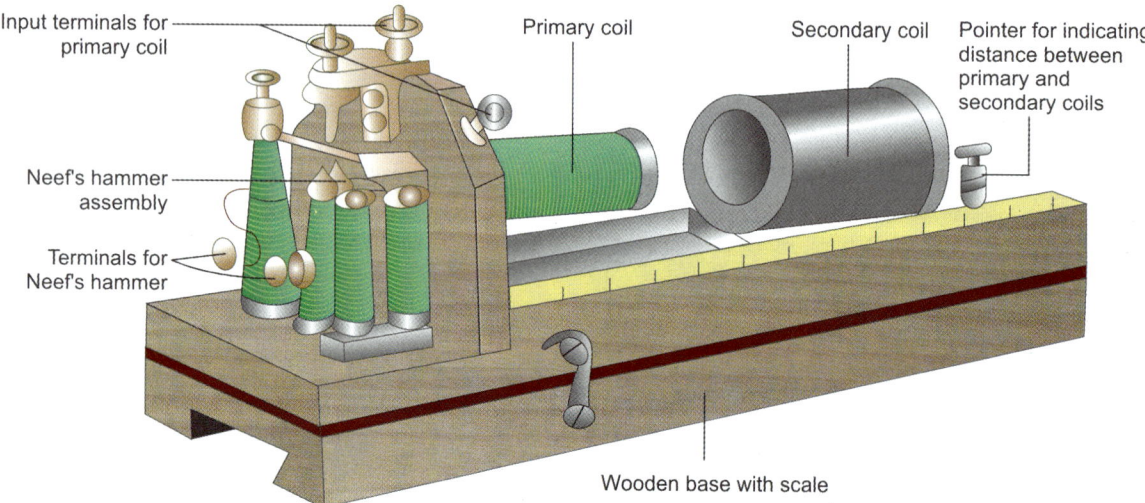

Fig. 2.2.6: The Du Bois–Reymond induction coil (the output terminals of the secondary coil are not shown).

f. *Contact button:* It is fitted on the top of the kymograph body at the level of the striker. When the terminals are included in the primary circuit, this circuit is completed only when the striker touches the contact button. Thus, the contact block terminals **function as a simple key in the primary circuit**, their purpose being to **mark the point of stimulation** on the recording surface. As on each rotation of the drum, the contact button will be pressed in close succession at a precise interval of time.

g. *Sherrington's recording drum:* It is a 6″ × 6″ cylinder with a glazed paper wrapped around it, is firmly fixed on the shaft with the locking lever.

h. *Leveling screws*—these are provided at the base of the drum for adjusting the tilt of the cylinder toward or away from the writing lever (Fig. 2.2.7).

5. **Lucas chamber/Muscle trough (Fig. 2.2.8):**
   - It is a transparent Perspex bath, 6″ × 4″ × 2″, with a clamp and drain pipe.
   - The base has two holes plugged permanently with a cork used in pinning of the tissues.
   - It is used in experiments where the tissues can be immersed in the Ringer's solution.

6. **Isotonic muscle lever (the writing lever) (Fig. 2.2.9):**
   - An L-shaped writing lever is employed for recording muscle contraction.
   - It has a horizontal arm which bears holes and notches for hanging weights.
   - The writing point of the lever is made up of a triangular piece of photographic film.
   - The vertical arm of the lever is tied to the tendon of the muscle via a thread.

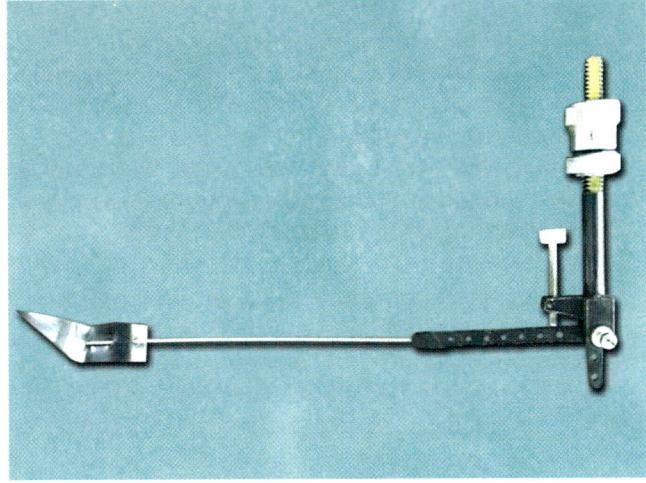

Fig. 2.2.9: Isotonic muscle lever.

   - A **screw** is provided with the vertical arm which can be moved up and down to bring the muscle into **free loaded** or **after loaded** condition.
   - **Ink-writing stylus:** *an ink-writing stylus (filled with ink) can be fitted on the writing lever. It is used to directly inscribe on the glazed paper without the need of "smoking" its surface.*

7. **Starling heart lever (Fig. 2.2.10):**
   - This lever is more sensitive than the writing lever and is used for recording the contractions of the frog's heart which are relatively weaker than skeletal muscle contractions.
   - The lever is supported by a fine adjustable nickel silver spring.
   - A hook is tied at one end of thread and is passed through the apex of the ventricle. The other end

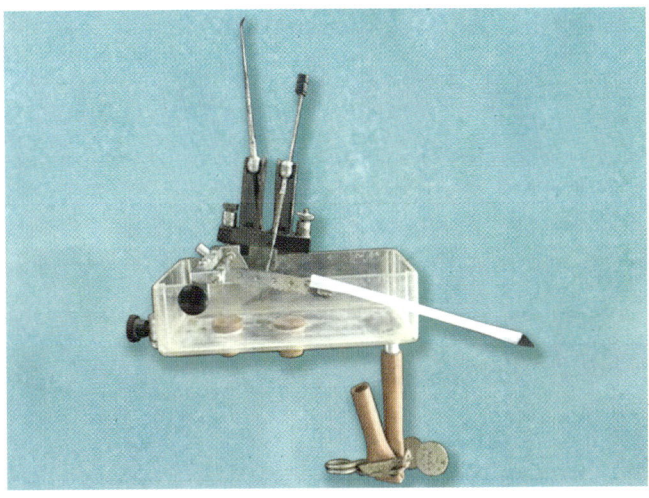

Fig. 2.2.8: Lucas chamber/Muscle trough.

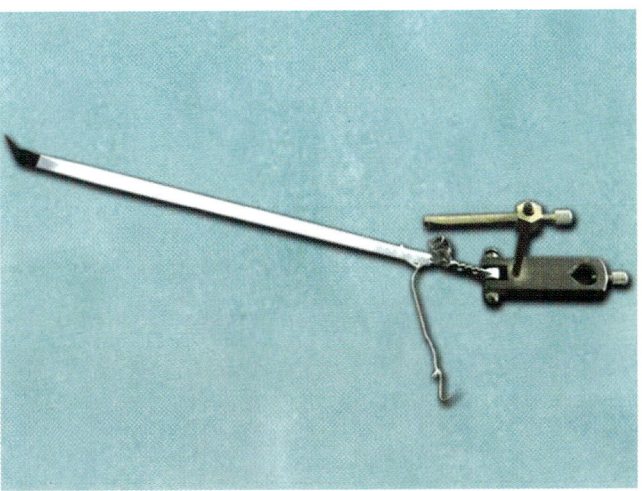

Fig. 2.2.10: Starling heart lever.

of the thread is tied to the lever to record the contractions of the ventricle.
- When the heart contracts, it pulls the lever down; when it relaxes, the spring pulls the lever back to its horizontal position.

8. **Isometric lever:** It consists of a holder, which carries a steel tension spring and a flat writing lever. This lever is used for recording isometric contractions.

9. **Variable interrupter (Fig. 2.2.11):**
    - It enables interruption of the primary circuit at a wider range of frequency which is more precisely adjustable than in the Neef's hammer.
    - The principle is similar to that of the Neef's hammer.
    - The variable frequency can be set with an adjusting screw.
    - Variable interrupter when used is connected in series with the induction coil.

10. **Time marking:** A time marking or a time tracing, is required on the recording surface in most of the experiments. The following types of time markers are employed:
    - *Tuning fork:* A tuning fork of 100 Hz is used in amphibian experiments. The tuning fork carrying a stylus on one of its prongs, is set into vibration and the stylus is gently touched to the smoked surface below the graph obtained. **The time interval between two crests (or two troughs) represents 0.01 second (n = 100).**
    - *Spring time marker:* It is used primarily for heart experiments. It usually gives time tracing for half seconds or quarter seconds. The writer makes vertical strokes at the desired time intervals.
    - *Electromagnetic time marker/signal marker:* It is used in the primary circuit. The lever of the signal marker moves with every make or break of the primary circuit and a vertical line is recorded (Fig. 2.2.12).

11. **Stimulating electrodes (Fig. 2.2.13):**
    - These are employed for delivering electrical stimuli to the tissues.
    - It consists of two insulated copper wires passing through a plastic body with a central hole for fixing it to the myograph board. The ends of the wire are bared of their insulation. They are quite simple to use.

12. **Student stimulator:** Electronic stimulators with a DC output of 0–15 volts are available. The various stimulus parameters, i.e. volts, pulse duration, pulse frequency, mode of operation (single; repetitive, 1–100/second; or an external trigger) is controlled by means of knobs provided on the equipment.

13. **Smoking:** A piece of white paper is properly pasted on the drum. The drum is then placed on the horizontal arm of the smoking stand. A burner is put on and the drum is rotated slowly to obtain a thin and uniformly black layer of soot. The paper will get burnt, if it does not fit evenly and tightly around the cylinder or if the flame is played on a stationary cylinder.

14. **Varnishing:** This is done to fix the recording on a smoked paper. Labeling of the recording is done before the paper is cut and taken out of the drum. The paper is then dipped in the 2% solution of resin or methylated spirit. The paper is then taken out and hung till it is completely dry. This procedure provides a permanent record.

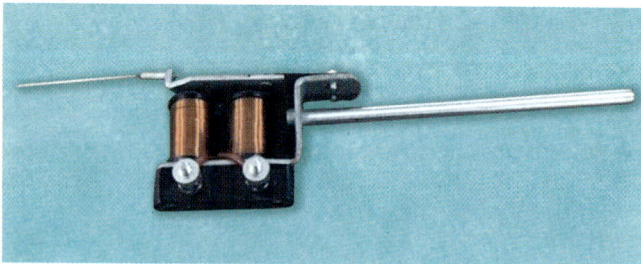

Fig. 2.2.12: Time/signal marker.

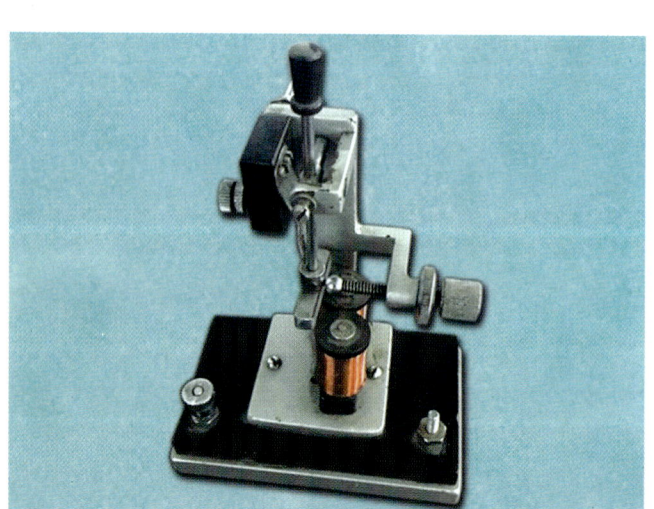

Fig. 2.2.11: Variable interrupter.

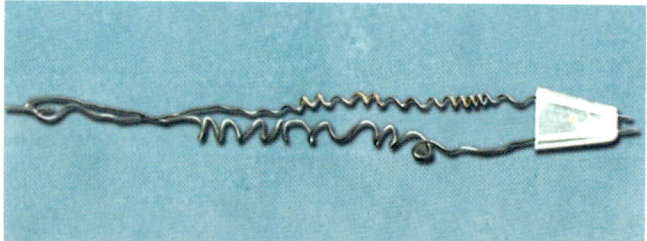

Fig. 2.2.13: Stimulating electrodes.

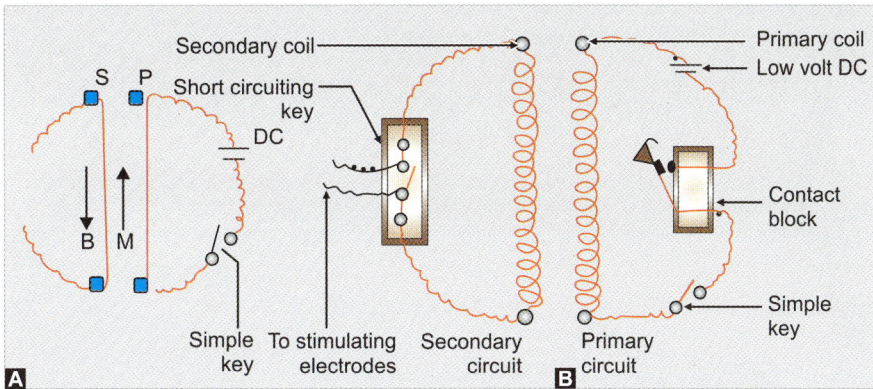

Figs. 2.2.14A and B: (A) Genesis of induced current. Flow of direct current (DC) in wire P causes induced (faradic) current in a nearby wire (S—secondary) only at make or break of DC. Arrows show the direction of induced current at make (M) and break (B) of DC; (B) Circuit for electrical stimulation of frog's nerve or muscle. The contact block makes and breaks the primary circuit by the striker of the rotating drum. The circuit can also be completed by tapping the spring with a finger.

ELECTRICAL CONNECTIONS

Figures 2.2.14A and B illustrates the connections required for obtaining induced current stimuli (induction shocks). Low-resistance cotton-covered copper wire or ordinary flex wire is wound round a pencil to give coiled wire pieces.
- **Circuit for single "make" and "break" stimuli:**
  - *Primary circuit:* Low voltage mains (battery, etc.), simple key and primary coil connected in series.
  - *Secondary circuit:* Secondary coil, short-circuiting key and stimulating electrodes are connected as shown in Figure 2.2.14B.
- **Taking kymograph in circuit:**
  - *Primary circuit:* Low volts, simple key, primary coil and contact block of drum are connected in series.
  - *Secondary circuit:* As above. The drum terminals are taken in the primary circuit when one wants to mark the point of stimulation or when two successive stimuli are needed.
- **Taking Neef's hammer, variable interrupter or vibrating reed in circuit:**
  - *Primary circuit:* Low volts, simple key, Neef's hammer of induction coil or vibrating reed or variable interrupter and primary coil.
  - *Secondary circuit* is as above. This circuit is used for getting repeated stimuli, such as for producing tetanus or for stimulating the vagus nerve.

ARRANGING THE APPARATUS

Place the induction coil just in front of you, the kymograph just beyond it, the simple key on the right side and the short-circuiting key on the left.

The muscle trough should be placed to the left of the induction coil so that the writing lever is at a tangent to the surface of the cylinder. This will allow you to see the writing point and the graph being obtained without unnecessary bending and twisting.

TROUBLESHOOTING

If after making the required connections, there is no response, try to locate the fault in a step-by-step fashion.
- Check the galvanic current by holding one end of a piece of wire on one terminal and brushing its free end on the other terminal. Sparking indicates a good current. A voltmeter will indicate the voltage.
- Check the simple key and the contact block terminals in a similar fashion. Switch on the drum; each time the striker touches the contact spring, there is sparking. This checks out the primary circuit.
- **Secondary circuit:** "Open" (i.e. switch off) the short-circuiting key and place the electrodes on the nerve muscle preparation and switch on the drum. If the leg muscles twitch with each shock, the stimulus is reaching the electrodes. If the stimulation of the nerve does not give a response, put the electrodes directly on the muscle belly; if the muscle contracts with each shock, the nerve has been damaged.

STUDENT PHYSIOGRAPH

The **"student physiograph"** consists of (Fig. 2.2.15):
1. **The main console:** The main console has the following:
   - *Chart drive:* The multispeed chart drive can provide paper speed ranging from 0.25 mm/s to 100 mm/s. The paper, 70 mm in width, is fed through a slot under the writing pens.
   - *Pen recording system:* Two recording pens are provided, the upper for the main recording channel and the lower for synchronized time/event recording.

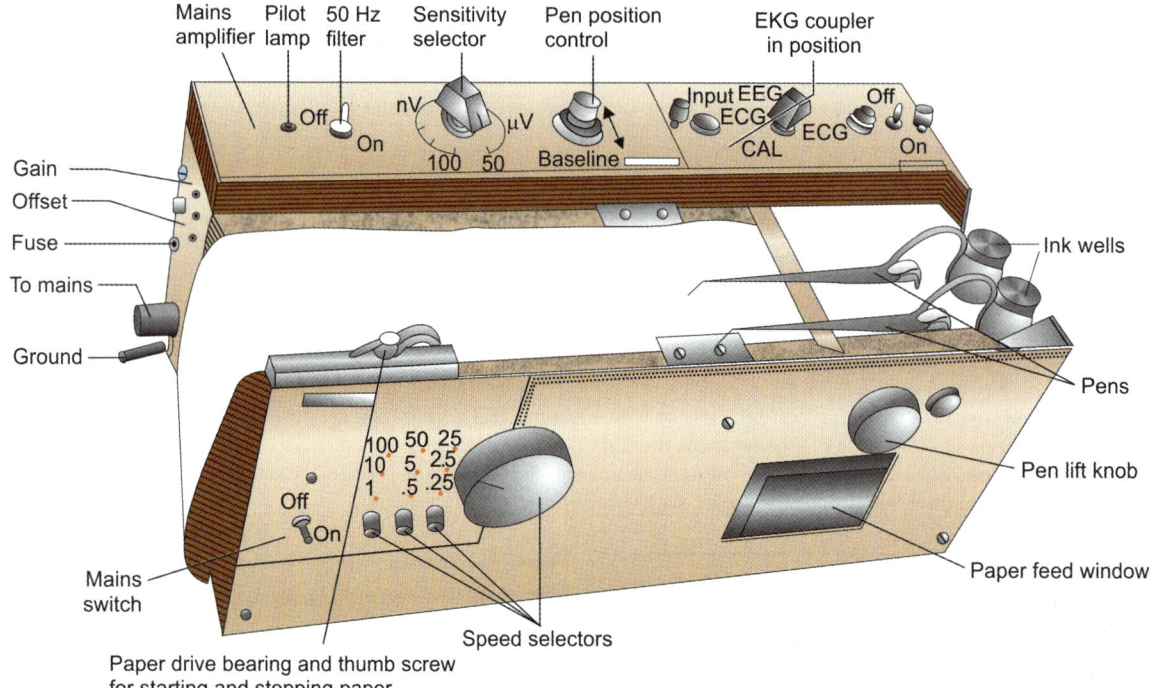

Fig. 2.2.15: Student physiograph.
(ECG/EKG: electrocardiogram; EEG: electroencephalogram)

- *The main amplifier:* The main amplifier which is common to all couplers is fitted in the console.
  Three screwdriver adjustments are provided on the side of the console. Once adjusted they do not normally require adjustments. The side of the console also has IN and OUT jacks. The OUT jack of one physiograph connected to the IN jack of another unit connects them in tandem and both units will record simultaneously from the same experimental set-up. Another input jack takes the synchronized event/time marker of the electronic stimulator.
- *Coupler housing:* Different interchangeable couplers can be plugged into the coupler housing. An appropriate transducer is to be connected to the coupler in use.
2. **Couplers:** The following couplers are available for use with the physiograph:
    - *Biopotential coupler:* The biopotential coupler is designed to record **electrocardiogram (ECG), electroencephalogram (EEG), electromyogram (EMG), sensory and motor nerve conduction velocities in humans, movements of the eyes (electronystagmogram)** and so on.
    - *Electrocardiogram (EKG):* The coupler is used for recording clinical EKG (ECG). There is a knob for selecting various leads—I, II, III, aVR, aVL, aVF, V, CR, CL and CF. There is another knob for calibration.
    - *Strain gage coupler:* This coupler records activity from various strain gage transducers (pressure–volume, volume and muscle–force transducers).
    - *Pulse-respiration coupler:* This coupler is employed for recording arterial pulse with a photoelectric pulse transducer and respiratory movements with a respiration belt transducer.
    - *Temperature coupler:* This coupler is used for recording rectal or surface temperature. For such recordings, the transducer has to be calibrated within the desired temperature range using a water bath.
3. **Stimulator:** The electronic stimulator can be used in two modes:
    a. To stimulate the tissue and to energize either a time base or act as an event marker.
    b. To provide electrical stimuli of up to 30 volts as a single pulse or as two successive stimuli with predetermined intervals ranging from 5 m/sec to 250 m/sec or as repeated stimuli with frequencies ranging from 0.5/s to 100/s. The electrical stimuli provided by the stimulator are rectilinear with a fixed pulse width of 0.5 m/sec.
4. **Transducers:** The wide range of transducers convert one form of energy into another, electrical energy, in this case:
    - *Pressure–volume transducer:* It is used for recording pressures from –50 mm Hg to 250 mm Hg and small changes in volume.

- *Volume transducer:* It is used for recording minute changes in volume.
- *Muscle-force transducer:* Employed for recording all muscle activity, heart activity, force, etc.
- *Pulse transducer:* Used for recording pulsations from any artery.
- *Respiration transducer:* Employed for recording respiratory movements.
- *Temperature transducer:* Used for recording surface or core temperature.

Student physiograph has the following **advantages** over the electromechanical devices:

- Many more parameters can be recorded on a single apparatus through the use of couplers, matching transducers and pickups.
- The group experiment concept permits more than one physiograph to be used independently or interconnected to each other in tandem for the same experimental set-up.
- Though, the controls are kept to a few, only the sensitivity and accuracy of these devices are high.

Steps for the Use of the Physiograph

1. Put the stack of paper in the paper receptacle. Lift the pens by turning the lift knob clockwise. Fold the paper end into a V and with the fingers of one hand pass it through the slot in the console top and then pull it out from the slot with the other hand. Slide the paper under the two Perspex guides and then under the ball bearing after lifting the latter by using the thumb screw.
2. From the mains switch on the console on the OFF position plug in the desired coupler. It is important to remember that a coupler should not be plugged in or removed while the mains switch is ON. Select the standard speed on 25 mm/s.
3. Apply the electrodes on the subject's arms and legs. Connect the electrodes through lead wires to the 5-pin junction box and the latter to the EKG coupler.
4. Switch ON the mains console and then the coupler. Adjust the sensitivity on the main amplifier to 1 mV. Adjust pen position to center. Put the lead selector control on the coupler to CAL position for calibration. Run the paper and press and release the CAL push button on the coupler three or four times while adjusting the CAL control so that 1 mV may produce a deflection of the pen by 1 cm. Stop paper.
5. Move the lead selector control to lead I position and record 6–8 ECG complexes. Stop paper; move the control to lead II and take recording. Continue this process till all the leads have been obtained.

QUESTIONS

Q.1. What is the function of primary and secondary keys?
Q.2. What is the difference between primary and secondary coils?
Q.3. Name the various keys and their functions.
Q.4. What is the function of induction coil?
Q.5. What are the characteristics of an ideal stimulus?
Q.6. Why induced current is used to stimulate the living tissue?
Q.7. What is the function of Neef's hammer?
Q.8. What are the factors affecting the strength of induced current.
Q.9. How is time interval calculated from the time tracing?
Q.10. What are the various functions of student physiography? Name the various couplers used.
Q.11. Why is it important to use induced current for the experiment?

Section 2: Amphibian (Frog) Experiments

STUDY NOTES

Date ....

CHAPTER 2.3

Dissection of Gastrocnemius Muscle-Sciatic Nerve Preparation of Frog

AIM

Dissection of gastrocnemius nerve muscle preparation (Fig. 2.3.1).

APPARATUS

1. Pithing needle, scissors, forceps and bone cutter.
2. Wooden dissection board, amphibian Ringer's solution and cotton wool.

Amphibian Ringer's Solution

The composition of amphibian Ringer's solution is as given below:
1. **Sodium chloride (0.6%):** Maintains isotonicity and required for generation of action potential.
2. **Calcium chloride (0.012%):** Maintains the excitability of the living tissue.
3. **Potassium chloride (0.014%):** Maintains the resting membrane potential.
4. **Sodium bicarbonate (0.02%):** Maintains optimal pH.

PROCEDURE

1. **Stunning:** Holding the frog gently and firmly, by its waist give a sudden strong blow on its head by striking against the edge of the table. This renders the frog unconscious.

> **NOTE**
> No anesthesia is used as it may suppress the excitability of the nerve, neuromuscular junction or muscle.

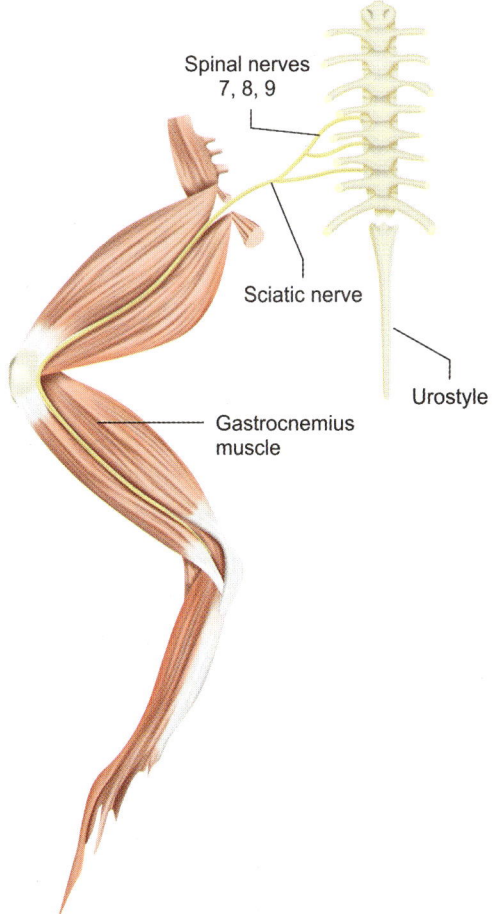

Fig. 2.3.1: Nerve-muscle preparation.

2. **Pithing:** The purpose of pithing is to destroy the brain and spinal cord so that the animal neither feels pain nor there are any reflexes present or voluntary movements during the dissection.
   - Hold the animal in your left hand and flex its head with your index finger. Ventroflexing of the head helps to locate the triangular depression which marks the point where the pithing needle has to be inserted.
   - Demarcate the point exactly in the center of the line joining the two tympanic membranes. There is a depression, where a sharp-pointed ***pithing needle*** should be pushed in. Thereafter, it is pushed downward into the vertebral canal.
   - The pithing needle is rotated in all possible directions to destroy the spinal cord properly.
   - When the spinal cord is destroyed and pithing is effectively complete then the limbs become flaccid, neither feels pain nor does it move its limb during dissection and shows loss of conjunctival and corneal reflexes. Destroying the brain alone is not sufficient as the spinal reflexes may interfere with muscle contractions.
   - Bring out the needle from the spinal cord. The frog is ready for dissection now.
3. **Dissection:**
   - Cut through the skin with scissors completely all around the trunk just below the forelimbs. Seize the skin in a duster and strip off the skin down to the toes.
   - Place the frog on the myograph board on its abdomen.
   - Pick up the tip of the urostyle with the forceps and cut the pelvic girdle on its either side, taking care not to injure the sciatic nerve.
   - Lift up the urostyle and cut 2 cm long piece of vertebral column above and below the exit of sciatic nerves. This piece of vertebral column is retained to keep the nerve stretched over the stimulating electrodes. It also provides a rigid body to prevent nerve injury during accidental rough handling.
   - Using a bone forceps, cut and divide this piece of vertebral column into two pieces. Lift each piece with forceps and snip away the nerves going to nearby tissues, taking care not to injure the sciatic nerves which can be seen disappearing into the thigh muscles.
   - Expose the sciatic nerve in the thigh between the muscles and gently separate the nerve from the thigh muscle. Use a glass rod to handle the nerve, identify, dissect and cut the gastrocnemius tendon from its attachment. Tie a thread around the tendon.
   - *Using any metal object will stimulate the nerve and cause the contraction of the muscle. Repeated contact with metal objects will lead to muscle fatigue.*
   - Free the muscle from the tibia. Cut off the tibia-fibula below the knee joint and the femur close to the knee joint. Remove all redundant muscle other than the gastrocnemius. The knee joint is kept intact as it is required to fix the nerve muscle preparation to the myograph board. Moreover the nerve may get injured in the process of cutting the knee joint.
   - The nerve-muscle preparation is now ready. Keep it immersed in frog's Ringer's solution till the commencement of the experiment.

PRECAUTIONS

1. Take care to cause minimum injury to the nerve-muscle preparation.
2. The nerve should never be subjected to stretching or be repeatedly touched by a metal object.
3. Keep moistening the nerve-muscle preparation with amphibian Ringer's solution to prevent drying.
4. Do not use forceps or other metallic objects to handle the nerve-muscle preparation.

QUESTIONS

Q.1. What is the composition and function of amphibian Ringer's solution?
Q.2. Why a small piece of vertebral column is retained at the end of a sciatic nerve?
Q.3. Why the intact knee joint is retained with the nerve-muscle preparation?
Q.4. Why the frog is not anesthetized?
Q.5. What is the purpose behind doing stunning and pithing of frog?
Q.6. Why the sciatic nerve should not come in contact with any metal objects during dissection?
Q.7. How will you know that the frog has been effectively pithed or not?
Q.8. Why is the head ventroflexed during pithing?
Q.9. Why is it not sufficient to destroy the brain alone?

STUDY NOTES

Date ....

CHAPTER 2.4

Simple Muscle Twitch

AIM

To demonstrate the effect of a single induced current shock to the nerve-muscle preparation and to calculate the time period of the various phases obtained.

THEORY

A single adequate stimulus applied to the sciatic nerve results in a sharp, momentary contraction of the muscle, followed immediately by its relaxation. This response is called a *simple muscle twitch (SMT)*.

The contraction does not begin immediately upon application of the stimulus. A period between the point of stimulus and the onset of contraction is called as the **latent period (LP)**. The **contraction period (CP)** is the period between the onset of contraction to the point that corresponds to the peak of contraction. The **relaxation period (RP)** is the period from the peak of contraction to the end of relaxation (Fig. 2.4.1). The wave obtained at the end of the response is called as the **physiological curve**. It is due to the inertia of the lever.

Causes of latent period: The latent period is due to the time taken by:
1. Action potential to travel along the nerve to the neuromuscular junction.
2. Release of neurotransmitter (acetylcholine) and its binding to the receptors.
3. Excitation contraction coupling.
4. Viscosity of the muscle.
5. Inertia of the lever system, which has to be overcome before contractions can be recorded.

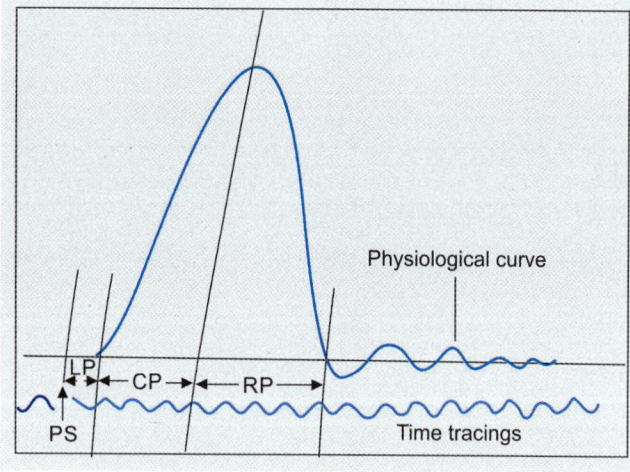

Fig. 2.4.1: Simple muscle twitch.
(PS: point of stimulation; LP: latent period; CP: contraction period; RP: relaxation period)

APPARATUS

1. Dubois-Reymond induction coil, simple key and short-circuiting key.
2. Kymograph (drum); cylinder with smoked paper or glazed paper with ink-writing stylus.
3. Myograph board, stimulating electrodes, hooks and weights.
4. Tuning fork (100 Hz), dividers, pins, thread, amphibian Ringer's solution and nerve-muscle preparation.

Speed of the drum: 640 mm/sec (fastest)
Strength of the stimulus: Minimal (threshold).

PROCEDURE

1. Set up the primary and secondary circuits. **Include the drum in the primary circuit** to obtain a single induction shock with every revolution of the cylinder. Since the minimal stimulus is desired, the distance between the primary and secondary coils is adjusted to obtain the contraction only at "break".
2. Mount the preparation on the myograph board and tie its thread to the hook. Adjust the lever so that it is horizontal and has a weight hung on it to prevent overshoot during the recording.
3. Support the vertical arm of the lever with the afterload screw (This screw will support the load until the activated muscle exerts a force sufficient to lift the load).
4. Reposition the cylinder, so that the recording can be properly obtained. Set the drum in motion and record the baseline. The primary key should be closed and the short circuiting key is open and the drum is set into motion. By releasing the tap key (in the primary circuit), nerve is stimulated by a single break shock.
5. **Mark the point of stimulus:** Bring the striker in contact with the contact button and mark the point of stimulus by manually raising the writing lever over the drum.
6. A simple muscle curve is obtained on the drum (Fig. 2.4.2).

> **NOTE**
> The points to be marked manually are: Point of stimulus, point of onset of contraction, point of beginning of relaxation, point of completion of relaxation before removing the drum from the circuit. The writing point moves in an arc-like fashion.

7. **Recording the time tracing:** The drum is restarted at the same speed and the vibrations of tuning fork with known frequency are recorded (100 vibrations per second). The vibrations should be recorded below the baseline. The distance between the top of two waves measures 0.01 second.
8. The time intervals are measured by calculating the number of waves and then by multiplying by 0.01 seconds.
9. Observe and study the simple muscle curve and note the duration of the different phases. The durations of various phases are given in Table 2.4.1.

Table 2.4.1: Calculated durations of various phases in simple muscle twitch.

Latent period (AB)	0.01 second
Contraction period (BC)	0.04 second
Relaxation period (CD)	0.05 second
Total simple muscle twitch duration in the frog's gastrocnemius muscle	0.1 second

CORRELATION OF SIMPLE MUSCLE TWITCH AND ACTION POTENTIAL ON THE SAME TIME SCALE

When the muscle action potential and the simple muscle twitch are plotted on the same time scale the twitch starts 2 ms after the start of depolarization of the membrane before repolarization is complete (Fig. 2.4.3).

PRECAUTIONS

1. The nerve-muscle preparation should be stimulated briefly by a single induction shock.
2. Care should be taken to mark the point of stimulus.
3. Time tracing should be taken just below the graph.

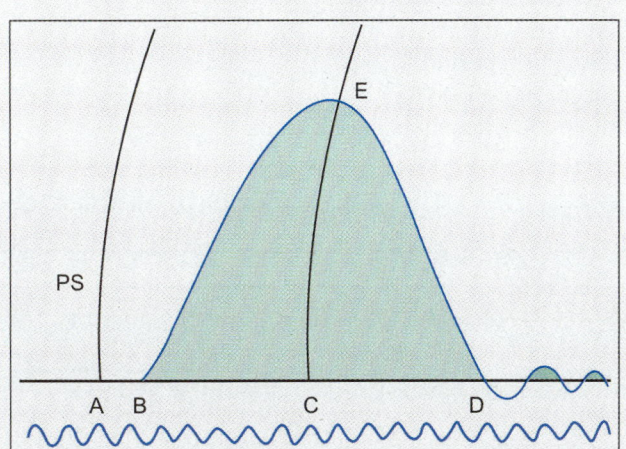

Fig. 2.4.2: Simple muscle twitch. PS: point of stimulation; AB: latent period; BC: contraction period; CD: relaxation period; BE: contraction phase; ED: relaxation phase. Tuning fork = 100 Hz.

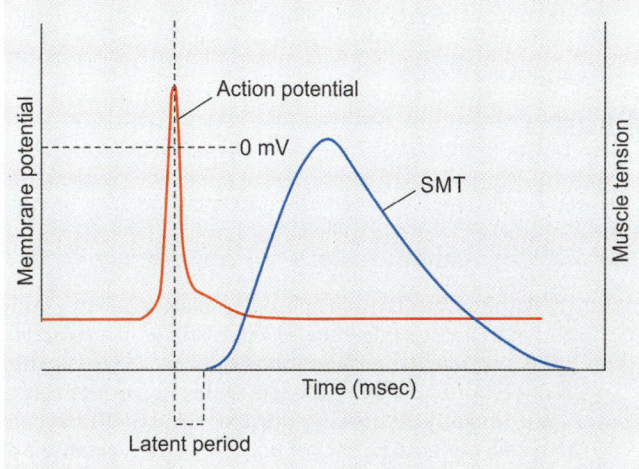

Fig. 2.4.3: Correlation of simple muscle twitch and action potential on the same time scale.

QUESTIONS

Q.1. What type of nerve is the sciatic nerve? Why does its stimulation cause muscle contraction? Is the muscle twitch recorded by you a normal physiological event?

The sciatic nerve is a mixed nerve. When the nerve fiber is stimulated, the action potential is generated which travels down the nerve up to neuromuscular junction where acetylcholine is released. The acetylcholine binds to the nicotinic receptors present on the postsynaptic membrane. This in turn leads to the generation of action potential in the sarcolemma of all the muscle fibers innervated resulting in excitation contraction coupling. Under normal physiological conditions a simple muscle twitch is not produced in the body except in the case of a tic.

Q.2. Why is the kymograph included in the primary circuit?

The drum is taken in the primary circuit for two reasons—firstly, to obtain a single induction shock (the "make"—induced current is the effective stimulus), and, secondly, to mark the point of stimulation.

Q.3. What are the causes of latent period?

Q.4. What type of muscle contraction is recorded in this experiment?

The muscle contraction recorded in this experiment is the *isotonic* (same tension) type. The distance the lever moves indicates the degree of shortening. The muscle does external work since it moves the load to a certain distance, the tension remaining the same.

Q.5. What is isometric contraction? Do such contractions occur in the body?

Muscles consist not only of *contractile components* (contractile proteins), but also *elastic* and *viscous elements* (elastic fibers, tendons, connective tissue sheaths, blood vessels, etc.), which are arranged *in series* with the contractile components. Therefore, if both the ends of a muscle are rigidly fixed, it is possible for the muscle fibers to contract without an appreciable shortening of the *muscle as a whole*, though there is development of tension. Such a contraction is called *isometric* ("same measure" or length) (The myofibrils do contract and shorten and in doing so, they stretch the in-series elastic elements. There are "parallel" elastic elements also in the muscle).

> **NOTE**
> Even during isotonic recording of an afterloaded muscle here, there is an initial period of isometric contraction during which the tension is rising, until it exceeds the load and shortening of the muscle occurs and the load is lifted.

Both isotonic and isometric contractions occur in the body and even in the same muscles. For example, in attempting to lift a car, muscles generate great tension or force but they cannot shorten. However, the same muscles can lift a lighter load. Similarly, antigravity muscles (i.e. muscles, which maintain our posture against gravity), such as extensors of the back, hips and knees contract isometrically to maintain the erect posture, but they can shorten to cause movements at these joints.

Q.6. What are the factors, which determine the height of the simple muscle curve?
1. Strength of stimulus
2. Initial length of muscle fibers (preload)
3. Type of loading
4. Temperature
5. Type of muscle fibers in the muscle
6. Inertia of the lever system: Greater is the instrumental inertia and lower is the height of the twitch curve.
7. Magnification of the lever: The magnification by the lever depends on the ratio of the lengths of the vertical and horizontal arms. This is, of course, fixed in a given lever. A longer horizontal arm will cause greater magnification.

> **NOTE**
> The frequency of stimulation, determines the force of contraction. In the present context, however, we have employed a single stimulus.

Q.7. Which properties of muscle are demonstrated in this experiment?

The important properties demonstrated in this experiment include excitability, contractility, relaxation and conductivity.

Q.8. What is a physiological curve?

Q.9. Can the duration of different phases of simple muscle twitch be determined, if no time tracings are taken?

Yes, this can be determined, if we know the speed of the drum accurately.

Q.10. What is the function of the load suspended from the lever?
- It prevents the overshooting of the lever from the drum so that the complete graph is recorded on the drum.
- It also overcomes the inertia of the lever.
- It keeps the lever horizontal.

Q.11. What are the criteria of an ideal lever?

An ideal lever should not have any momentum. It should be weightless so that there is no resistance.

OBSERVATION AND RESULT

Write down the duration of:
Latent period (LP) ....
Contraction period (CP) ....
Relaxation period (RP) ....
Simple muscle twitch ....
....
....
....

INTERPRETATION

....
....
....
....
....

STUDY NOTES

Teacher's Signature

CHAPTER 2.5

Effect of Temperature on Simple Muscle Twitch

AIM

To demonstrate the effect of temperature on muscle contraction.

THEORY

When there is change in the surrounding temperature (Ringer's solution), there is a change in the amplitude and the duration of different phases of simple muscle twitch (SMT) (Fig. 2.5.1). These changes are seen because of the changes in the viscosity and the metabolism of the living tissue with charge in temperature. There is also a change in the conduction velocity of the sciatic nerve.

APPARATUS

- Same as in SMT except Lucas chamber is used instead of myograph board (*Refer* Chapter 2.4).
- Cold (10–15°C) and warm (38–40°C) Ringer's solution
- Thermometer.

Speed of the drum: 640 mm/sec (fastest)
Stimulus: Maximal

PROCEDURE

1. Arrange the same apparatus as used for recording SMT, except that Lucas chamber is used in place of myograph board. With the muscle immersed in amphibian Ringer's solution at room temperature record a SMT.
2. Replace the solution with amphibian Ringer's solution at 38–40°C, wait for about five minutes and record another SMT, taking care that the point of stimulus, strength of the stimulus and the baseline remains same.
3. Replace the hot Ringer's solution with cold Ringer at 10–15°C and record another SMT after waiting for about 5 minutes.
4. The points of stimulation, peaks of curve and the ends of the curves are marked.
5. A time tracing of known frequency (100 Hz) is marked on the drum.
6. Remove the paper and label your graph appropriately indicating the temperature for each twitch. Tabulate your

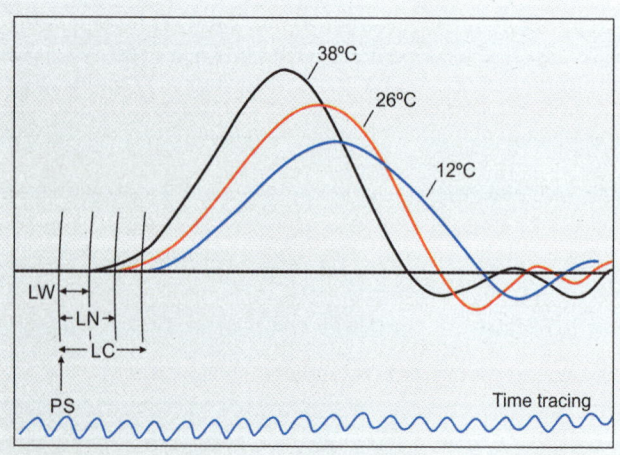

Fig. 2.5.1: Effect of temperature on simple muscle twitch (SMT). (PS: point of stimulation; LW, LN and LC: Latent periods of warm, normal at room temperature and cold Ringer's solutions respectively)

Chapter 2.5: Effect of Temperature on Simple Muscle Twitch

results, indicating the height of each curve in centimeters and the durations of various time periods.

PRECAUTIONS

1. The muscle must be immersed in the amphibian Ringer's solution at various temperatures for at least 5 minutes before taking the recording.
2. Temperature of warm Ringer's solution should not exceed 42°C as the proteins get denatured beyond this temperature.
3. Effect of warm Ringer's solution should be recorded before that of cold Ringer's solution. Cold Ringer's solution slows down the metabolic activity of the muscle thereby delaying the recovery process.
4. Baseline, the point of stimulus and strength of stimulus should be the same in all the three tracings to facilitate comparison.
5. Compare the three muscle curves recorded at three different temperatures with respect to durations of latent period, contraction phase, relaxation phase and height of contraction.

PHYSIOCLINICAL SIGNIFICANCE

The warm up exercises performed before any athletic activity enhances the performance. Also if the environmental temperature is increased within the physiological limits, the efficiency of skeletal muscle contraction increases (especially during exercise).

QUESTIONS

Q.1. What is the effect of moderately high temperature on the muscle twitch?
Warm Ringer (40°C) increases the excitability and hastens various metabolic processes in the muscle; it also decreases the viscosity. The total twitch duration decreases with decrease in latent period (LP), contraction period (CP) and relaxation period (RP). The speed of contraction increases, as is evident from the steep slope of the contraction phase; relaxation is also faster. Also due to the increase in enzymatic and chemical activities inside the muscle the height of contraction increases.

Q.2. What is the effect of low temperature on muscle contraction?
Cold has opposite effects due to slowing down of chemical processes and increase in viscosity. If the temperature is reduced to 0°C or below, the excitability is lost.

Induced hypothermia produced by cooling the skin or blood, where the core temperature can be reduced to about 25°C, is frequently employed in patients during operations on the brain or heart.

Q.3. What is rigor mortis and what is its importance?
Rigor mortis, in which there is shortening and rigidity of muscles, occurs some hours after death. The rigidity is due to loss of all the ATP, which is required for detachment of cross-bridges, which are fixed to actin filaments in an abnormal and resistant manner. Depending on the environmental temperature and other factors, the rigidity disappears after some hours due to destruction of muscle proteins by enzymes released from cellular lysosomes. The appearance and disappearance of rigidity and other factors help a forensic expert in fixing the time of death.

Q.4. Is "all-or-none law" being violated in this experiment?
No, in this experiment, the temperature is changing hence the law is not valid. It is valid only when all the physiological conditions, e.g. environmental temperature are kept constant.

Q.5. What is heat rigor?
High temperature, (45–50°C and above) causes coagulation of muscle proteins, the muscle shortens and goes into an irreversible state called **"heat rigor"**.

Q.6. Why the effect of warm Ringer's solution should be taken before that of cold Ringer?

Q.7. Why should temperature above 42°C not to be taken?

Q.8. Write the physiological significance of this experiment.

OBSERVATION AND RESULT

Recording of effect of temperature on simple muscle twitch.				
Temperature	Amplitude	Latent period	Contraction period	Relaxation period
Normal				
Warm (38°)				
Cold (12°)				

INTERPRETATION

....
....
....
....
....

Section 2: Amphibian (Frog) Experiments

STUDY NOTES

Teacher's Signature

Date ....

CHAPTER 2.6

Conduction Velocity of Sciatic Nerve of Frog

AIM

To determine the velocity of nerve impulse of frog's sciatic nerve.

THEORY

Conduction velocity of a nerve is defined as the distance traveled by the nerve impulse per unit time.

Two most important determinants of nerve conduction velocity are:
1. Diameter of nerve fiber
2. Myelination of nerve.

PRINCIPLE

The conduction velocity is calculated by dividing the distance between the two points of stimulation with the difference in the latent period of the two simple muscle twitches (SMTs).

APPARATUS

1. Same as in SMT (Refer Chapter 2.4).
2. Reversing key (instead of short-circuiting key).
3. Two pair of electrodes labeled as "A" and "B".
Speed of the drum: 640 mm/s (fastest)
Strength of stimulus: Minimal

PROCEDURE

1. Set up the nerve-muscle preparation as used to record a SMT.
2. The "A" electrode is kept on the vertebral end of the nerve and the "B" electrode is kept at muscle end.
3. Record the baseline. A SMT is recorded by stimulating "A" electrode first. This point of stimulus is marked as "P". This curve is labeled as "V" curve.
4. Keeping the baseline, point of stimulus and strength of stimulus unchanged, then "B" electrode is stimulated with the help of reversing key and an SMT is recorded. This curve is labeled as "M" curve.
5. A time tracing is taken with a tuning-fork of frequency of 100 Hz. The distance is measured between the midpoints of the two pair of electrodes ("d" in cm).
6. The difference in the two latent periods determines the time taken for the impulse to be conducted from the vertebral end of the nerve to the muscle end (Fig. 2.6.1).

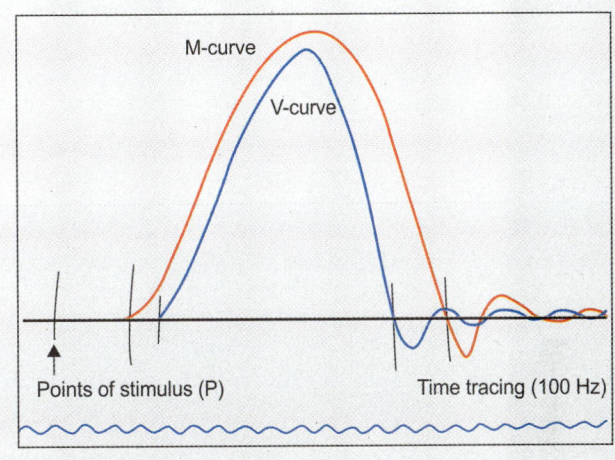

Fig. 2.6.1: Determination of nerve conduction velocity in frog (M-curve: simple muscle twitch following stimulation of the nerve near the muscle end; V-curve: simple muscle twitch following stimulation of nerve near vertebral end).

CALCULATION OF VELOCITY

Conduction velocity of a nerve (expressed as cm/s)

$$= \frac{\text{Distance (``d'') traveled in cm}}{\text{Time (``t'') taken by nerve impulse to travel from one point to another in seconds}}$$

Express it in m/s.

> **NOTE**
> The normal conduction velocity of frog nerve = 40–60 m/s.

PRECAUTIONS

1. Same as for SMT (*Refer* Chapter 2.4).
2. The baseline, point of stimulation and strength should be same for all the recordings.
3. The distance traveled should be measured accurately by taking the distance between the midpoint of two pairs of electrodes.
4. The difference in the latent period should be measured accurately.

PHYSIOCLINICAL SIGNIFICANCE

Refer Chapter 3.15.

QUESTIONS

Q.1. What is the normal conduction velocity of Frog's Sciatic nerve?

Q.2. What are the factors, which affect the velocity of conduction of nerve impulses?
1. **Diameter of nerve fiber:** In general, the greater the diameter of the nerve fiber, the greater is its conduction velocity.
2. **Presence of myelin sheath:** In myelinated fibers, the nerve impulse jumps from one node of Ranvier to the next, a process called saltatory conduction (Ionic fluxes occur only at the nodes).
3. **Temperature:** It also affects the conduction velocity, warming increasing it while cooling decreasing the velocity.

Q.3. Why the distance traveled by nerve impulse is measured from the midpoints of the two electrodes?
As the electrode has two limbs and it is not known which limb is anode or cathode. Thus, the distance is measured from the midpoints of two limbs of the electrodes.

Q.4. How are nerve fibers classified?
Refer Chapter 3.15.

Q.5. What is the physioclinical significance of this practical?
Determination of conduction velocity helps in assessing.
1. Extent of damage to the nerve fiber.
2. Recovery of the nerve fiber after damage.

OBSERVATION AND RESULT

....
....
....
....
....

INTERPRETATION

....
....
....
....
....

STUDY NOTES

Teacher's Signature

Date ....

CHAPTER 2.7

Effect of Two Successive Stimuli (of Same Strength) on Skeletal Muscle Contraction

AIM

To demonstrate the effect of two successive stimuli (of same strength) on Frog's nerve-muscle preparation.

THEORY

When two successive stimuli (maximal/supramaximal stimuli) are applied to the skeletal muscle, the response to the second stimulus depends upon how soon it has been given after the first stimulus. Since the contractile machinery does not have a refractory period, the effects in response to two successive stimuli given before muscle relaxation can be added up. The magnitude of the contraction in response to the second stimulus is greater than the first. This phenomenon is called the "Beneficial Effect" as the first stimulus becomes beneficial for the second one.

The interval between the two stimuli can be varied by appropriately separating the two prongs of the "striker".

APPARATUS

Same as in simple muscle twitch (SMT) (*Refer* Chapter 2.4).
Speed of the drum: 640 mm/s (fastest)
Strength of stimulus: Maximal/supramaximal.

PROCEDURE

1. Set up a nerve-muscle preparation and a stimulation unit to supply maximal/supramaximal stimuli and record an SMT using maximal/supramaximal stimulus.
2. Separate the projecting strikers, so that they strike the contact button in close succession. Adjust the distance between the strikers, so that the 2nd stimulus would fall during:
    - First half of the latent period
    - Second half of latent period
    - In the contraction period
    - In the relaxation period
    - Immediately after the relaxation period of the first SMT.
3. Record the all above muscle contractions using the same stimulus strength.
4. Write your observation in terms of whether the response of the two stimuli is fused or discrete and what is the change in the height of contraction.

PRECAUTIONS

1. Care should be taken to gradually increase the distance between the contact arms (strikers).
2. Point of stimulus should be marked for both the SMT.
3. The applied stimuli should be of maximal/supramaximal strength.

PHYSIOCLINICAL SIGNIFICANCE

The response obtained from a successive stimulus is greater than that from the first stimulus. This phenomenon is called as beneficial effect.

The second stimulus gets benefitted from the changes produced in the muscle due to the first stimulus (Fig. 2.7.1).

Chapter 2.7: Effect of Two Successive Stimuli (of Same Strength) on Skeletal Muscle Contraction

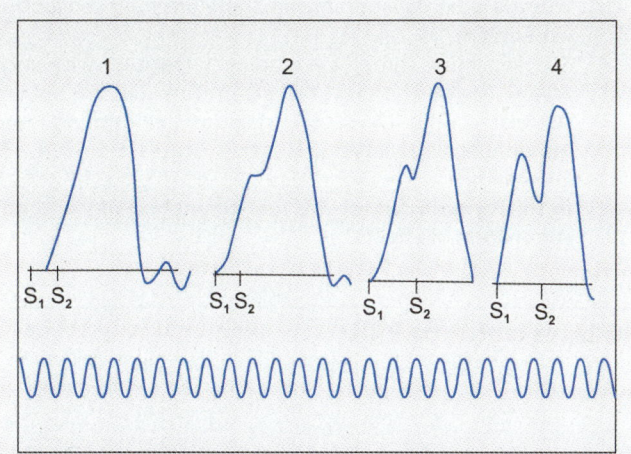

Fig. 2.7.1: Effect of two successive stimuli on muscle contraction given during different phases of muscle contraction.

The mechanism of beneficial effect:
1. In a single twitch, the Ca^{2+} released from the terminal cisterns into the sarcoplasm is rapidly mopped up during relaxation. When there is no relaxation or incomplete relaxation, some Ca^{2+} remains in the sarcoplasm for a longer time and this, together with additional Ca^{2+} released by the second stimulus, increases the duration of the active state. The prolonged active state increases the amount of stretch on the series elastic elements of the muscle, so that more force is transmitted to the recording system (or to the bones in the intact animal), thus increasing the height of the curve.
2. Decrease in the viscosity of the muscle resulting from the first contraction decreases the elastic inertia of the muscle, which may contribute to beneficial effect.
3. Some increase in H^+ ion concentration may be contributing to the beneficial effect.
4. A slight increase in temperature also contributes to the beneficial effect.

QUESTIONS

Q.1. What is refractory period? Is it the same in all the excitable tissues?

After a tissue has responded electrically to an effective stimulus, there is a very brief interval of time, called the *refractory period*, during which the tissue loses its excitability, i.e. it does not respond to a second stimulus. It is divided into absolute refractory period (ARP) and relative refractory period (RRP). During ARP, the tissue does not respond to another stimulus howsoever strong it may be; while during RRP, the tissue responds to a stronger than usual stimulus.

The muscle and nerve fibers are refractory during their action potentials (APs). The ARP corresponds to most of the spike potential, while the RRP coincides with its later part. The AP in skeletal muscle lasts only for 3–5 ms (i.e.

early half of latent period of a twitch), but the mechanical response, which starts just before the end of AP, lasts much longer (300–400 ms). Since the contractile machinery has no refractoriness, the effects of two or more stimuli can be added up.

In contrast, the cardiac muscle is refractory throughout its contraction phase, which lasts almost as long as its action potential (i.e. 200–300 ms) (Fig. 2.7.2).

In nerve fibers, the refractory period, which corresponds to the spike potential, lasts for **1–2 ms** (Fig. 2.7.3).

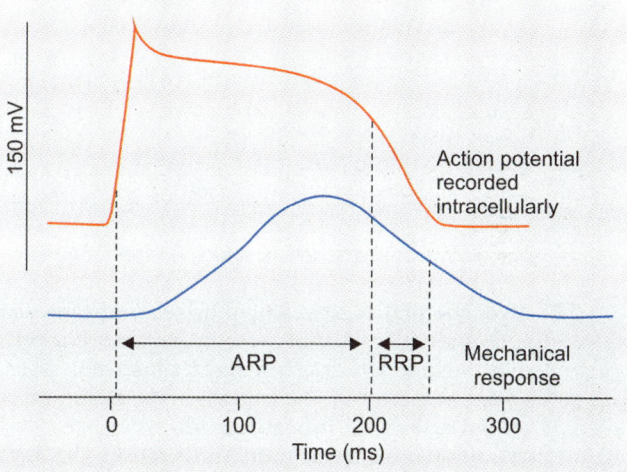

Fig. 2.7.2: Relationship between mechanical response and action potential in cardiac (ventricular) muscle.
(ARP: absolute refractory period; RRP: relative refractory period)

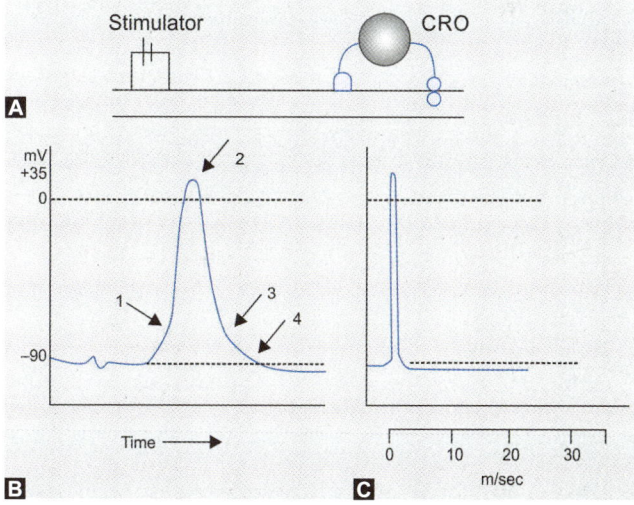

Figs. 2.7.3A to C: Diagram of action potential in a thick mammalian myelinated nerve fiber. (A) Method or recording monophasic action potential; (B) Action potential drawn with time distortion to show its various components. Arrows: 1—firing level, 2—overshoot and start of repolarization (positive part of action potential), 3—repolarization slows down, 4—beginning of after-depolarization; (C) Action potential drawn without time distortion, showing the typical spike.
(CRO: Cathode ray oscilloscope)

Q.2. Describe the graphs obtained when the second stimulus is applied during different phases of the simple muscle twitch resulting from the first stimulus.

- **Latent period:** As the early half of this corresponds to ARP, a second stimulus applied during this period has no effect. The muscle responds only to the first stimulus and the graph obtained is similar to that obtained with a single stimulus. If the second stimulus falls during the latter half of latent period, the effects of the two are added up and the graph obtained is of higher amplitude.
- **Contraction phase:** When the second stimulus is applied during the contraction phase, the muscle continues its contraction and the graph obtained shows an increase in the force of contraction—an effect called *"summation of contractions"* or *"wave summation"*, which is due to beneficial effect.
- **Relaxation phase:** When the second stimulus arrives during relaxation phase, the relaxation is arrested and another contraction results, the force of contraction being more due to beneficial effect. This phenomenon is sometimes called *"superposition"* or *"imposition"* of waves.
- **After the first twitch:** When the second stimulus is applied after the relaxation is complete, there is another response and two twitches are obtained, the second being more forceful. The increase in the height of the second curve is due to beneficial effect.

Q.3. What is beneficial effect and what is its cause?

Beneficial effect: The effects of two successive stimuli described above mean that the contraction produced by the first stimulus is somehow beneficial for the second contraction, due to which is the muscle contracts with greater force.

Q.4. Why are maximal/supramaximal stimuli employed for this experiment?

Supramaximal stimuli are employed, because with such a stimulus, all the motor fibers in the sciatic nerve are stimulated. Thus, the second stimulus cannot bring more motor fibers into action and thereby increase the force of contraction.

Q.5. In this experiment, do we see summation of stimuli or summation of effects?

It is the summation of effects that we see here.

OBSERVATION AND RESULT

INTERPRETATION

STUDY NOTES

CHAPTER 2.8

Effect of Increasing Strength of Stimulus on Skeletal Muscle Contraction

AIM

To study the effect of increasing strength of stimulus on skeletal muscle contraction on stationary drum.

THEORY

Single "make" and "break" stimuli of successively increasing strength, from subthreshold to supramaximal, are applied to the sciatic nerve and their effect on force of muscle contraction is recorded separately on a stationary drum.

The different types of stimuli that can be applied to an excitable tissue are:
- **Subthreshold stimulus:** The stimulus below the threshold that does not produce a response (also called the **subminimal stimulus**).
- **Threshold stimulus/minimal stimulus:** It is defined as minimum strength of stimulus that is required to produce a response.
- **Submaximal stimulus:** The stimulus between threshold and maximal stimulus.
- **Maximal stimulus:** The stimulus that produces maximum response.
- **Supramaximal stimulus:** The stimulus that is stronger than the maximal stimulus, which when applied causes no further increase in the magnitude of contraction.

NOTE
Supramaximal stimuli are avoided in physiological studies because they are susceptible to cause disturbances in the state of living tissues by outlasting the duration of application.

By stimulating a muscle with increasing strength of stimulus, more and more motor units are recruited leading to increase in amplitude of contraction.

APPARATUS

Same as for simple muscle twitch (SMT) (*Refer* Chapter 2.4).
Speed of the drum: stationary
Strength of the stimuli: variable

PROCEDURE

1. Set up a nerve-muscle preparation and a circuit for obtaining single "make" and "break" stimuli. **Exclude the drum from the primary circuit a**nd do not connect it to the mains AC supply. Include an electromagnetic signal marker in series with primary circuit.
2. Engage the gear at the "N" (neutral) position and keep the writing point away from the drum.
3. The secondary coil is moved farthest to the primary coil.
4. Give induced shocks. If no response is obtained (Fig. 2.8.1), the secondary coil is moved gradually toward the primary coil each time by 1 cm. Press and release the key and look for contraction at "make" and "break".
5. The procedure is repeated till there is a response (contraction) at break shock. Record the contraction on the smoked drum. The distance (in centimeter) between primary and secondary coil is measured and noted. The writing point is made to touch the drum now to obtain the recording.
6. Move the secondary coil closer to the primary coil each time by 1 cm and rotating the drum, manually record the contractions at both "make" and "break".

Chapter 2.8: Effect of Increasing Strength of Stimulus on Skeletal Muscle Contraction

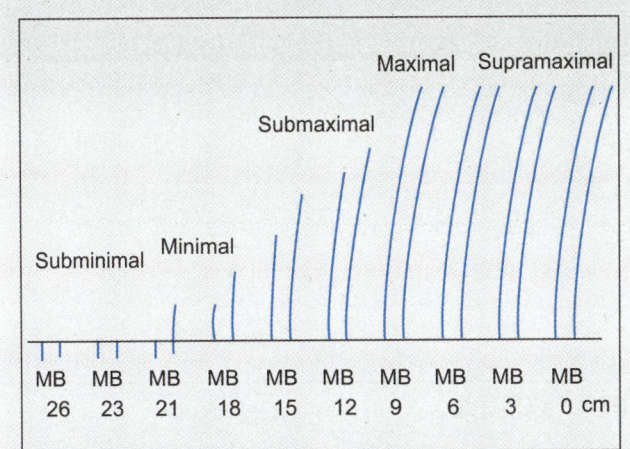

Fig. 2.8.1: Effect of increasing the strength of stimulus on the force of contraction of skeletal muscle. The points of stimulation of subthreshold stimuli are marked below the baseline. The first response appeared with a **break stimulus**, with the secondary coil 21 cm away from the primary coil.

7. Repeat the procedure till there is no further increase in height of contraction due to increase in strength of stimulus. The distance between the primary and secondary coil for each stimulus is noted (Fig. 2.8.1).
8. Label the responses "M" (for "make" stimulus), "B" (for "break" stimulus) and indicate the distance between primary and secondary coil, in centimeter, below each pair of responses.
9. Move the secondary coil to the position where the strength of the induced shock is reduced to just below the threshold stimulus. Now rapidly switch the simple key ON and OFF a few times until the effects of these stimuli are summated and a contraction results.

NOTE
One should wait for at least 15 seconds between make and break shocks. This is to avoid the beneficial effect.

PRECAUTIONS

1. The drum should be excluded from the primary circuit.
2. Ensure that there is sufficient time between two successive stimuli to avoid beneficial effect.
3. The writing point should not be removed from the cylinder during the experiment, so that it presses on the paper with the same force each time a stimulus is applied.
4. To prevent fatigue, unnecessary repeated stimulation should be avoided.

PHYSIOCLINICAL SIGNIFICANCE

Gradation of muscular activity is brought about in the following ways:
1. **Number of motor units in operation:** With minimum activity, only a few motor units are in action. With increasing effort, more and more motor units are recruited into activity, a phenomenon called *"multiple motor unit summation"*.
2. **Frequency of nerve impulses:** As the impulse frequency increases, its effects are summated (wave summation) and the muscle tension increases.
3. **Synchronization of impulses:** Different motor units are, at any one time, in different phases of activity—some contracting and others relaxing; algebraic summation occurs and the muscle gives a steady but weak pull. With increasing synchronization, the force increases.
4. **Initial length of muscle fibers:** Up to an optimal limit, greater the initial length of muscle fibers (i.e. before they contract), greater is the force of contraction. This, however, is not the usual method of varying the force of contraction in the body.
5. **Warming up:** It is a complex mechanism, which increases muscle performance.

QUESTIONS

Q.1. What is a motor unit?
A single anterior horn cell (alpha motor neuron), its axon and all its branches and all the muscle fibers innervated by this neuron are called a *motor unit*.

Q.2. What are the different grades (in terms of strength) of stimuli?

Q.3. Which stimulus is the threshold stimulus in your experiment?
The minimum intensity of induced shock that would activate enough motor units to cause contraction of the muscle at "break".

Q.4. Why does the force of contraction increase when the strength of stimuli, in the submaximal range, is gradually increased?
The sciatic nerve contains motor fibers of varying excitability. Subthreshold stimuli fail to excite any, while a threshold stimulus excites a few motor units and the muscle gives a weak contraction. As the strength of the stimuli is increased, more and more fibers are recruited into activity and the force of contraction goes on increasing. This phenomenon is called *quantal* or *multifiber summation*.

Q.5. Why does the force of contraction not increase after the strength of stimulus is increased beyond the maximal level?
A maximal stimulus is that which excites all the motor fibers and therefore, all the motor units are already contracting

to their maximum extent (all-or-none law; see below). As a result, any further increase in the strength of the stimuli (supramaximal stimuli) has no effect in increasing the force of contraction.

Q.6. What is "all-or-none" law? How is it applicable to excitable tissues?

The *"all-or-none" law* states that under the same experimental conditions, a "unit tissue" responds to its maximum possible extent (or does not respond at all, if the stimulus is subthreshold), whatever the strength of stimulus as long as it is at or above the threshold level. This law is applicable to single nerve fiber, single skeletal muscle fiber, a motor unit and the heart as a whole. However, the skeletal muscle as a whole does not obey the "all-or-none" law. This law relates to the strength of the stimulus and the response.

Q.7. How is the force of muscle contraction graded (varied) in the intact body?

OBSERVATION AND RESULT

Measure the amplitude of contractions in centimeter and the distance between the primary and secondary coil. Note down the findings in Table 2.8.1.

Table 2.8.1: Measurement of amplitude of contractions and distance between primary and secondary coil in centimeter.

Sl. No.	Distance between primary and secondary coil (in cm)	Amplitude of contraction (in cm)
1		
2		
3		
4		
5		
6		

INTERPRETATION

....
....
....
....
....

STUDY NOTES

CHAPTER 2.9

Genesis of Tetanus

AIM

To demonstrate the effect of increasing frequency of stimuli on skeletal muscle contraction (Genesis of Tetanus).

THEORY

Instead of applying two successive stimuli (as was done in the last experiment), if many successive stimuli of maximum strength are applied to the skeletal muscle, the response of the muscle depends on the frequency of stimulation as explained in Figure 2.9.1.

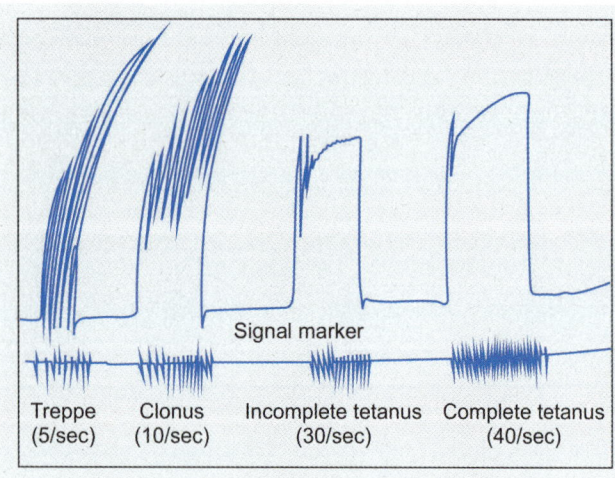

Fig. 2.9.1: Genesis of tetanus.

Treppe/Staircase Phenomenon

When a skeletal muscle is stimulated with multiple successive stimuli given **at the end of relaxation phase** of a simple muscle twitch, there is a progressive increase in the amplitude of successive contractions till a stage is reached where no further increase in the height of contraction is seen. This is known as Treppe or Staircase phenomenon. Treppe (German word for staircase) can also be demonstrated in cardiac muscle, which, however, cannot be tetanized due to its long refractory period. Treppe should not be confused with summation of contractions and tetanus.

Clonus

When repeated maximal stimulations are given and the frequency is such that successive stimuli **fall in the mid relaxation phase** due to the previous stimulus, the muscle relaxes but not completely. This response is called as clonus. It should not be confused with clinical clonus seen in upper motor neuron lesions.

Tetanus

It is defined as the continuous (sustained) state of contraction. It results when multiple successive maximal stimuli are falling **during the contraction phase** due to the previous stimulus so that the activation of contractile mechanism occurs repeatedly before the muscle gets time to relax.

In **complete tetanus**, there is complete fusion of contractions and there is no relaxation. Here all the fibers contract maximally and the tension developed is approximately four times greater than that developed during individual twitch contraction.

In **incomplete tetanus**, the contractions do not completely fuse but there are phases of partial relaxation.

APPARATUS

1. Same as for simple muscle twitch (SMT) (*Refer* Chapter 2.4).
2. Electromagnetic signal marker
3. Variable interrupter/Neef's hammer.

Speed of the drum: 12.5 mm/sec
Strength of stimuli: maximal

PROCEDURE

1. Exclude the drum from the primary circuit.
2. Include variable interrupter to provide 5–25 stimuli/sec or Neef's hammer in its place to provide 40 or more stimuli/sec, as and when required.
3. Engage the gear lever at 12.5 mm/sec speed (medium speed).
4. Set up a nerve–muscle preparation and stimulate it with gradually increasing frequencies, *for a few seconds each time*.
5. Note the effect by gradually increasing the frequency of stimuli of 5, 10, 25 and 40 stimuli per second.
6. If a state of complete tetanus is not obtained by variable interrupter, the Neef's hammer is used instead.

CALCULATION OF TETANIZING FREQUENCY

The *"tetanizing"* or *"fusion"* frequency is that rate of stimulation of a muscle at which there is complete fusion of individual contractions to produce tetanus.

$$\text{Tetanizing frequency} = \frac{1}{\text{Contraction period}}$$

If contraction period is 10 m/sec, frequency greater than 1/10 ms, i.e. 100/s will cause summation. This is the **tetanizing frequency**.

PRECAUTIONS

1. Do not include the drum in the circuit.
2. While stimulating the preparation, go from lower to higher frequency.
3. Neef's hammer should be included in the primary circuit, if tetanizing frequency is not achieved.
4. Do not connect Neef's hammer and variable interrupter simultaneously into the primary circuit.

PHYSIOCLINICAL SIGNIFICANCE

Voluntary and reflex movements depend on the *nature of discharge from the motor neurons*—
- Number of activated neurons
- Frequency of their firing
- Their synchronicity.

Basically, all contractions are tetanic in nature. Weak contractions result from low-frequency firing. When one group is firing, the others are silent and vice versa. Algebraic summation occurs. Thus, the individual variations are evened out and a smooth contraction results. The erect posture of our body is maintained due to sustained (tetanic) contraction of the antigravity muscles.

QUESTIONS

Q.1. What is "tetanizing" or "fusion" frequency? How is it calculated?

Q.2. What is "treppe" or "staircase effect"?

Q.3. How does the tension developed during a complete tetanus vary from that of a simple muscle twitch?

The tension developed during a complete tetanus is four times more than that of a simple muscle twitch. The tension developed by a muscle depends on the active state of the contractile components; and how much tension is transmitted to the recording system (or to the bone) depends on the amount of stretch (laxity or tautness) exerted on the series elastic components (SEC) of the muscle, as already explained.

During one twitch contraction, enough Ca^{2+} is released to engage all the myosin heads to the actin sites, but it is removed quickly from the cytoplasm and relaxation occurs. Because of the quick removal, the peak tension is not achieved. With repeated stimuli, Ca^{2+} remains longer in the cytoplasm, increasing the duration of the active state (due to continuous recycling of myosin heads). This increases the amount of stretch on the SEC and the tension developed rises. Up to physiological limit, greater the frequency of stimulation, greater is the tension developed.

Q.4. What is meant by the term "genesis of tetanus"? Can you demonstrate tetanus in your body?

The term refers to the "generation" or production, of tetanus by gradually increasing the frequency of stimulation of the nerve–muscle preparation until tetanus results.

Tetanus is a smooth and sustained contraction of a muscle, without reference to the frequency of stimulation. If you make a strong fist, your forearm muscles will contract tetanically.

The term tetanus should not be confused with a disease called tetanus. In this condition, there are widespread convulsions in the body due to tetanus toxin released by the infecting bacteria. Vaccination is a common practice to provide immunity against this disease.

Section 2: Amphibian (Frog) Experiments

Q.5. What is the nature of muscle contractions in the body? Are they simple twitches, subtetanic or tetanic contractions?

Q.6. How is tetanus different from tetany?
Tetany is the condition of exaggerated neuromuscular excitability, which occurs due to decrease in ionized Ca^{2+}, which in turn causes increased membrane permeability to Na^+. Skeletal muscle spasms and cramps are seen in the extremities.

Q.7. Why the cardiac muscle cannot be tetanized?

Q.8. Write examples of slow and fast muscles and their relative tetanizable frequencies.

Q.9. Write the factors affecting tetanizing frequency.
The factors that affect are:
1. *Type of the muscle:* Slow muscles (muscles of back and soleus muscle) have low tetanizing frequency as they produce slow sustained contraction (have longer contraction period), while the fast muscle (small muscles of hand and extraocular muscles) have greater tetanizing frequency as the contraction period is less.
2. *Strength of stimulation.*
3. *Temperature:* At high temperature, the contraction period decreases, hence higher is the tetanizing frequency.

Q.10. Draw the graphs showing relationship between frequency of stimuli and type of curve obtained.

OBSERVATION AND RESULT

....
....
....
....
....

INTERPRETATION

....
....
....
....
....

STUDY NOTES

Date ....

CHAPTER 2.10

Genesis of Fatigue

AIM

To demonstrate the phenomenon of fatigue in nerve muscle preparation.

THEORY

When the muscle is stimulated repeatedly for a prolonged period of time, it loses its physiological property of contraction and there occurs a decrease in the working capacity. This phenomenon of temporary decrease in the working capacity of a living tissue is called as **fatigue**. However, it regains its property of contraction after some time. It is a **reversible** phenomenon.

Causes of Fatigue

1. Lack of nutrition.
2. Accumulation of waste metabolites and interference with neuromuscular transmission by substances like pyruvic and lactic acids and breakdown products of ATP.
3. Depletion of acetylcholine from the motor nerve endings.

APPARATUS

Same as in simple muscle twitch (SMT) (*Refer* Chapter 2.4).
Speed of the drum: 640 mm/sec (fastest)
Strength of stimuli: maximal

PROCEDURE

1. Set up the apparatus and circuit as for the SMT.
2. Draw a baseline and mark the point of stimulation.
3. On a fast moving drum, repeatedly stimulate the nerve and record the 1st, 2nd and 3rd contractions, keeping the point of stimulation same.
4. Stop the drum and move the writing lever away from the drum taking care that the point of stimulation does not change. By pressing the tap key, stimulate the nerve repeatedly so that the nerve muscle preparation is stimulated once during each revolution.
5. Record every 10th contraction by applying the writing lever to the drum. This should be done till the muscle contractions are too weak to be recorded.
6. Place the stimulating electrodes directly on the muscle and record the response. Label this contraction DS (direct stimulation) as shown in Figure 2.10.1.
7. Rest the nerve muscle preparation for 5 minutes. During this time, keep pouring fresh Ringer's solution.
8. After changing the point of stimulus on the same baseline, stimulate the nerve and record the recovery of the muscle.
9. Observe the change in amplitude and duration of the various phases of the first three contractions and the following contractions. The first few contractions increase in amplitude due to **beneficial effect**.

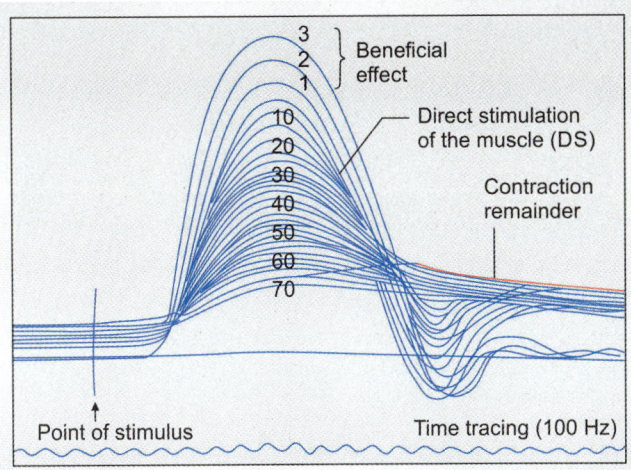

Fig. 2.10.1: Phenomenon of fatigue.

As stimulation is continued, there is a progressive increase in latent period and a decrease in amplitude. The rise of tension is slower and relaxation is more gradual and incomplete.

Finally, the muscle fails to contract altogether and the lever does not return to the baseline, i.e. the muscle remains in a state of partial contraction called **contraction remainder**.

10. After the muscle undergoes fatigue through stimulation of its nerve, it responds briskly to **direct stimulation**. After a variable period, the muscle responds once again to stimulation of its nerve.

PRECAUTIONS

1. The point of stimulus and the baseline should remain unchanged for recording the fatigue curve.
2. For recording the effect of direct stimulation, put the electrodes directly on the muscle.
3. Rest the preparation for 5 minutes and keep pouring fresh Ringer's solution in order to record the response of the muscle after recovery.

PHYSIOCLINICAL SIGNIFICANCE

Site of fatigue: The only three possible sites are—the nerve fiber, the neuromuscular junction (NMJ) and the muscle fiber. The fact that the nerve is practically not fatigable and that direct stimulation of the muscle causes contraction, indicates, by exclusion, that NMJ is the seat of fatigue in this *in vitro* preparation, which has no blood supply.

It can be shown that **nerve is not the site of fatigue** by arranging two nerve muscle preparation (N1 and N2) in such a manner that both are stimulated simultaneously. A piece of ice is kept on the nerve just before the NMJ on the N2 preparation. This will block the transmission of the nerve impulses. Both the preparations are stimulated till the N1 muscle does not contract, i.e. the preparation is fatigued. The ice piece is removed from the N2 preparation and again both the preparations are stimulated. N1 will not respond but N2 will show the response.

Alternatively, this can be also proved by bringing the nerve of a fresh preparation in contact with the nerve of the fatigued preparation. The second muscle responds to every induction shock while the first one does not—the first nerve merely acting as an electrical conductor. Recording of action potentials from the first nerve can also show that it is not the seat of fatigue (If direct stimulation of muscle is continued, fatigue occurs due to exhaustion of glycogen. There is no recovery from fatigue in this case).

QUESTIONS

Q.1. What is the site and cause of fatigue in the isolated nerve–muscle preparation? Justify.

Q.2. What is the first site of fatigue in intact body?
It is the synapse in the brain.

Q.3. How is fatigue studied in man and what is its cause?
Fatigue in man is studied by using a *Mosso's ergograph* in which work is performed by a finger or thumb in lifting a weight.

Q.4. What is contraction remainder and what is its cause?
When fatigue sets in, the muscle is unable to relax fully and remains in a state of partial contraction called *contraction remainder*. Since, ATP is involved in the removal of Ca^{2+} ions from the cytoplasm causing relaxation, a decrease of ATP and accumulation of metabolites appear to be responsible for the inability of all the myosin heads to disengage from the active sites on actin filaments (compare with Rigor mortis).

Q.5. What is the medical relevance of fatigue?
An athlete runs initial part of the race slowly because speeding up in the initial part will lead to early setting of fatigue as anaerobic metabolism will lead to accumulation of lactic acid and waste metabolites.

Q.6. What are the causes of recovery from fatigue?
- Removal of waste metabolites
- Supply of nutrition (fresh Ringer's solution)
- Resynthesis of acetylcholine help in recovery from fatigue.

Q.7. How will you prove that nerve is not the first site of fatigue?

Section 2: Amphibian (Frog) Experiments

OBSERVATION AND RESULT

No. of contraction	Latent period (seconds)	Contraction period (seconds)	Relaxation period (seconds)	Height of contraction (centimeters)
1				
2				
3				
10				
20				
30				
40				
50				
60				
70				
Direct stimulation of the muscle				

INTERPRETATION

....
....
....
....
....

STUDY NOTES

Teacher's Signature

Date ....

CHAPTER 2.11

Effect of Load on Skeletal Muscle Contraction (Freeload and Afterload)

AIM

To demonstrate the effect of load on skeletal muscle contraction and compare the work done in free- and after-loaded conditions.

THEORY

A load can act on a muscle either before it starts to contract (**freeloading/preload**) or after the contraction has started (**afterloading**). Using successively increasing loads (weights), muscle contractions are recorded in these two conditions. The work done by the muscle for each weight can then be calculated. Load at which maximum work is done is called **optimal load.**

The performance of the muscle is measured in terms of work done during isotonic muscle contraction.

APPARATUS

1. Same as in simple muscle twitch (SMT) (*Refer* Chapter 2.4).
2. Weights (10, 20, 30, 40 and 50 g).

Speed of the drum: Fastest/stationary
Strength of the stimulus: Minimal

PROCEDURE

Recording on a Moving Drum (Speed 640 mm/s) (Fig. 2.11.1)

1. Set-up your experiment as for SMT (Chapter 2.4). Draw a baseline and mark the point of stimulation. Hang 10 g weight on the lever about an inch from the fulcrum.

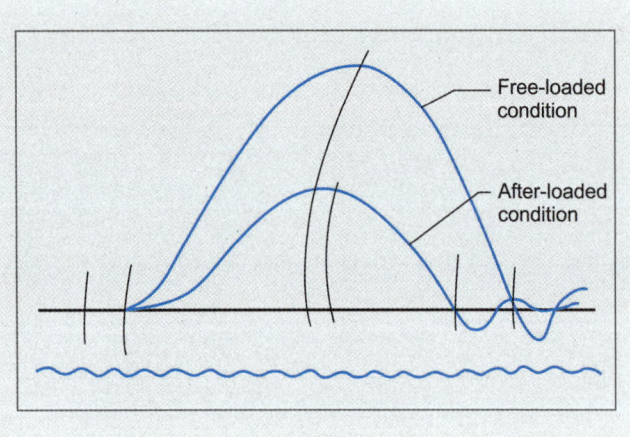

Fig. 2.11.1: Effect of load on muscle contraction on a moving drum.

2. **Afterloaded condition:**
   a. Ensure that the afterload screw is touching and supports the vertical arm of the lever, so that the weight does not act on the muscle and stretch it. The weight acts on the muscle after the onset of muscle contraction. This is called the afterloaded condition.
   b. Record a single SMT at a drum speed of 640 mm/sec and mark the point of stimulation.
   c. Without changing the point of stimulation and strength of stimulus, record the subsequent contractions by adding 10 g each time and label the curves (10, 20, 30...g) accordingly.
   d. Repeat the procedure till the muscle is unable to lift the weight any more.

3. **Freeloaded condition (preload):**
   a. Remove all the weights from the hanger and withdraw the afterload screw right up to the frame of the lever, so that it will no longer support the vertical arm of the lever. The weight will now act freely on the muscle even when the muscle is not contracting, i.e. it stretches the muscle before it starts contracting. This is a freeloaded condition.
   b. Record the first and subsequent contractions as explained above using different weights. Each time when more weight is added on the hanger, the lever sags down more and more, thus stretching the muscle more. The drum has to be lowered to bring the writing point to the same baseline.
   c. Repeat the procedure till the muscle is unable to lift the weight any more.

> **NOTE**
> On a moving drum, the free- and afterloaded contractions may be recorded separately on the same baseline, keeping the point of stimulus and strength of stimulus the same (Fig. 2.11.1). One can record the height, the speed of shortening and various periods of each contraction curve.

Recording on a Stationary Drum

1. **Freeloaded condition (preload) (Fig. 2.11.2A):**
   a. Withdraw the afterload screw from the fulcrum. In this free loaded condition, the lever comes down as the muscle is stretched by the weight and thus, the baseline shifts down more and more on adding subsequent weights.
   b. Record the contractions by rotating the cylinder forward manually by 1 cm each time using the neutral gear.
   c. Subsequently add weights by 10 g and record the contraction till the muscle is not able to lift the load any more.

2. **Afterloaded condition (Fig. 2.11.2B):**
   a. Set up the apparatus as to record the SMT. Do not include the drum in the circuit.
   b. Hang 10 g weight from the lever and adjust the lever in the afterloaded position.
   c. Record the muscle contraction by giving electrical stimulus. The contraction is recorded as curved vertical line.
   d. After each contraction rotate the drum manually by 1 cm each time by using the neutral gear. After setting the new position again put in a gear to avoid free movement of the drum.
   e. Subsequently add weights in steps of 10 g and record the contractions till the muscle is not able to lift the load any more.

Afterloading: As the load increases, the latent period increases due to lever inertia. The height decreases because the muscle has to lift greater loads. The contraction period decreases due to decrease in the duration of active state, while the relaxation period decreases because the load hastens the return of the lever to the baseline.

Freeloading: The latent period decreases for a few contractions then it may increase a little or remain unchanged. The height (force) of contraction increases for the first few contractions (up to a physiological limit), then it starts decreasing. The speed of contraction also increases as can be seen from the slope of the curve. Since the duration of the active state does not change, the contraction time does not change. The relaxation period decreases because the load hastens the return of the lever.

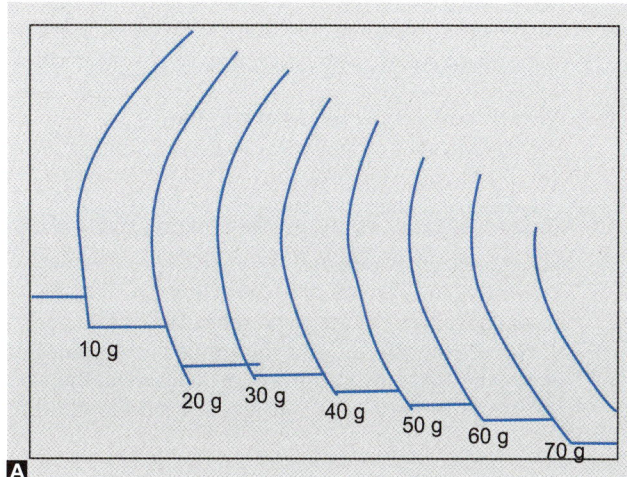
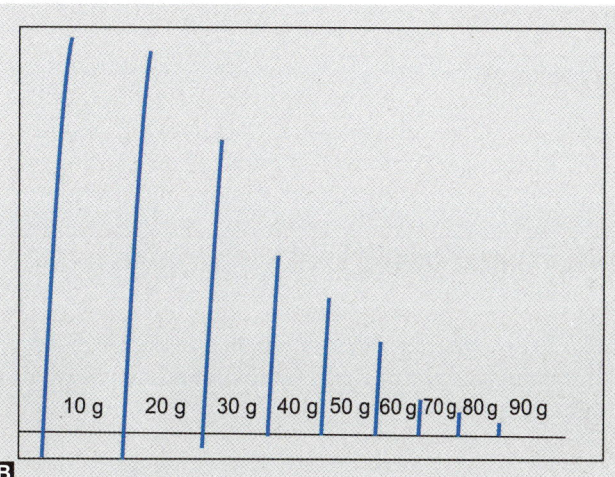

Figs. 2.11.2A and B: Effect of load on muscle contraction on a stationary drum. (A) Freeload; (B) Afterload.

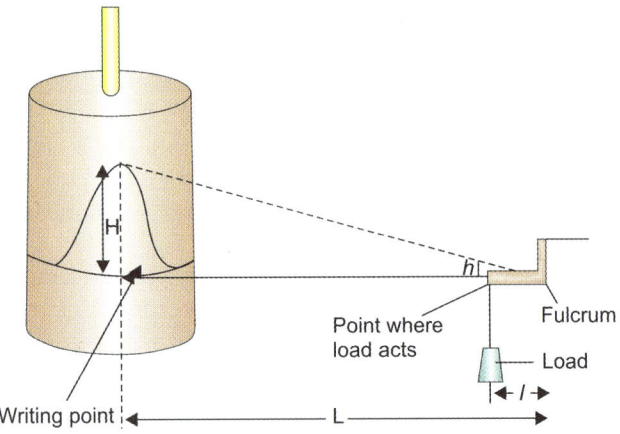

Fig. 2.11.3: Calculation of work done.
(H: Height of contraction; L: Distance between fulcrum and writing point of lever; l: Distance between fulcrum and point where the load acts; h: actual height to which the weight has been lifted).

In the stationary drum the height of contraction can also be noted. In freeloaded condition, the lever comes down as the muscle is stretched by the weight, so the baseline shifts down more and more on adding subsequent weights.

CALCULATION OF WORK DONE

Work done = Force (W) × Displacement (h)
W = Load lifted in g and h = actual height to which the weight has been lifted in centimeter.
$$h = l/L \times H$$
Where;
l = Distance between the fulcrum and the point where the load acts
L = Distance between the fulcrum and the writing point of lever
H = Height of contraction curve for each load
Work done (W) = Force (load) × l/L × H in g/cm
Multiply with 981 to express the result in ergs (Fig. 2.11.3).

PRECAUTIONS

1. Same as in simple muscle twitch (SMT) (*Refer* Chapter 2.4).
2. Do not change the point of stimulus (for recording on a moving drum) and strength of stimulating current.

PHYSIOCLINICAL SIGNIFICANCE

- When some muscular work is done the muscles are slightly stretched in order to obtain maximum effect.
- Stretching and warm-ups by athletes probably serve the same purpose.

QUESTIONS

Q.1. What is meant by the terms "tension" and "load"?
Tension is the force exerted by a contracting muscle on an object.
Load is the force exerted by the weight of an object on a contracting muscle, i.e. it is the resistance offered to muscle shortening.
Thus, *muscle tension and load are opposing forces.*

> **NOTE**
> To lift a load, the muscle tension must exceed the load. If the load is greater than the muscle tension, the load will not be lifted and no external work will be done.

Q.2. Define resting length, initial length, equilibrium length and optimal length of a muscle.
Resting length: The length of the muscle in the body **at rest** at which the **active tension is maximum**.
Initial length: The length of the muscle just before the onset of contraction.
Equilibrium length: Length of the relaxed muscle cut from its bony attachment.
Optimal length: The length of a muscle at which the active tension is maximum.

Q.3. Why the work done is more in freeloaded condition than in an afterloaded condition?
The gradual stretching of the muscle during freeloading increases the initial length of the muscle fibers which increases its force of contraction and work efficiency.

Q.4. What is optimum load?

Q.5. What is meant by "afterloaded" and "freeloaded" contractions?

Q.6. How would you ascertain whether a twitch has been recorded in the "afterloaded" or "freeloaded" condition?
After the muscle twitch is over, a few waves or oscillations are recorded. These are not a part of muscle contraction, but a result of muscle elasticity and jerking of the lever due to its momentum. These waves are called *physiological* or *shatter waves*. If the muscle is in the afterloaded state, the shatter waves appear mainly above the baseline, but if it is freeloaded (or preloaded), the waves are recorded mainly below the baseline.

Q.7. What is Starling's law and what is its basis?
The **Starling's law** (or Frank–Starling law) states that "Within the physiological limit the force of contraction is directly proportional to the initial length of the muscle fiber".
[In the case of heart, the diastolic filling determines the initial length (preload) of muscle].

The length of the muscle fibers determines the degree of overlap between myosin and actin filaments. At optimal sarcomere length (2.2 μm) maximum crossbridges are present between the myosin and actin filament. Therefore, maximum force is obtained when the preload (initial

Chapter 2.11: Effect of Load on Skeletal Muscle Contraction (Freeload and Afterload)

length) is set at this sarcomere length of 2.2 μm. At shorter lengths, actin filaments bump into each other and decrease the overlap. When overstretched, the thin filaments are pulled out, thus decreasing the overlap. In both cases, force obtained is decreased.

Q.8. Do freeloaded and afterloaded contractions occur in the body?

Varying the preload (i.e. the initial length) is not an important method of varying the force of contraction of muscles because the muscle length generally depend on the type of motor activity being performed. But, if it is possible to stretch the muscles, more force can be obtained, as is done by weight lifters who allow the weight to stretch their muscles before they lift the weight with a sudden effort.

Q.9. What is the physioclinical significance of this practical?

Q.10. Write the freeloaded and afterloaded conditions of cardiac muscle *in vivo*.

In vivo the end-diastolic volume represents the preload of the cardiac muscle and peripheral resistance constitutes the afterload.

OBSERVATION AND RESULT

....
....
....
....
....

INTERPRETATION

....
....
....
....
....

Section 2: Amphibian (Frog) Experiments

STUDY NOTES

Teacher's Signature

Date ....

CHAPTER 2.12

Recording of a Normal Cardiogram of Frog's Heart and Effect of Temperature on it

AIM

To record a normal cardiogram of frog's heart and the effect of temperature on it.

THEORY

The frog's heart consists of two atria and one ventricle. **Sinus venosus** is the pacemaker of frog's heart and the impulse travels from sinus venosus to the atria and then to the ventricle. Electrical events in the heart precede the mechanical contractions. The different mechanical events recorded are atrial systole, atrial diastole and ventricular systole followed by ventricular diastole. The recording obtained by the various **mechanical events** of the frog's heart is known as **cardiogram**.

NORMAL CARDIOGRAM

The cardiogram is a record of the mechanical activity of the heart, while electrocardiogram is a record of the electrical activity of the heart. In this and the following experiments, the mechanical events of the heart will be recorded with a Starling's heart lever (Fig. 2.12.1).

APPARATUS

1. Myograph board
2. Lucas chamber
3. Dissection apparatus
4. Amphibian Ringer's solution (cold and warm)
5. Kymograph with drum
6. Starling's heart lever

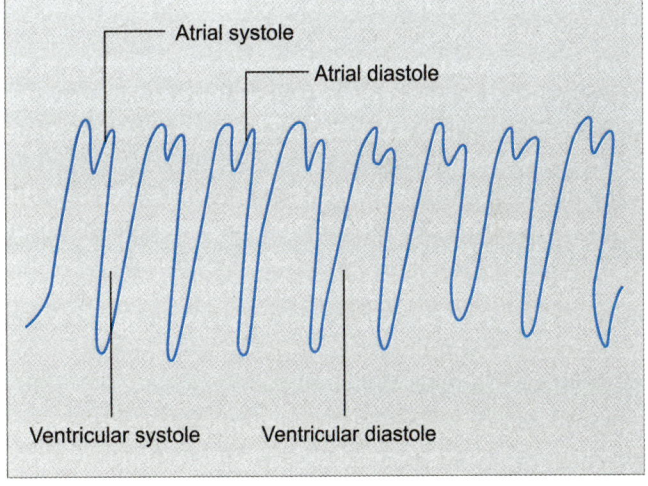

Fig. 2.12.1: Normal cardiogram of frog's heart.

7. Time/signal marker
8. Dropper, thread, cotton wool and pins.

Speed of the drum: 2.5 mm/sec

PROCEDURE

Exposure of the Frog's Heart

1. Stun and pith a frog and lay it on its back in a dissection tray. Using a scissors, incise the skin in the midline from xiphisternum to the jaw. Extend the lower end of this cut laterally and remove both pieces of skin. The anterior chest wall is now exposed.
2. Give a horizontal cut in the muscles at the level of xiphisternum (do not cut through the abdominal wall,

otherwise the viscera will spill out). Using bone forceps and scissors, cut through the pectoral girdles and remove the chest wall in one piece. The heart will now be revealed beating in its pericardial sac. Slit through the pericardium and remove it right up to the base of the heart. Removal of pericardium is important as it will help to support the heart firmly from the apex and the variables which are used will come in direct contact with the heart muscle.

3. By inserting a pin through the bulbous (base), *fix the base of the heart to the myograph board so that the contracting heart is not pulled from both the ends and the recording is not affected.*
4. Examine the heart carefully (Fig. 2.12.2). There is **one ventricle,** separated from the **two atria** by the atrioventricular groove and **bulbus arteriosus** which arises from the ventricle and divides into two aortae.
5. Lift the ventricle up and find behind it the **sinus venosus** with the two venae cavae emptying into it.
   - A careful observation will reveal the **white crescentic line** between the sinus venosus and right atrium. This is the site of the Remak's and Bidder's ganglia of the vagus nerves.
   - The color of the ventricle becomes pale during systole as blood is forced out of it. Feel the hardening of the ventricle when it contracts. There are no valves in the frog's heart.
   - **Sequence of heartbeats:** The contractions of the **four units** of the heart are progressive. The sinus leads off, followed by the atria, ventricle and bulbus in that order. The rate of the heart depends on the frequency of the sinus, as it is the pacemaker.

Recording of Normal Cardiogram

1. Transfer the frog to the Lucas chamber. Fit the Starling's heart lever on the vertical rod of the stand directly above the heart and pass the sharp hook of the bent pin through the apex of the ventricle, taking care not to puncture its cavity.
2. Lift the heart gently by raising the lever and adjust its position, so that its movements are satisfactory and its mean position is horizontal.

> **NOTE**
> During systole, the lever is pulled down, while during diastole the spring of the lever pulled up to its former position.

3. Move the stand carrying the preparation and the lever, so that the lever is at a tangent to the cylinder and the writing point is lightly touching the cylinder surface. Record the cardiac activity for about 15 cm on the paper, with the drum moving at a **speed of 2.5 mm/s.**
4. Take the time tracing every 5 seconds with the help of time signal marker below the graph obtained.
5. Note the number of peaks recorded and calculate the frog's heart rate.

> **NOTE**
> Normal heart rate of frog varies from 30/minute to 50/minute.

Effect of Temperature on Frog's Cardiogram (Fig. 2.12.3)

1. Pour amphibian Ringer's solution at room temperature on the heart fixed in the Lucas chamber; note the temperature of the Ringer's solution. With the drum running at slow speed (2.5 mm/sec) pour Ringer's solution warmed to about 40°C on the heart, until there is an obvious increase in its rate and force.
2. Stop the kymograph and pour Ringer's solution at room temperature on the heart till it resumes the previous rate and force.
3. Then again record the effect of cold Ringer's solution at about 10°C in the same manner.
4. Take the time tracing every 5 seconds with the help of time signal marker below the graph obtained. Label your tracing, indicating with arrows, the points where hot and cold Ringer's solution was applied. Calculate the heart rate at these temperatures and enter the data in your workbook.

> **NOTE**
> - At high temperature, there is an increase in the metabolic activity of the pacemaker cells which generates more cardiac impulses per unit time, thus increasing the **heart rate and height of contraction**. Increased metabolic activity of the working cells of the atria and ventricle and decrease in the viscosity increase the **force of contraction**.
> - Cold has the opposite effects due to decrease in the metabolic activity.

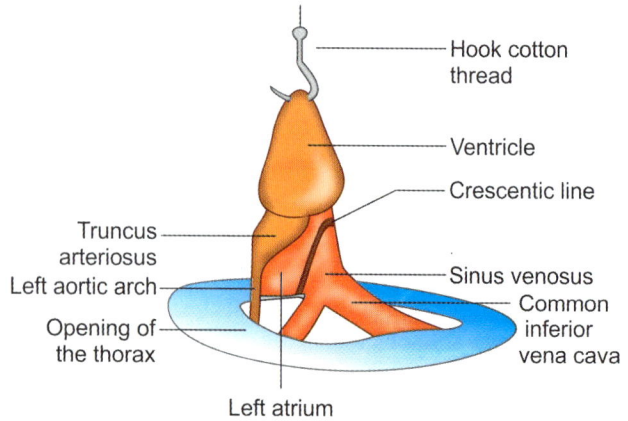

Fig. 2.12.2: Frog's heart.

Chapter 2.12: Recording of a Normal Cardiogram of Frog's Heart and Effect of Temperature on it 147

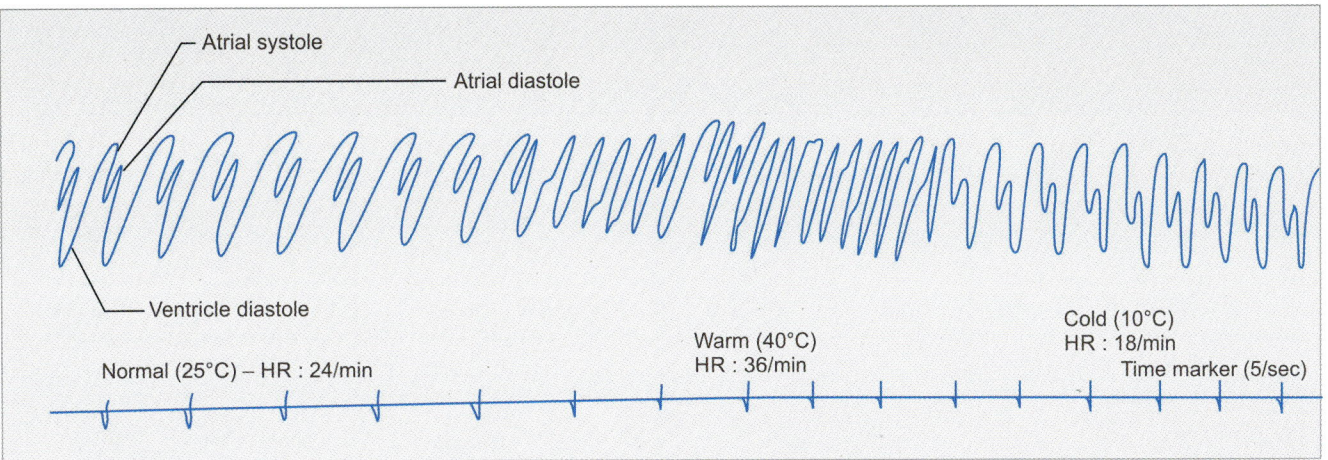

Fig. 2.12.3: Effect of temperature on cardiogram.

PRECAUTIONS

1. Care should be taken not to damage the heart during dissection.
2. Pericardium should be removed before fixing the heart on the myograph board.
3. Record the normal cardiogram before recording the effect of warm and cold Ringer's solution.
4. The temperature of warm Ringer's solution should not be more than 42°C.
5. Effect of warm Ringer's solution should be recorded before the effect of cold Ringer's solution.
6. Do not puncture the ventricle while passing the pin through its apex.

PHYSIOCLINICAL SIGNIFICANCE

This practical shows that heart rate changes in the human body with change in internal body temperature, e.g. exercise, fever and hypothermia.

QUESTIONS

Q.1. Why is frog's heart used for the study of properties of heart?
The frog heart continues to beat even after the chest is opened. It obtains an adequate supply of oxygen directly from the blood in its chambers and from the atmosphere (it has no coronary circulation). Its rate is sufficiently slow to allow observation of its sequence. Also, it continues to function over a wide range of temperature. The properties which can be studied include excitability, automaticity, rhythmicity, contractility, conductivity, refractoriness and all-or-none law.

Q.2. Describe the graph obtained by you.
The downstroke of the tracing represents systole and the upstroke diastole. There is atrial systole followed by atrial diastole, then ventricular systole (this is the strongest of the four contracting units) is followed by diastole (contraction of sinus may also be recorded). The heart rate is beats/min and the rhythm is regular).

Q.3. What is the mechanism of action of hot and cold Ringer's solution on frog's heart?
Q.4. What is the physioclinical significance of this practical?
Q.5. Why it is important to fix the base of the heart?
Q.6. Why it is necessary to remove the pericardium?
Q.7. What will happen if only the ventricle is warmed?
Warming of ventricles increases only the height of the contraction but the rhythm remains unchanged.

OBSERVATION AND RESULT

Recording of effect of temperature on frog's cardiogram.

	Heart rate (beats/min)	Height of contraction (cm)
Normal (°C)		
Warm Ringer's solution (.....°C)		
Cold Ringer's solution (.....°C)		

INTERPRETATION

....
....
....
....
....

STUDY NOTES

CHAPTER 2.13

Properties of Cardiac Muscle

AIM

To study the properties of frog's heart.

THEORY

1. The following properties will be studied in a **beating heart**:
   a. Autorhythmicity
   b. Extrasystole and compensatory pause
   c. Refractory period.
2. The following properties will be studied in a **quiescent heart (after Stannius ligatures)**:
   a. Summation of subminimal stimuli.
   b. All-or-none law
   c. Staircase phenomenon.

APPARATUS

1. Same as in recording of normal cardiogram (*Refer* Chapter 2.12)
2. Induction coil
3. Wire electrodes and signal marker.

Speed of the drum: 2.5 mm/sec (Slow)

PROPERTIES IN A BEATING HEART

1. **Extrasystole:** When the heart is stimulated [by an impulse other than that originates from the sinoatrial (SA) node] during late diastole (relative refractory period), the heart muscle may contract. This contraction comes earlier than the normally expected contraction. This is called extrasystole.
2. **Compensatory pause:** The pause (silence) following the extrasystole is known as compensatory pause. This is because the next normal impulse coming from the SA node reaches in the absolute refractory period of extrasystole and hence fails to evoke a response. The response which follows the compensatory pause is of greater magnitude than the previous one because of the accumulation of calcium ions during the pause.
3. **Refractory period:** The cardiac muscle has a long refractory period. This is because the action potential of cardiac muscle has a long duration of about 300 ms. During much of the action potential (about 250 ms), the cell is completely refractory to further stimulation, i.e. it is unable to fire no matter how strongly it is stimulated. This unresponsive state is called as **absolute refractory period.** During the latter part of action potential (about 50 ms), the cell is able to fire a second action potential provided a stronger than a normal stimulus is given. This period is called as **relative refractory period.** The cardiac muscle action potential duration is almost equal to the duration of mechanical activity. Therefore, the mechanical responses of cardiac muscle **cannot be summated or tetanized.**

PROCEDURE

1. Set up the experiment as for recording a normal cardiogram.
2. Apply electrodes on the ventricle of heart.
3. The distance between primary and secondary coil is so adjusted that a minimal stimulus is obtained.
4. Use the electromagnetic signal marker to indicate the application of stimulus.
5. A few normal beats are recorded.
6. A "break" shock is applied by opening the short circuiting key and thereafter the primary key.

7. Stimulate the ventricle during the different phases of the cardiac cycle, i.e. systole, early and late diastole and record the effects.
8. The graph is labeled properly to show the systole and diastole in the cardiogram, point of application of extra stimulus, extrasystole and compensatory pause. A time tracing is also taken.

> **NOTE**
> When the stimulus falls during any part of systole, it has no effect (Figs. 2.13.1A to E); the heart continues to beat as before. But when the stimulus falls during diastole, the heart contracts immediately. This extra contraction is called **extrasystole** or **premature beat**, is followed by a pause called **"compensatory pause"**. Duration of normal contraction, the extrasystole and compensatory pause is equal to two normal cardiac cycles.

This experiment also shows the properties of **excitability, contractility, autorhythmicity** and **conductivity** (stimulation of any part causes contraction of the rest of the heart).

PROPERTIES IN A QUIESCENT HEART (AFTER STANNIUS LIGATURES)

1. **Effect of Stannius ligature:**
   - *First Stannius ligature:* When a ligature is applied over the sinoauricular junction and tied, the conduction of impulse from sinus venosus to atria is blocked. Therefore, atria and ventricle stop beating, but the sinus venosus continues to beat. After sometime, the atria start to generate their own impulses at a slower rate and the atria and ventricle start contracting. This is **atrial rhythm**.
   - *Second Stannius ligature:* When a ligature is applied between the atria and ventricle and tied, the transmission of cardiac impulse is blocked from the atria to the ventricle. The ventricle stops beating whereas the atria continue to beat. After sometime, the ventricle starts generating its own impulses and starts beating at a rate of 15–40 beats/min. This is called **idioventricular rhythm.**
2. **All-or-none law:** It is applicable to the whole heart as it acts as a **functional syncytium** because of the presence of gap junctions. Therefore, with threshold stimulus the heart will contract to its maximum and it will not respond if the stimulus is below the threshold.
3. **Staircase phenomenon:** It refers to the successive increase in the first few cardiac contractions after the silent heart has started to beat. It is because of the **beneficial effect** of the previous contraction (accumulation of calcium ions).
4. **Summation of subminimal stimuli:** A subminimal stimulus generates a graded potential which can be summated because it does not have any refractory period. More than one subminimal stimuli add together and may take the membrane potential to the firing level so as to generate an action potential.

PROCEDURE

Effect of Stannius Ligature

1. Set up the experiment as for recording a normal cardiogram.
2. Pass a ligature thread under the truncus arteriosus and the atria, bring its ends to the dorsum of the heart. Ensure that the ligature thread is placed at the junction of sinus venosus and atria (on the white crescentic line). This is **First Stannius ligature**.
3. Record some normal beats, stop the drum, then tie the thread with a single knot over the white crescentic line.
4. If it has been applied properly, the sinus will continue to beat as before, while the atria and ventricle will stop during diastole after one or two beats (Fig. 2.13.1B). They will begin to beat after a variable period of 10–20 minutes at a slower rate. This is **atrial rhythm**. Record this activity. Stop the drum and tie the second Stannius ligature.
5. **Second Stannius ligature:** Tie a tight ligature between the atria and ventricle, the ventricle immediately stops contracting, while the sinus and atria continue to beat at their own different rates (the first Stannius ligature is still in place). The drum is restarted and the recording is taken when the ventricle has stopped beating.
6. The drum is again stopped. Wait for some time till the ventricle starts contracting. This is **idioventricular rhythm.** And the contractions are recorded.
7. The time tracing is recorded. The rate of the three rhythms—sinus rhythm, atrial rhythm and idioventricular rhythm is calculated (Fig. 2.13.1B).
8. **Summation of Subminimal Stimuli:**
   a. The primary and secondary coils are kept at the farthest distance and then they are gradually brought closer till the break shock is produced.
   b. The secondary coil is now moved a little away from the primary coil so as to find a stimulus that just fails to produce a contraction of the heart.
   c. Apply this stimulus several times at the interval of 0.5–1 second till the ventricle shows contraction. The 10th–20th stimulus generally gives a full contraction. Each subminimal stimulus produces some changes in the heart muscle, making it more excitable to the successive stimulus. Once the summation of potential changes induced by subminimal stimuli reaches to threshold, the ventricle contracts as shown in Figure 2.13.1E.

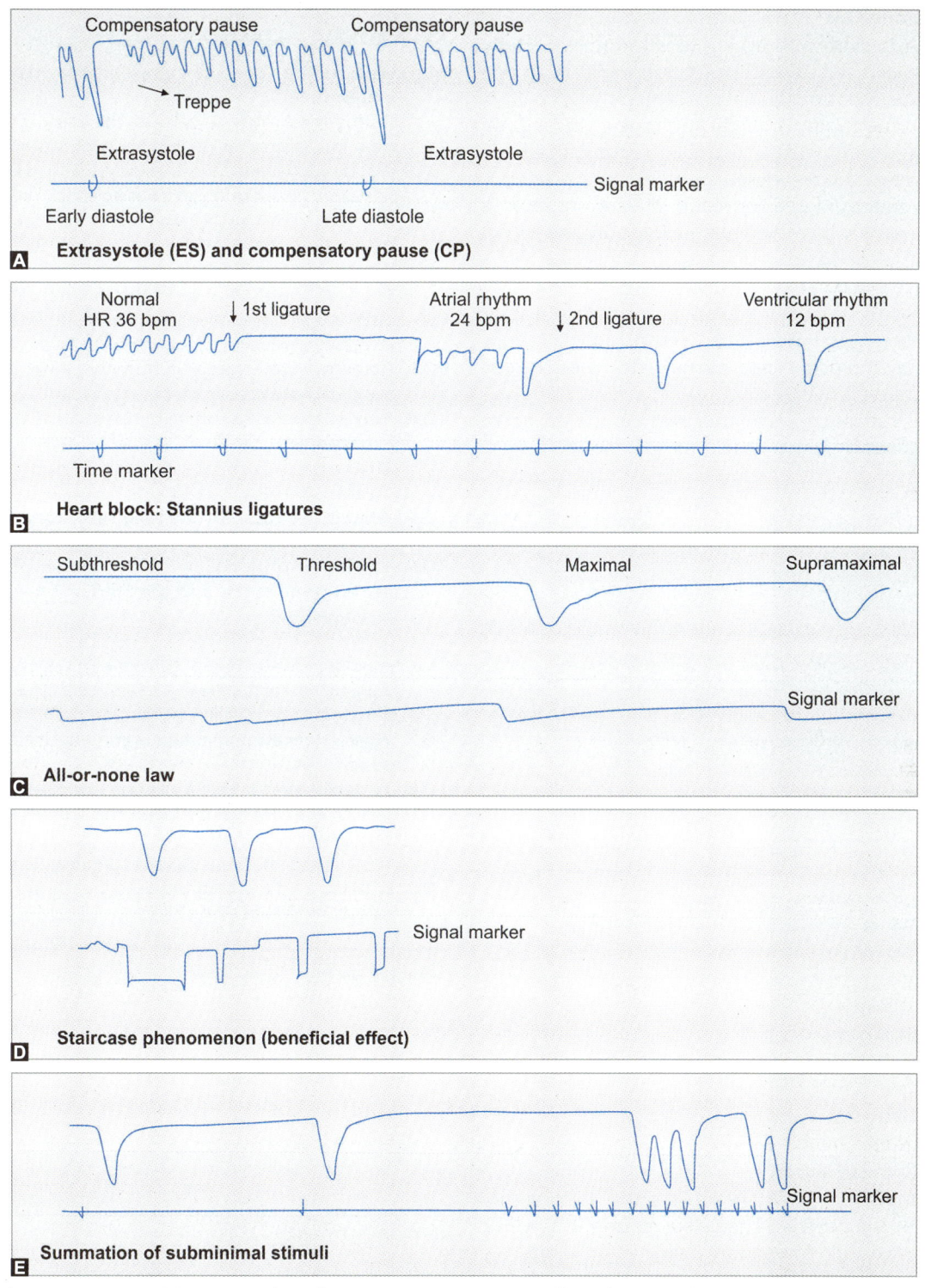

Figs. 2.13.1A to E: (A) Extrasystole and compensatory pause; (B) Effect of Stannius ligatures; (C) All-or-none law; (D) Staircase phenomenon (beneficial effect); (E) Summation of subminimal stimuli.
(HR: heart rate; bpm: beats per minute)

9. **All-or-none Law:**
   a. Starting with subthreshold stimuli, gradually increase the strength of stimuli until there is a contraction (threshold response).
   b. Continue to apply single stimulus of increasing strength, allowing at least 30 second intervals between each response.
   c. Note that though the strength of each stimulus is successively increased but the force of contraction remains the same.
10. **Staircase Effect:**
    a. Three to four **threshold** stimuli are given one after the other at an interval of 2–3 seconds, so that a new contraction occurs immediately after the previous relaxation is over.
    b. Note the successive increase in the force of contraction of the ventricle due to **beneficial** effect.

PRECAUTIONS

1. To study the phenomena of extrasystole and compensatory pause, the stimulus has to be applied during late diastole.
2. To study the staircase phenomenon, the ventricle should be stimulated repeatedly after every 2 seconds.
3. For studying the summation of effects due to repeated subminimal stimuli, the stimuli (subthreshold) should be applied repeatedly after 0.5–1 seconds.

PHYSIOCLINICAL SIGNIFICANCE

Extrasystole: Extrasystoles are commonly seen in medical practice. The common causes are:
1. **Physiological causes**
   a. Smoking
   b. Excessive intake of tea or coffee
   c. Anxiety
   d. Lack of sleep.
2. **Pathological causes**
   a. Hyperthyroidism
   b. Hypoxia
   c. Electrolytes imbalance
   d. Myocardial damage
   e. Digitalis overdose, etc.

Some ectopic foci (from other than the normal site) in the atria or the ventricles generate an impulse, which causes an extrasystole (premature beat).

About **2–4 extrasystole/minute** are considered normal in humans. If the frequency of extrasystoles is >6/min, that may indicate some **pathological condition.**

Heart block: Whenever there is a stoppage of impulse transmission from atria to ventricle, it is called heart block. Three degrees of heart block can occur in humans (I, II and III degree).

QUESTIONS

Q.1. **What is the cause of compensatory pause after an extrasystole?**
During the extrasystole, when the usual cardiac impulse from the pacemaker reaches the ventricle, it finds that it is already contracting (due to extrasystole) and in the absolute refractory period (ARP), so it has no effect. The ventricle has, therefore, to wait for the next impulse from the sinus to arrive before it can contract—hence the brief pause.

Q.2. **What is "postextrasystolic potentiation"?**
The first contraction after the compensatory pause is often more forceful than the usual heartbeat. This is due to increased availability of intracellular calcium.

Q.3. **Do extrasystoles occur in humans? What is the normal frequency of extrasystole?**

Q.4. **How will you differentiate between atrial and ventricular extrasystole?**
Atrial and ventricular extrasystole can be distinguished with the help of an electrocardiogram (ECG).

Q.5. **What is the cause of the long refractory period of the cardiac muscle? What is its advantage?**

Q.6. **What is all-or-none law? Which tissues obey this law? Are all-or-none law and the Starling's law of the heart incompatible?**
For the all-or-none law to be applicable, all the experimental conditions are to be kept constant. This does not happen in Starling's law of the heart where the initial length of cardiac muscle changes resulting in increased force of contraction.

Q.7. **What is staircase phenomenon and what is its physiological basis?**

Q.8. **To demonstrate the all-or-none law phenomenon, why should the interval between the stimuli should be 30 seconds?**
This will prevent summation of stimuli or beneficial effect.

Q.9. **With the help of a diagram describe the properties of the cardiac muscle of a frog?**

OBSERVATION AND RESULT

....
....
....
....
....

INTERPRETATION

....
....
....
....
....

STUDY NOTES

Date ....

CHAPTER 2.14

Effect of Stimulation of Vagosympathetic Trunk and White Crescentic Line on Frog's Cardiogram

AIM

To study the effect of stimulation of vagosymapthetic trunk and white crescentic line (WCL) on frog's cardiogram.

THEORY

The vagosympathetic trunk contains preganglionic parasympathetic nerve fibers and postganglionic sympathetic fibers (in mammals, the two systems run separately), but there are many more vagal fibers than sympathetic. Therefore, vagal effects usually predominate.

The stimulation of vagal fibers decreases heart rate and conduction, but it has no effect on ventricular contraction.

The **white crescentic line** is formed by the postganglionic parasympathetic neurons located at the junction between sinus venosus and atria. Stimulation of WCL will have the same effect as the stimulation of vagal fibers.

APPARATUS

1. Same as in properties of cardiac muscle (*Refer* Chapter 2.13)
2. Stimulating electrodes
3. Signal marker.

PROCEDURE

1. **Exposure of vagosympathetic trunk:**
   a. Expose the heart as before. Identify the narrow strip of petrohyoid muscle which runs from the base of the skull to the hyoid bone, as it crosses a very shiny tendon.
   b. Lift up the lower border of the muscle and to find the vagosympathetic trunk and carotid vessels crossing the shiny tendon.
   c. Expose the other trunk also. Put loose ligatures around them, so that they can be lifted up for stimulation.
   d. Include the Neef's hammer (for repeated stimuli) and signal marker in the primary circuit.
2. **Stimulation of vagosympathetic trunk:** Record a few normal beats then stimulate the vagosympathetic trunk for 4–5 seconds with the help of Neef's Hammer. Note the stoppage of the heart during diastole. This is **vagal inhibition** (Figs. 2.14.1).
3. **Stimulation of WCL:** After normal beats are restored, stimulate the WCL for a few seconds and note cardiac inhibition as above. Repeat steps 2 and 3 on the other side (Fig. 2.14.2).
4. **Vagal escape:** After recording the vagal inhibition, continue the stimulation of vagus till the heart recovers automatically even on continuation of vagal stimulation. This is called as **vagal escape** (Fig. 2.14.1B).

PRECAUTIONS

1. The student should record the normal cardiogram before recording the effect of each variable.
2. The vagosymapthetic trunk should be identified by its anatomical landmark.

Chapter 2.14: Effect of Stimulation of Vagosympathetic Trunk and White Crescentic Line on Frog's Cardiogram

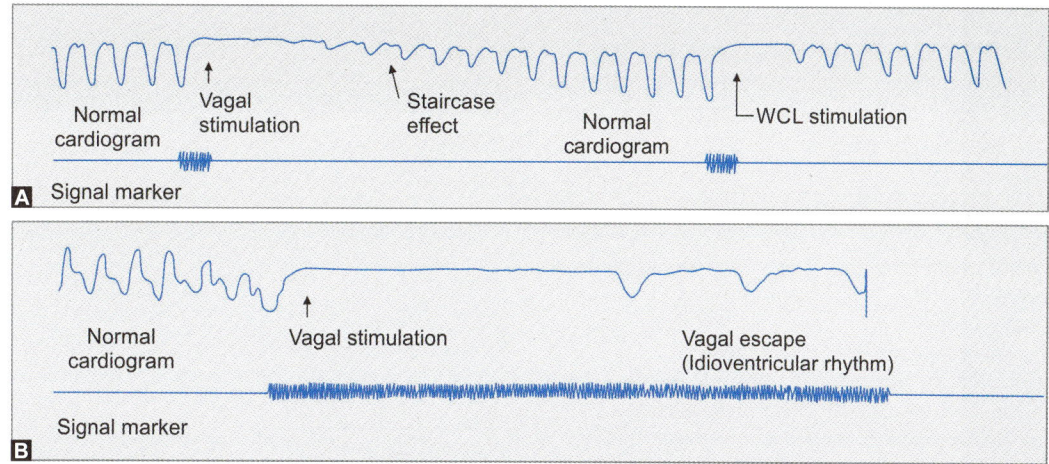

Figs. 2.14.1A and B: (A) Effect of stimulation of vagosympathetic trunk and white crescentic line (WCL); (B) Phenomenon of vagal escape.

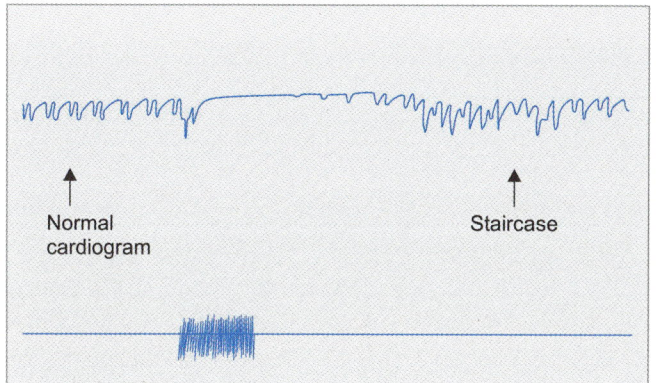

Fig. 2.14.2: Effect of white crescentic line (WCL) stimulation.

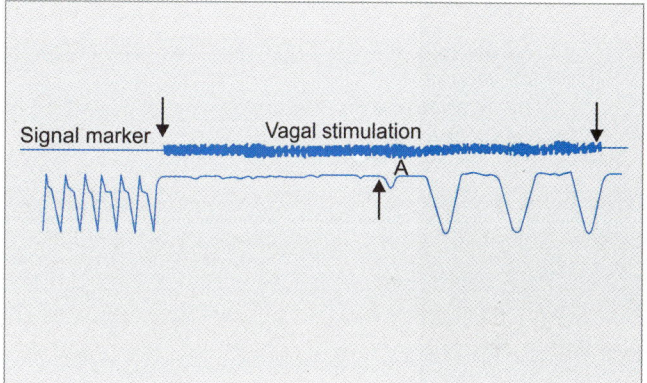

Fig. 2.14.3: Idioventricular rhythm after prolonged vagal stimulation.

3. A lower strength to a higher strength of stimuli should be used to study the effect of vagal stimulation on heart.
4. Label the recording properly to mark the start and termination of stimulation.

PHYSIOCLINICAL SIGNIFICANCE

1. Unlike the amphibian heart, the vagal and sympathetic fibers are separate in human beings, therefore, only parasympathetic effects are seen on stimulating the vagus. On continuous stimulation of the vagus, there results vagal escape (Figs. 2.14.2 and 2.14.3).
2. **Vagal tone** is the tonic inhibitory influence of the vagus on the human heart. When the heart is denervated (sympathetic and parasympathetic supply are cut), the intrinsic heart rate is 100–120/min, whereas the normal heart rate in humans is 60–100/min. This decrease in the heart rate is due to vagal tone.
3. **Vagal escape:** When the vagus (it supplies the ventricle in *amphibia*) is stimulated, the heart at first stops, but as the stimulation is continued, the heart escapes from this inhibitory effect and starts to beat once again—a phenomenon called vagal escape. The following factors are involved:
   a. *Idioventricular rhythm:* When the heart stops due to vagal stimulation, the ventricles start generating the impulse which is known as idioventricular rhythm. It is significantly lower than the normal heart rate (Fig. 2.14.3).
   b. *Depletion of acetylcholine:* On continuous stimulation of vagus, the acetylcholine released at the nerve endings is depleted after sometime. Therefore the effect of vagal stimulation on heart is temporary.
   c. When the vagosympthetic trunk is continuously stimulated, the sympathetic fibers are also activated. This **sympathetic effect** may overpower the vagal effect, thus releasing the ventricle from inhibition.

d. *Vasovagal syncope:* If there is a sudden stimulation of vagus nerve, there occurs a transient and sudden loss of consciousness. Strong emotions in humans may lead to vagal syncope, but the immediate vagal escape restores the heart beat.

QUESTIONS

Q.1. What type of nerve fibers are present in the vagosympathetic trunk?
Q.2. What is vagal tone?
Q.3. What is vagal escape and what is its cause?
Q.4. If both sympathetic and parasympathetic nerves to the heart are blocked, what is the effect on heart rate?
Q.5. Which nerve fibers constitute the white crescentic line?
Q.6. Describe the autonomic supply of mammalian heart.
Mammalian heart is supplied by both sympathetic and parasympathetic nervous system. The vagi supply fibers to the sinoatrial (SA) node, atrioventricular (AV) node and atrial muscles. No vagal fibers are distributed to ventricles. In some individuals, right vagus is dominant, whereas in others it is the left vagus.
The sympathetic fibers supply SA and AV node and muscles of atria and ventricles.

OBSERVATION AND RESULT

Describe the effects of the following on frog's heart

Vagal stimulation (short duration)	
Vagal stimulation (long duration)	
WCL stimulation	

INTERPRETATION

....
....
....
....
....

Chapter 2.14: Effect of Stimulation of Vagosympathetic Trunk and White Crescentic Line on Frog's Cardiogram

STUDY NOTES

Teacher's Signature

Date ....

CHAPTER 2.15

Effect of Variables on Intact Frog's Heart

AIM

To study the effect of variables on intact frog's heart.

THEORY

1. **Adrenaline:**
   a. It is a sympathomimetic agent.
   b. It acts on both α and β receptors on the target organs.
   c. In the heart it acts on β_1 receptors which on stimulation have a **positive chronotropic** and **inotropic effect**. In the cardiac muscle cells, it increases the permeability mainly to Ca^{2+} ions and, to some extent Na^+ ions. Influx of Na^+ in the pacemaker cells increases the slope of phase 4 of the action potential (AP) thus increasing the heart rate. The large influx of Ca^{2+} increases the force of contraction.
2. **Acetylcholine (ACh):** Acetylcholine acts on two types of receptors:
   a. *Muscarinic (M_2) receptors* are present on cardiac muscle, smooth muscle and exocrine glands including sweat glands. These are blocked by the drug atropine.
      - ACh acts directly on the pacemaker cells and increases the permeability to K^+ ions which causes more of these ions to move out. This results in hyperpolarization which decreases the slope of phase 4 of the AP thus decreasing the heart rate **(negative chronotropic effect)**.
      - When ACh acts directly on atria and ventricle it increases the permeability to K^+ ions; the K^+ efflux shortens phase 2 of AP which decreases the Ca^{2+} influx and, therefore, the force of contraction **(negative inotropic effect)**.
   b. *Nicotinic receptors* are present on motor end plates (blocked by curare, etc.) and on postganglionic neurons in autonomic ganglia. Hexamethonium (at autonomic ganglion) and tubocurarine (at neuromuscular junction) block these receptors.
3. **Atropine:**
   a. It is a parasympatholytic agent.
   b. It blocks the action of ACh on the muscarinic receptors.
   c. When applied on the heart after ACh, it has no effect, but when applied before ACh, atropine blocks the inhibitory action of ACh.
4. **Nicotine:**
   a. It acts through the nicotinic cholinergic receptors which are present in the neuromuscular end plates and in the peripheral autonomic ganglia.
   b. When applied to the frog's heart it acts on the parasympathetic ganglia located on the white crescentic line.
   c. In low concentrations, nicotine stimulates the postganglionic parasympathetic fibers causing bradycardia, while in high concentrations it blocks the ganglia **by causing persistent depolarization**.

APPARATUS

1. Same as in recording of normal cardiogram (*Refer* Chapter 2.12).
2. Adrenaline: 1 in 10,000
3. Acetylcholine: 1 in 100,000

4. Atropine 0.5%
5. Nicotine 0.5%.

PROCEDURE

1. **Effect of adrenaline:** Record few normal beats. Stop the drum and pour a few drops of 1 in 10,000 solution of adrenaline on the heart. Record the effect.
2. Stop the drum and wash the heart with Ringer's solution till the normal cardiogram reappears.
3. **Effect of acetylcholine:** Record a few normal beats then pour a few drops of 1 in 100,000 solution of acetylcholine. Record the effect.
4. As the heart is beating, apply 0.5% atropine solution. There will be no effect.
5. Stop the drum, wash with Ringer's solution.
6. Now study the effect of acetylcholine after applying atropine solution on the heart—the heart will not be inhibited this time.
7. **Effect of nicotine:** After washing with Ringer's solution when normal beats are restored, pour a few drops of 0.5% nicotine solution on the heart. Note that there is no effect.
8. Stimulate the vagosympathetic trunk and compare with the effect obtained before adding nicotine.
9. Stimulate the white crescentic line (WCL) and similarly compare the effect.
10. **Effect of atropine:** Wash the heart with Ringer's solution. When normal beats are restored, pour atropine on the heart. Note that there is no effect on the heart.
11. Stimulate the vagosympathetic trunk and compare with the effect obtained before adding nicotine.
12. Stimulate the WCL and similarly compare the effect (Figs. 2.15.1A to C).

PRECAUTIONS

1. The student should record the normal cardiogram before recording the effect of each variable.
2. The frog's heart should be rinsed with amphibian Ringer's solution between applications of various drugs.

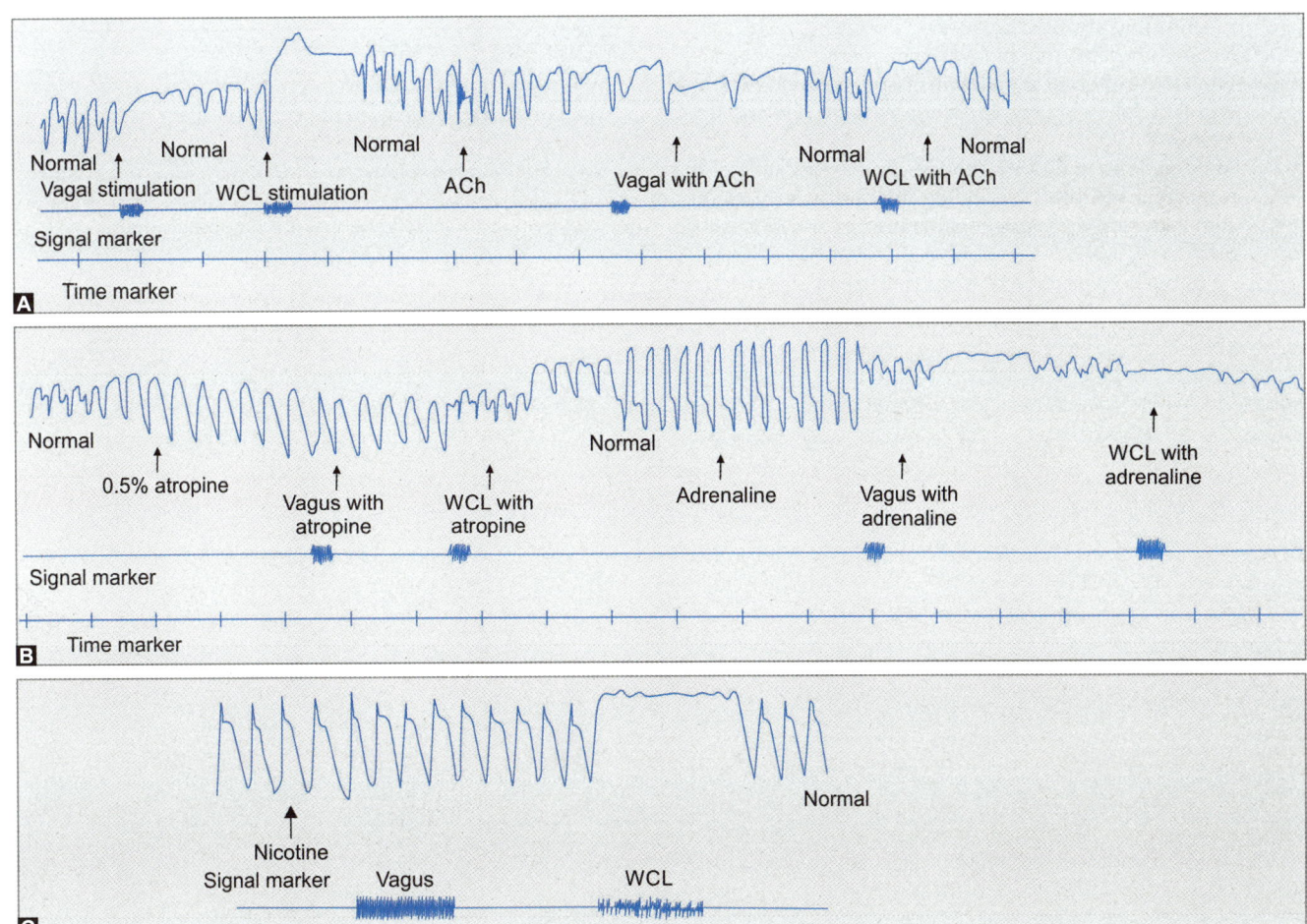

Figs. 2.15.1A to C: Effect of adrenaline, acetylcholine, nicotine and atropine on Frog's heart.
(WCL: white crescentic line; ACh: acetylcholine)

Section 2: Amphibian (Frog) Experiments

QUESTIONS

Q.1. What are the locations in the body where acetylcholine is released?

Acetylcholine is released at the following sites:
- Preganglionic sympathetic nerve endings (in the ganglia).
- Preganglionic and postganglionic parasympathetic nerve endings.
- Postganglionic sympathetic fibers supplying the sweat glands, pilomotor muscles and those supplying the blood vessels of skeletal muscles are cholinergic.
- Neuromuscular junctions of all skeletal muscle fibers.
- Many synapses in the CNS.

Q.2. How is acetylcholine inactivated in the body? What are anticholinesterases?

The enzyme *acetylcholinesterase (AChE)* catalyzes the hydrolysis of ACh to choline and acetate, which are reused. *Anticholinesterases* are drugs which inhibit the action of AChE, so that ACh is preserved at the site for a longer time. These drugs include physostigmine (eserine), neostigmine and diisopropylfluorophosphate (DFP), an ingredient of some pesticides and nerve gases. Neostigmine is used in the treatment of myasthenia gravis.

Q.3. What is the effect of local application of adrenaline, nicotine and atropine on the frog's heart?

Q.4. Name the agents that block the cholinergic receptors?

Q.5. What is the effect of stimulation of vagosympathetic trunk and WCL following the application of atropine and 0.5% nicotine?

After application of 0.5% atropine there is blockade of the muscarinic receptors located on the cardiac muscle. Thus stimulation on the vagosympathetic trunk and WCL will be ineffective.

About 0.5% nicotine when applied to frog's heart acts on the parasympathetic ganglia located on the WCL. Thus after application of nicotine:

a. Stimulation of vagosympathetic trunk will not cause inhibition of the heart.
b. WCL stimulation will cause inhibition of the heart.

Q.6. Explain how transient depolarization of neuron excites it whereas persistent depolarization inactivates it?

Transient depolarization brings the resting membrane potential toward the firing levels, whereas the persistent depolarization inactivates the Na$^+$ channels thus preventing the generation of action potentials.

OBSERVATION AND RESULT

Variables	Heart rate	Force of contraction
Adrenaline		
Acetylcholine		
Atropine		
Nicotine		

INTERPRETATION

....

....

....

....

....

STUDY NOTES

CHAPTER 2.16

Perfusion of Isolated Frog's Heart

AIM

To study the effect of variables on isolated frog's heart.

THEORY

The rate and force of contraction of heart is affected by different drugs and ions. These change the ionic composition of the myocardial cells and the nodal tissue either acting directly on ion channels or on different receptors. In this practical, the effect of various drugs and chemicals are being observed in isolated frog's heart.

APPARATUS

1. Amphibian Ringer–Locke's solution
2. Mariotte (perfusion) bottle
3. Syme's cannula
4. 1% $CaCl_2$, 1% NaCl and 1% KCl
5. Adrenaline: 1:100,000
6. Acetylcholine: 1:1000,000.

Composition of Amphibian Ringer–Locke Solution

The fluid required for perfusing the isolated heart of frog has the composition given in Table 2.16.1.

PROCEDURE

1. Expose the frog's heart and remove the pericardium. Pass a thread around the sinus. Make a small slit in the sinus, introduce a Syme's cannula into it and tie a knot around it.
2. Cut the aorta and other vessels and lift the cannula along with the heart. Fit a Starling's heart lever upside down on a stand and fix the cannula in a clamp directly above the heart lever. Connect the side arm of the cannula to a reservoir containing Ringer–Locke solution and raise the reservoir about 30 cm above the heart to provide a pressure head (Fig. 2.16.1).
3. Push the bent pin of the lever through the apex of the ventricle, make necessary adjustments and record a few beats.
4. After the tracing has stabilized, raise the reservoir to increase the perfusion pressure.
5. Add 1% NaCl solution via the side tube of the cannula and record its effects. Wash the heart with the perfusion fluid and study the effects of 1% KCl and 1% $CaCl_2$ solutions.
6. Wash the heart well with Ringer–Locke solution and study the effects of adrenalin and acetylcholine (Fig. 2.16.2 and Table 2.16.2).

Table 2.16.1: Composition of the amphibian Ringer-Locke's solution required for perfusing the isolated heart of frog.

NaCl	0.60 g
$CaCl_2$	0.012 g
KCl	0.014 g
$NaHCO_3$	0.01 g $NaHCO_3$
Na_2HPO_4	0.001 g dissolved before $CaCl_2$ is added
Glucose	0.1 g (to be added just before use)
Distilled water	To make it 100 mL

(NaCl: sodium chloride; $CaCl_2$: calcium chloride; KCl: potassium chloride; $NaHCO_3$: sodium bicarbonate; Na_2HPO_4: disodium phosphate)

> **NOTE**
> In this case, the upstroke is systole and the downstroke is diastole.

Chapter 2.16: Perfusion of Isolated Frog's Heart

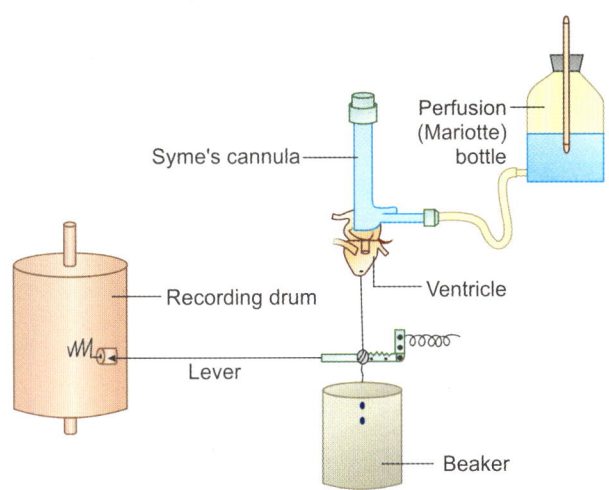

Fig. 2.16.1: Perfusion of frog's heart.

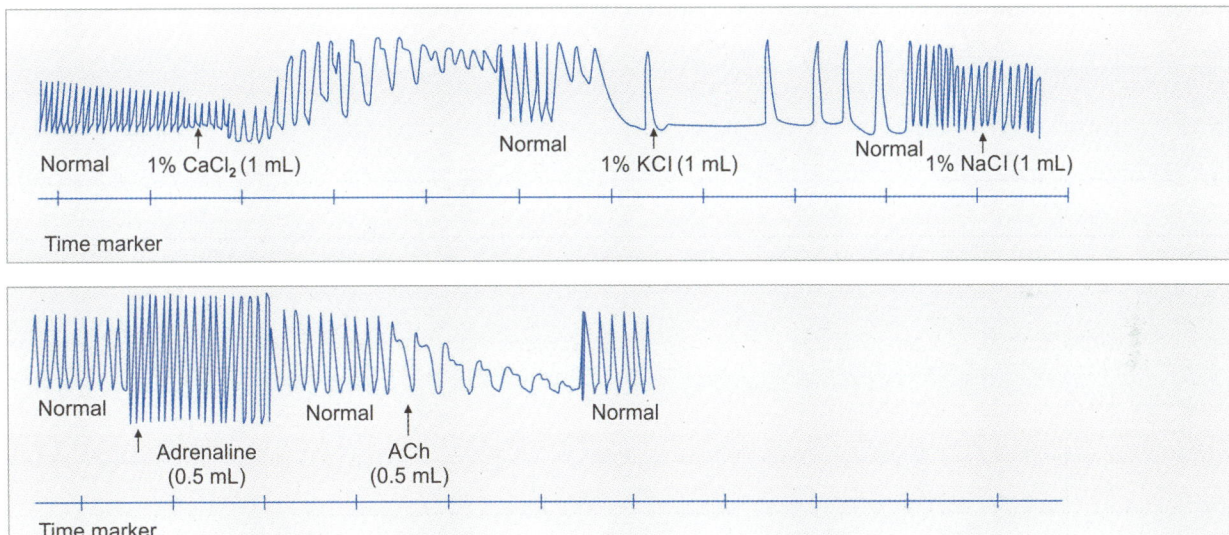

Fig. 2.16.2: Effect of variables on isolated frog's heart preparation.

Table 2.16.2: Effect and mechanism of variables on isolated frog's heart.		
Agent	**Heart rate**	**Force of contraction**
1. NaCl (1%)	No effect	There may be a decrease in the contractility as Na^+ competes with Ca^{2+}
2. KCl (1%)	↓ because of decrease in RMP of nodal tissue	↓ Finally the heart stops in diastole. This is because of decrease in RMP of atrial and ventricular muscles
3. $CaCl_2$ (1%)	No effect	Increase in ECF Ca^{2+} leading to increase in intracellular Ca^{2+}. Marked increase in Ca^{2+} in ECF may cause calcium rigor
4. Adrenaline	Increases, due to increased Na^+ entry in nodal tissues	Increases due to Ca^{2+} influx in myocardial fibers
5. Acetylcholine	Decreases, HR as K^+ efflux hyperpolarizes the nodal tissues	Decreases because of decrease in Ca^{2+} influx in myocardial fibers

(ECF: extracellular fluid; RMP: resting membrane potential)

QUESTIONS

Q.1. Describe the effects of various drugs and chemicals on frog's heart.
Q.2. What do you mean by calcium rigor?

STUDY NOTES

Section 3

Human Experiments

CHAPTERS

Unit 1: Cardiovascular System
3.1 Examination of Arterial (Radial) Pulse
3.2 Recording of Systemic Arterial Blood Pressure
3.3 Effect of Posture on Blood Pressure and Heart Rate
3.4 Effect of Exercise on Blood Pressure and Heart Rate
3.5 Recording and Interpretation of an Electrocardiogram
3.6 Cardiac Efficiency Tests

Unit 2: Respiratory System
3.7 Stethography
3.8 Spirometry: Lung Volumes and Capacities
3.9 Vitalography and Effect of Posture on Vital Capacity
3.10 Cardiopulmonary Resuscitation
3.11 Basal Metabolic Rate

Unit 3: Special Senses
3.12 Perimetry

Unit 4: Nervous System
3.13 Reaction Time (Visual and Auditory)
3.14 Electroencephalography
3.15 Electroneurodiagnostic Tests
    A. Nerve Conduction Study
    B. Electromyography
    C. Evoked potentials

3.16 Study of Human Fatigue by Mosso's Ergograph and Handgrip Dynamometer
3.17 Autonomic Function Tests

Unit 5: Reproductive System

3.18 Semen Analysis
3.19 Pregnancy Diagnostic Tests
3.20 Birth Control Methods

UNIT 1: CARDIOVASCULAR SYSTEM

Date ....

CHAPTER 3.1

Examination of Arterial (Radial) Pulse

AIM

Examination of arterial (radial) pulse.

THEORY

After each systole, the alternate expansion and recoil of the aorta sets up a pressure or pulse wave. This rhythmic pulsatile wave travels from segment to segment of the arterial tree and causes expansion and recoil of their walls which is felt as the **arterial pulse**.

Why is radial artery chosen?
The routine examination of arterial pulse is done on this artery, (called the "pulse") because:
- It is conveniently accessible as it is located in an exposed part of the body.
- The artery lies over the hard surface of the lower end of the radius.

The radial artery is palpated with the tips of three fingers compressing the vessel against the head of radius bone (Fig. 3.1.1). The subject's forearm should be slightly pronated and the wrist slightly flexed. The index finger (toward the heart) varies the pressure on the artery, the middle finger feels the pulse, while the ring finger prevents reflections of pulsations from the palmer arch of arteries. The radial pulse has to be examined under the following headings:
1. Rate
2. Rhythm
3. Volume
4. Condition of vessel wall

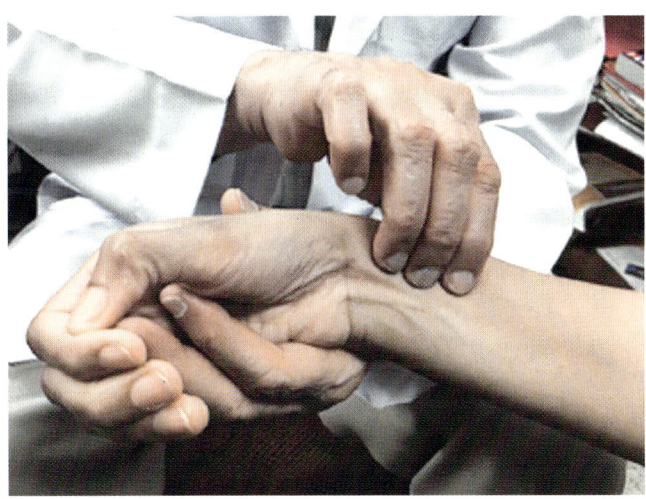

Fig. 3.1.1: Examination of radial pulse.

5. Radiofemoral delay
6. Equality on both sides
7. Character and form.

Rate of Pulse

The pulse rate is expressed as beats per minute. Normal pulse rate at rest averages about 60–90 beats/min.

> **NOTE**
> The pulse rate should be counted for full 1 minute.

The pulse rate should always be compared with the heart rate, as in some cases the pulse rate may be less than heart rate (**pulse deficit**).

Factors Affecting the Heart Rate (Pulse Rate)

1. **Tachycardia:** An increase in heart rate above 90 beats/min is called tachycardia.

   Physiological causes:
   a. Emotional excitement, nervousness and apprehension.
   b. Muscular exercise.
   c. In newborns: The heart rate may be 120–150 beats/min; it gradually decreases during infancy and childhood.
   d. Sex: The rate is comparatively higher in females; there may be tachycardia during pregnancy.
   e. Diurnal variations: Higher rates are seen in the evening and may exceed 100 beats/min.

   Pathological causes:
   a. Fever due to any cause: For every 1°C rise in temperature, the heart rate increases by about 10–14 beats/min. The raised temperature acts directly on the sinoatrial (SA) node and generates more action potentials per unit time.
   b. Thyrotoxicosis: Increased metabolism of SA node generates more action potentials.
   c. Atrial flutter and fibrillation: The pulse is fast and irregular.
   d. Paroxysmal atrial tachycardia: Sudden onset and sudden offset are characteristic features.
   e. Circulatory shock: The pulse is fast and weak (thready pulse).

2. **Bradycardia:** A decrease in heart rate below 60 beats/min is called bradycardia.

   Physiological causes:
   a. Athletes: The resting heart rate may be 50–55 beats/min; it is due to increased vagal tone.
   b. Sleep and meditation: The rate may be below 55 beats/min during deep meditation.
   c. The rate may be below 60 beats/min under **basal conditions**, i.e. before a person gets out of bed after a good night's sleep.

   Pathological causes:
   a. Myxedema: Hyposecretion of thyroid hormone is commonly associated with low pulse rates.
   b. Heart block: The rate depends on the degree of heart block. In complete heart block, the ventricular rate may be 30–40 beats/min (idioventricular rhythm).
   c. General weakness and debility following prolonged illness.
   d. Drugs: Treatment with drugs such as digitalis and propranolol.

Rhythm

The normal pulse waves follow at regular intervals, i.e. the rhythm is regular. It can be either:

Regularly irregular: Irregularity of pulse occurring at regular intervals, e.g. in extrasystoles (premature ectopic beats)

Irregularly irregular: Irregularity of pulse seen at irregular intervals, e.g. atrial fibrillation.

The pulse rate normally increases during deep inspiration and decreases during deep expiration. When this happens during quiet breathing, it is called **sinus arrhythmia**, which is due to irradiation of impulses from the inspiratory center to the cardiac center.

Volume

The "volume" of the pulse refers to the amplitude of the movement or expansion of the artery during the passage of pulse wave. It is a rough guide to the pulse pressure. It can be:

Low volume pulse (thin, thready pulse) of low stroke volume seen in **shock**.

High volume pulse of hyperkinetic circulation seen in:
- Pregnancy, exercise
- Fever
- Anemia
- Thyrotoxicosis.

Condition of the Vessel Wall

The index finger is used to obliterate the flow of blood and ring finger should be used to empty the blood vessel. The middle finger is then used to palpate the vessel wall. The emptied vessel should then be rolled against the underlying bone. In young individuals, the "empty" artery is so compliant that it cannot be felt as a separate structure. However, the vessel becomes palpable in old age and is felt as a cord-like structure due to atherosclerosis and calcification.

Radiofemoral Delay

When the femoral artery and the radial artery are palpated simultaneously the two pulses normally beat together, i.e. there is no delay between occurrence of the pulse in femoral and radial artery. Radiofemoral delay is seen in **coarctation of the aorta**.

Equality on the Two Sides

The arterial pulse of one side is always compared with that of the other side for all of its features described above. Normally, there is no difference between the two.

Character or Form

Character or form refers to the waveform of the pulse, i.e. whether the individual pulse wave has a normal rise, maintenance or fall (its contours) as the pulse is being palpated. The character should be evaluated at the right carotid artery, i.e. the pulse closest to the heart and least subjected to distortion and damping in the arterial tree. Since the contours of the pulse waves cannot usually be clearly felt by palpation, one has to record the pulse with an electronic transducer (**Dudgeon's sphygmograph** used to be employed in the past).

Normal Character of Arterial Pulse

The normal pulse wave (Figs. 3.1.2A to C) shows the following components:
- **Percussion wave or the anacrotic limb:** This is the sharp upstroke. It is due to expansion of the artery due to ventricular systole and corresponds to the maximum ejection phase.
- **Catacrotic limb:** The down stroke is called the catacrotic limb which has the following two components:
  - *Tidal wave:* This predicrotic wave is due to elasticity of aorta. It is sometimes recorded soon after the peak of the tracing.
  - *Dicrotic notch and wave:* These are seen on the descending limb. The notch, the negative wave, is due to recoil of the elastic aorta that causes the blood column to momentarily sweep back towards the heart. The reverse flow closes the aortic valve and rebounds from it to cause the positive dicrotic wave.

The systolic and diastolic phases of the ventricle can be indicated on the arterial pulse tracing. The maximum ejection phase lasts from the beginning of upstroke to the peak of percussion wave, while the reduced ejection phase lasts from the peak to the dicrotic notch. Thus, systole is approximately from the beginning of upstroke to the dicrotic notch.

Abnormal Character of Arterial Pulse:

- **Anacrotic pulse (pulsus parvus or slow-rising pulse):** It is a small (parvus = small), weak, pulse which rises slowly and has a delayed peak. The weak upstroke is due to decreased stroke volume and a narrow pulse pressure. It is seen especially in **aortic stenosis.**
- **Dicrotic pulse:** There are two palpable waves, one in systole and the other in diastole. It is seen most commonly in low stroke volume.
- **Corrigan's, water hammer or collapsing pulse:** It is characterized by an abrupt rise and a sudden fall of the pulse wave in early diastole. It is seen most commonly in **aortic regurgitation** in which the incompetent valve cannot close properly to prevent backflow of blood from the aorta back into the ventricle. The rapid upstroke is due to greatly increased and vigorous stroke volume while the collapsing is caused by two factors—the diastolic "run-off" of blood back into the left ventricle and the rapid "run-off" of blood toward the periphery due to low peripheral resistance resulting from arteriolar dilatation.
- **Alternating pulse (pulsus alternans):** The pulse beats are regular but alternately large and small in amplitude, i.e. strong and weak beats. It is seen in **left ventricular failure** when the ventricle is severely diseased.
- **Pulsus paradoxus:** Normally there is a slight fall of blood pressure (by 8–10 mm Hg) during inspiration. The term "pulsus paradoxus" describes the marked decrease in blood pressure which occurs on deep inspiration in patients with **large pericardial effusion** or **severe asthma**. It is an accentuation of normal physiological fall in systolic pressure. The paradox is that while the pulse may not be felt at the wrist, heart sounds may still be heard at the precordium.
- **Thready pulse:** Thin, thready pulse is characterized by **low volume and increased pulse rate**. It is seen in **shock** and is due to decrease in stroke volume.

Examine all other peripheral arterial pulses: For example, **brachial**—at the elbow; **carotid**—in the neck; **femoral**—in the groin; **popliteal**—popliteal fossa; **posterior tibial**—behind medial malleolus; and **dorsalis pedis**—on the dorsum of the foot at the midpoint between medial and lateral malleoli, at the base of the first metatarsal bone. The volume of each is compared with the other side.

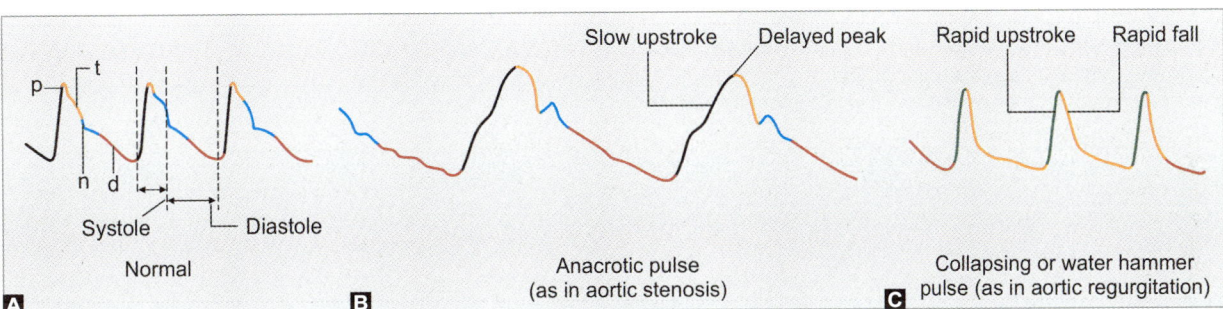

Figs. 3.1.2A to C: Sphygmogram: An arterial pulse tracing (A) Normal pulse tracing, p: percussion wave, t: tidal wave, d: dicrotic notch, n: dicrotic wave; (B) Anacrotic pulse tracing in aortic stenosis—showing a gradual upstroke and slow descent; (C) Water hammer (Corrigan's) pulse—showing rapid upstroke and descent.

COMMENTS

Since the arteries are not perfectly elastic, the pulse wave is gradually dampened as it progresses along the vessels. With the great reduction of pressure in the arterioles, the damping effect is great and little pulsations may be seen in the capillaries. However, if the arterioles dilate, as they do in hot weather and after exercise, the pulsations reaching the capillaries are greater and may be transmitted to the venules. Similarly, when the pulse pressure is greatly increased as in aortic regurgitation, the pulsations are seen in the capillaries. Properly applied pressure on a nail-bed or on the mucosa of the lip (with a glass slide) will show alternate flushing of the blanched margin.

PRECAUTIONS

1. The pulse should be examined after the subject has relaxed for at least 5 minutes.
2. The forearm of the subject should be semi-pronated and the wrist should be slightly flexed.
3. The pulse rate should be counted for complete 1 minute.
4. To detect radiofemoral delay the femoral artery should be examined simultaneously with the radial artery.
5. Pulses of both sides should be examined and compared.
6. While examining the radial pulse three fingers should be used.
7. All the peripheral pulses should be examined.

Objective Structured Practical Examination

Aim: To examine the radial artery of the subject provided.
Procedural steps: See text above.
Checklist:

1. Stand on the subject's right side and explain the procedure. (Y/N)
2. Hold the subject's right hand in a semi-pronated and slightly flexed position. Then place three middle fingers on the radial artery and compress it slightly against the bone. (Y/N)
3. Note the rhythm, volume and character of the pulse. Count the rate for 1 minute and note the result. (Y/N)
4. Compress the artery with the proximal finger and try to roll the artery against the bone with the other two fingers. (Y/N)
5. Compare the equality of pulses in both arms. Count the heart rate to see if there is any pulse deficit. (Y/N)

QUESTIONS

Q.1. Why is radial artery chosen?
Q.2. List the various precautions taken during radial pulse examination.
Q.3. Why are three fingers used for radial pulse examination?
Q.4. How much is the normal pulse rate and what determines the pulse rate?
Q.5. Define sinus arrhythmia.
Q.6. What is tachycardia and what are its causes?
Q.7. What is bradycardia and what are its causes?
Q.8. What is pulse deficit?
   Normally, the pulse rate and the ventricular rate (as determined by auscultation at the heart) are identical. However, in the case of extrasystoles (premature beats) and atrial fibrillation, some of the ventricular beats are too weak to be felt at the radial artery so that the heart rate is higher than the radial pulse rate—a condition called **pulse deficit**.
Q.9. Examine the arterial pulse in the subject provided and comment on your findings.
Q.10. List some different types of abnormal pulse.
Q.11. What are the causes of high volume and low volume pulse?
Q.12. What is the cause of bradycardia in trained athletes?

OBSERVATION AND RESULT

....
....
....
....
....

INTERPRETATION

....
....
....
....
....

STUDY NOTES

Date ....

CHAPTER 3.2

Recording of Systemic Arterial Blood Pressure

AIM

To record the systemic arterial blood pressure.

INTRODUCTION

The term **blood pressure** (BP) refers to the pressure exerted by the blood as it presses against and attempts to stretch the walls of the blood vessels.

The BP is not steady throughout the cardiac cycle but fluctuating, i.e. it is pulsatile. The various **components** of BP are as follows:

1. **Systolic blood pressure (SBP):** The maximum pressure reached during the maximum ejection phase of systole is called **systolic blood pressure (SBP)**. Normal range is 100–140 mm Hg. According to new guidelines of Joint National Committee (JNC): Normal BP: <120/80 mm Hg (Table 3.2.1).
2. **Diastolic blood pressure (DBP):** The minimum pressure reached during diastole is called **diastolic blood pressure (DBP)**. Normal range is 60–90 mm Hg

Table 3.2.1: JNC 7 Classification of HTN

BP classification	Systolic blood pressure (mm Hg)	Diastolic blood pressure (mm Hg)
Normal	<120	and <80
Prehypertension	120–139	or 80–89
Stage 1 hypertension	140–159	or 90–99
Stage 2 hypertension	≥160	or ≥100

(JNC: Joint National Committee; HTN: Hypertension)

3. **Pulse pressure (PP):** It is the difference between SBP and DBP, the average PP being about 40 mm Hg. Normal range is 30–60 mm Hg.
4. **Mean arterial pressure (MAP):** It is the average pressure during the cardiac cycle. Since the duration of systole is shorter than that of diastole, the MAP is slightly less than the average of SBP and DBP. Normal range is 90–100 mm Hg.
MAP is calculated as:
$$MAP = DBP + 1/3\ PP$$
There are two methods for measurement of systemic arterial blood pressure:

1. **Direct method:** The direct method of recording BP in which an artery is punctured with a cannula connected to a manometer. It measures the end pressure which is sum of **lateral pressure and pressure due to kinetic energy.**
Disadvantage: This method is not safe and convenient in clinical practice as it is an invasive procedure and involves high-risk of infections.

> **NOTE**
> These days, direct method is used in research work in animals and during cardiac and arterial catheterization in man.

2. **Indirect Method**

Principle

The brachial artery is first compressed by inflating a rubber bag (connected to a manometer) placed around the arm. When the rubber bag is inflated the air pressure in the cuff overcomes the arterial pressure and obliterates the arterial

Chapter 3.2: Recording of Systemic Arterial Blood Pressure

lumen leading to stoppage of blood flow. The pressure is then slowly released which initiates the turbulent flow of blood through the obstructed segment of the artery which can be studied by:
- **Palpatory method:** Feeling the radial pulse.
- **Oscillatory method:** Observing the oscillations of the mercury column.
- **Auscultatory method:** Listening to the sounds produced in the part of the artery just below the obstructed segment.

> **NOTE**
> The BP can also be measured in femoral artery by indirect method.

APPARATUS

Stethoscope (Steth = Chest, Scope = To Inspect) (Fig. 3.2.1)

Stethoscope was invented by **René Laennec** in 1819. The instrument has the following three parts:
1. **Chest piece:** The chest piece has—
   - A bell
   - A flat diaphragm
2. **Rubber tubing:** In the commonly used stethoscope, a single soft-rubber pressure tube (inner diameter 3 mm) leads from the chest piece to a metal Y-shaped connector. The diaphragm is used to hear high-pitched sounds while the bell is used to hear low-pitched sounds.
3. **Ear frame:** It consists of two curved metallic tubes. The upper ends of the tubes are curved so that they correspond to the curve of the external auditory meatus, i.e. they are directed forward and downward. Two plastic knobs threaded over the ends of the tubes fit snugly in the ear. The ear frame is connected to the chest piece by means of rubber tubing.

Sphygmomanometer

Different types of BP instruments (e.g. mercury sphygmomanometer, aneroid and digital BP apparatus) are in use, but the one in common use is the mercury sphygmomanometer (Fig. 3.2.2). It consists of the following parts:
1. **Mercury manometer:** The manometer is a graduated in vertical glass tube, having markings from 0 to 300 mm Hg, each division representing 2 mm Hg. The lower end of the glass is connected to a mercury reservoir and the upper end is closed with the help of metal cap. The mercury column rises and falls in the glass tube lumen with increase or decrease of pressure in the reservoir, respectively.
2. **Rubber bag; Riva–Rocci cuff:** The "cuff" as it is usually called, consist of an inflatable rubber bag, 24 cm × 12 cm which is fitted with two rubber tubes—(1) one connecting it to the mercury reservoir and (2) the other to a rubber bulb (air pump). The bag is enclosed in a long strip of inelastic cloth with a long tapering free end. The cloth covering keeps the rubber bag in position around the arm when pressure is being measured. In some cuffs, two Velcro strips are provided in appropriate locations for the same purpose (Figs. 3.2.3A and B).

   The rubber bag is 12 cm wide which is enough to form a pressure cone that reaches the underlying artery even in a thick arm. As per the **Thumb rule**:
   - The **width** of the bag should be **20% more than the diameter** of the arm.
   - And the **length** should cover **two-thirds of the arm circumference**.

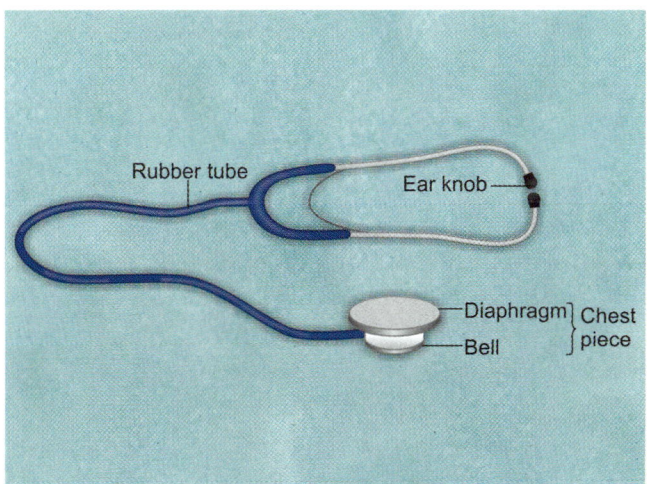

Fig. 3.2.1: Stethoscope.

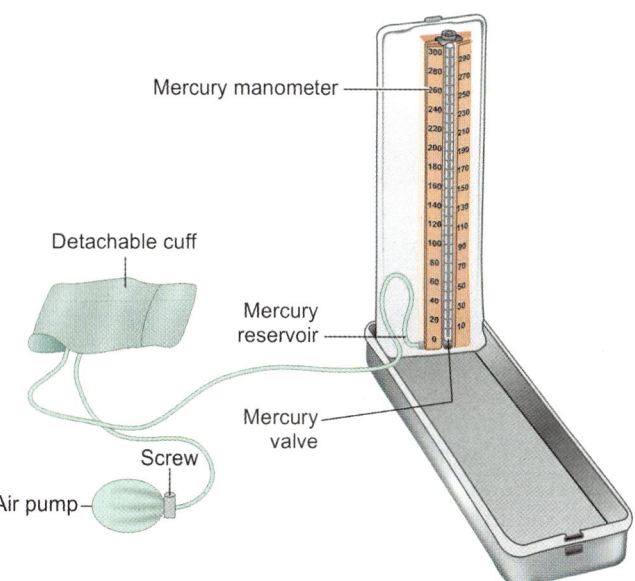

Fig. 3.2.2: Sphygmomanometer.

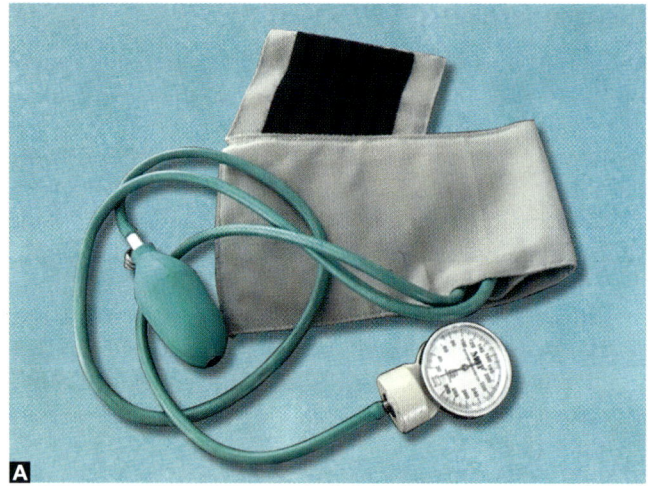

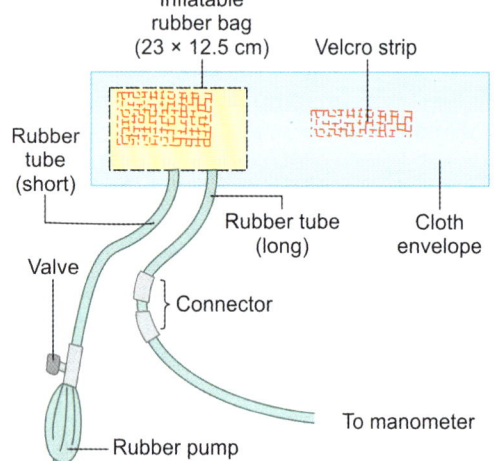

Figs. 3.2.3A and B: (A) Aneroid sphygmomanometer; (B) Riva–Rocci cuff.

The recommended width of the bag in different age groups is as under:

- *Infants (below 1 year):* 2.5 cm
- *Below 4 years:* 5 cm
- *Below 8 years:* 8 cm
- *Adults:* 12 cm.

> **NOTE**
> The problem of miscuffling (inappropriate size of the cuff) constitutes the most frequent error in the recording of BP. In order to prevent that the **American Heart Association guidelines** specify that the proper cuff should have a **bladder length (rubber bag) of 80%** and a width of at least **40% of arm circumference.** It is also to be remembered that BP measurement error is greater with an undersized cuff than it is with an oversized cuff.

3. **Air pump (rubber bulb):** It is an oval-shaped rubber bulb of a size that conveniently fits into one's fist. It has a one-way valve at its free end and a leak valve with a knurled screw, at the other end from where the rubber tube leading to the cuff is attached. The cuff can be inflated by turning the leak valve screw clockwise and alternately compressing and releasing the bulb. Deflation of the bag is achieved by turning this screw anticlockwise.

> **NOTE**
> Since the criteria for classification of hypertension are based on BP reading taken in seated subjects in doctor's clinic. It is preferable to take BP measurements in sitting position. However, BP can also be measured in supine position if the patient is very sick or in standing position (to detect orthostatic hypertension). It is to be remembered that BP measured are not the same in seated and supine position.

Aneroid manometer: In this manometer, metal bellows, mechanical links and a calibrated dial replace the mercury manometer. However, it should be calibrated against a mercury manometer from time to time.

> **NOTE**
> Although mercury sphygmomanometer is the "gold standard" for taking BP measurements. However, because of the environmental issues other types of devices (e.g. aneroid sphygmomanometer/ digital electronic pressure transducers) are increasingly being used.

PROCEDURE

Palpatory Method (Riva–Rocci, 1896)

1. Make the subject sit or lie in supine and allow 5 minutes for mental and physical relaxation (Fig. 3.2.4).
2. Open the lid of the apparatus. Release the lock on the mercury reservoir and check that the mercury is at the zero level. If it is above zero, subtract the difference from the final reading. If it is below zero, add the required amount of mercury to bring it to zero level.
3. Place the cuff around the upper arm with the center of the bag lying over the brachial artery keeping its lower

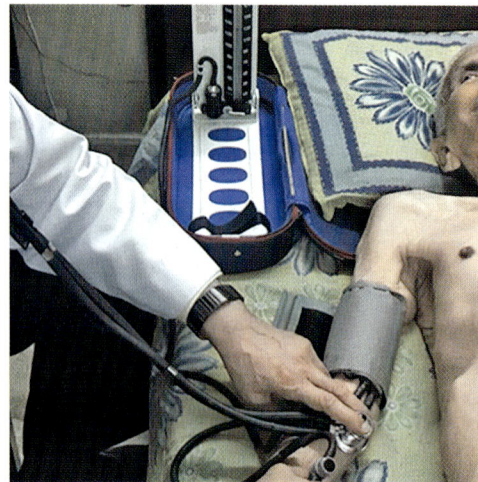

Fig. 3.2.4: Recording of blood pressure (BP) in supine position.

edge about 3 cm above the elbow (antecubital fossa). The cuff should neither be too tight nor very loose. It should be ensured that the arm is at the level of the heart.
4. Palpate the radial artery at the wrist and feel its pulsations with the tips of your fingers. Keeping your fingers on the pulse, hold the air bulb in the palm of your other hand and tighten the leak valve screw with your thumb and fingers.
5. Inflate the cuff slowly until the pulsations disappear; note the reading then raise the pressure for another 30–40 mm Hg.
6. Open the leak valve and control it so that the pressure gradually falls in steps of 2–4 mm Hg. Note the reading when the pulse just reappears. **The pressure at which the pulse is first felt is the SBP** (it corresponds to the time when at the peak of each systole, small amounts of blood start to flow through the compressed segment of the brachial artery). Deflate the bag quickly to bring the mercury to the zero level.

> **NOTE**
> It is easier to detect the reappearance of radial pulse than its disappearance. The first 2–3 beats being feeble may be missed so that the actual SBP is 4–6 mm Hg higher than the recorded value.

7. Record the pressure in the other arm. Take three readings in each arm, deflating the cuff for a few minutes between each determination.

Advantages of Palpatory Method

This method avoids the pitfall of the auscultatory method in missing the auscultatory gap.

Disadvantages of Palpatory Method

- This method measures only SBP. The DBP cannot be measured.
- This method lacks accuracy because the SBP measured by it is lower than the actual value by 4–6 mm Hg. It assumes that the first escape of blood under the cuff will cause pulsations in the peripheral artery (radial in this case). Definite pulsation may not occur until the cuff pressure has been reduced by 6–8 mm Hg.

Oscillatory Method

When the cuff pressure is raised and then lowered, oscillations appear which become maximum and then disappear. The appearance of oscillations represent the SBP while their disappearance represents the DBP.

Auscultatory Method

> **NOTE**
> Before recording the BP by the auscultatory method, it should always be first recorded by the palpatory method so as to avoid missing the auscultatory gap.

> **NOTE**
> Ordinarily no sounds are heard when the chest piece of a stethoscope is applied over the brachial (or any other) artery. However, if the cuff pressure is raised above the expected SBP and then gradually lowered, a series of sounds called **Korotkoff sounds** are heard over the artery just below the cuff.

1. Place the cuff over the upper arm as described earlier and record the BP by the palpatory method.
2. Locate the brachial artery in the antecubital fossa just medial to the tendon of the biceps.
3. Place the chest piece of the stethoscope on this point and keep it in position.

> **NOTE**
> The chest piece should not rub against the cuff, rubber tubes or the skin in this area because these disturbing noises will interfere with auscultation of sounds.

4. Inflate the cuff rapidly by using the rubber bulb. Raise the pressure to 40–50 mm Hg above the systolic level as determined by the palpatory method.
5. Lower the pressure gradually until a clear, sharp and tapping sound is heard. Continue to lower the pressure and try to note a change in the character of the sounds.

   These sounds are called Korotkoff sounds and show the following phases (Fig. 3.2.5):
   - **Phase I:** This phase starts with a faint tapping sound when a jet of blood is able to cross the previously obstructed artery. As the pressure is lowered, the sounds continue as sharp and clear taps. This phase lasts for 10–12 mm Hg fall in pressure.

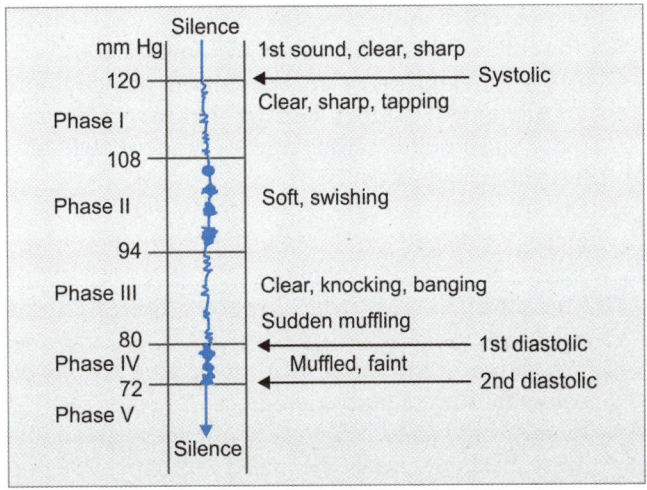

Fig. 3.2.5: Phases of Korotkoff sounds showing the changes in their character during each phase as the mercury column is gradually lowered. Systolic pressure: First appearance of sounds. Diastolic pressure: Sudden muffling of sounds.

> **NOTE**
> **Criterion of systolic pressure:** The level at which the first sound is heard, is taken as the SBP.

- **Phase II:** The sounds become murmurish and remain so during the next 10–14 mm Hg fall in pressure.
- **Phase III:** The sound becomes clearer and louder that continue for the next 12–14 mm Hg pressure.
- **Phase IV:** The sound becomes muffled in character lasting for next 5 mm Hg fall in pressure.
- **Phase V:** This phase begins when the Korotkoff sounds disappear completely.

> **NOTE**
> The level at which the sound disappears is marked as DBP. In children and in patients with severe hypertension muffling (phase IV) rather than the disappearance (phase V) of sound is marked as DBP.

6. Take three readings with the auscultatory method.

PRECAUTIONS

1. The subject should be physically and mentally relaxed. He/she should be assured and rested for 5 minutes or so to avoid the condition of **"white coat hypertension"** (i.e. some people have higher BP readings in the clinician's office than during their normal daytime activity).
2. The sphygmomanometer should be checked for zero error if any.
3. The arm, with the cuff wrapped around it, should be kept at the level of the heart to avoid the influence of gravity. The cuff tubing should not rub against the chest piece of the stethoscope.
4. The cuff should neither be too tight nor too loose.
5. The cuff should not be left inflated with high pressure for any length of time because the discomfort and reflex spasm of the artery and its branches will give false high readings.
6. Do not apply pressure on the artery with the chest piece as this may produce partial obstruction of the artery and a fake low reading.
7. Check the pulse rate at the time of recording BP as the HR affects the BP.
8. The palpatory method must always be employed before the auscultatory method.
9. In suspected and known cases of hypertension, the pressure should always be raised well above 200 mm Hg or above the level estimated by palpatory method.
10. In obese subjects, a cuff that is wider than the standard should be used. Similarly, when measuring the pressures in the thigh, the cuff should be wider because the thick layer of fat in the obese or the large amounts of tissues in the thigh dissipates some of the cuff pressure, thus giving false high results (the BP may be recorded with the cuff on the forearm while palpating and auscultating the radial artery).

Objective Structured Practical Examination–I

Aim: To record the BP of the subject provided by the palpatory method.
Procedural steps: See text above.
Checklist:
1. Check the zero reading of the manometer. Explain the procedure. Expose the arm up to the shoulder. (Y/N)
2. Wrap the cuff firmly around the upper arm, keeping its lower edge about 3 cm above the elbow and its middle lying over the brachial artery. (Y/N)
3. Keep the BP apparatus at the level of the heart. Open the stopcock between the two limbs of the mercury manometer. (Y/N)
4. Palpate the brachial artery and mark its position. Then hold the rubber bulb in the right hand, close the leak valve screw and inflate the cuff slowly until the radial pulse disappears. (Y/N)
5. Release the pressure in the cuff slowly till the radial pulse reappears. Note the reading. (Y/N)

Objective Structured Practical Examination–II

Aim: To record the BP of the subject provided by the auscultatory method.
Procedural steps: See text above.
Checklist:
1. Check the BP apparatus and stethoscope and expose the upper arm. (Y/N)
2. Record the BP by the palpatory method. (Y/N)
3. Correctly locate the lower end of the brachial artery. Then apply the ear pieces of the stethoscope to the ears and place its chest piece over the brachial artery. (Y/N)
4. Inflate the cuff rapidly and raise the mercury column to a high level. (Y/N)
5. Lower the pressure slowly in steps of 2–3 mm Hg till systolic and diastolic pressures are recorded, note the readings. (Y/N)

QUESTIONS

Q.1. What is mean arterial pressure and what is its significance?
Mean arterial pressure (MAP) is the average pressure during the cardiac cycle.
Significance of mean arterial pressure
MAP of about 95 mm Hg provides the pressure head or the **driving force** (vis-a-tergo) for the flow of blood through the arteries, capillaries and veins, etc. The MAP in medium-sized arteries (e.g. radial) is about 90 mm Hg. Thus, most viscera, muscles and other tissues are perfused at a relatively high pressure. Mean pressure of about 85–80 mm Hg at the start of arterioles falls to about 32 mm Hg at their capillary ends

(thus, maximum fall in pressure occurs in the arterioles). The pressure then continues to fall progressively till it reaches zero in the right atrium. The pressure gradient of about 95 mm Hg is responsible for the **circulation of blood and tissue perfusion.**

Q.2. What is pulse pressure and what is its significance?
Pulse pressure is the difference between SBP and DBP, the average PP being about 40 mm Hg. Other factors remaining unchanged, the magnitude of PP indicates the stroke volume. Thus, it provides information about the condition of CVS. For example, conditions, such as atherosclerosis (hardening of blood vessels) and patent ductus arteriosus generally increase the PP. The normal ratio of SBP to DBP and to PP is about 3:2:1.

Q.3. Name the precautions that you will observe while recording blood pressure.

Q.4. What are the advantages and disadvantages of palpatory method of recording blood pressure?

Q.5. What will be the effect of using a wrong sized blood pressure cuff in different age groups or a standard cuff in a very obese person?
If an over- or undersized cuff is used, the reading will be higher than actual because more pressure would be required in the cuff to overcome tissue resistance and to form a cone of pressure.

When a standard cuff is used in an obese individual, the reading will be higher than actual because of loss of pressure in overcoming tissue resistance.

Q.6. What are Korotkoff sounds and how are they produced?
Normally, the blood flow through the arteries is laminar or streamline and no sounds are heard when a stethoscope is placed on them. When the cuff pressure is raised above the expected SBP and then gradually lowered, a time comes, when at the peak of each systole, the intra-arterial pressure just exceeds the cuff (extra-arterial) pressure. But, in between these peaks, the artery is still constricted. Now, it is known that constriction of an artery increases the velocity of blood flow through the constricted part. Thus, when the small amounts of blood are jetted through the partially constricted artery, their velocity increases and then exceed the critical velocity. This produces **intermittent turbulence** that in turn produces Korotkoff sounds (beyond the constriction) which have a staccato quality (tapping intermittent sounds).

When the cuff pressure is near the diastolic level, the artery is still partially constricted, but **the turbulent flow is now continuous rather than intermittent** and sounds from continuous turbulent flow have a muffled quality rather than a tapping or staccato quality. As the cuff pressure further falls, the blood flow becomes laminar once again and the sounds disappear. The change in the character of sounds during early phases is related to the degree of turbulence.

Q.7. What is auscultatory gap and what is its significance?
In some patients of hypertension, there may be a gap in the Korotkoff sounds. As the mercury is lowered, a few faint sounds are heard which soon disappear only to reappear once again at a lower pressure. This brief interruption which may range from 40 to 60 mm Hg is called **"auscultatory" or "silent" gap**. If the mercury column is raised to this gap and then the pressure lowered, one may miss the first appearance of sounds which indicate SBP and thus record a false low SBP.

To avoid this mistake, the BP should always be recorded by the palpatory method first. Then during auscultatory method, the mercury column must be raised 30–40 mm Hg above the level found by palpatory method.

Q.8. When recording blood pressure, why should the upper arm with the cuff wrapped around its kept at the level of the heart?
The force of gravity exerts an important effect on the BP readings. The degree of its effect varies with the vertical distance above and below the level of the heart.

Q.9. What are the physiological variations in blood pressure?
Normally, variations in BP occur as mentioned here:
1. Age
2. Sex
3. Body build and obesity
4. **Diurnal variations:** The BP is lowest under basal conditions, the peak being seen in the late afternoon, mainly in the systolic level. The SP shows a significant fall during sleep.
5. **Emotional stress:** Hypertension is a natural response to pain and stress in nonhypertensive individuals. The SP rises during anger, apprehension, excitement, etc. Some hypertensives because of nervousness have higher BP in the clinician's office than during their normal daytime activity—a condition which has been called **white coat hypertension**.
6. Posture
7. Muscular exercise.
8. **Sleep:** The BP, both systolic and diastolic, tend to be low during the early restful stage of sleep, especially SBP which may fall by 15–20 mm Hg due to general relaxation, decrease in sympathetic tone, etc. Meditation has the same effect.
9. Pregnancy.

Q.10. How is arterial blood pressure maintained and controlled?
Establishing and maintaining blood pressure
There are five basic factors involved in establishing and maintaining systemic arterial BP. They include: (1) pumping action of the heart, (2) peripheral resistance, (3) elasticity of large blood vessels, (4) the volume of circulating blood and (5) the viscosity of blood.

Q.11. How is blood pressure regulated on short-term, intermediate term and long-term basis?
The BP regulatory mechanisms may be divided into: Short-term, intermediate-term and long-term processes. Short-term regulation is mainly neural while long-term regulation is hormonal.
1. *Short-term regulation of blood pressure:* This mechanism is **lifesaving** and functions from moment-to-moment and minute-to-minute (e.g. sudden standing from supine position may decrease the BP significantly and cause fainting. It involves baroreceptors, chemoreceptors and central nervous system (CNS) ischemic response.
2. *Intermediate term regulation of blood pressure:* This mechanism is **life-sustaining** and functions from day-to-day and from week-to-week. It involves movement of

tissue fluid into circulation by **capillary fluid shift** and **stress relaxation** of vessels.

3. *Long-term regulation of blood pressure:* This mechanism is **life-stabilizing** and functions over months and years. It involves **renal body fluids volume system** because the kidney is the major organ that regulates extracellular and thus intracellular fluid volume. The hormones involved include: Renin-angiotensin-aldosterone, catecholamines, vasopressin (ADH), ANP and nitric oxide (NO).

> **NOTE**
> The sinoaortic baroreceptors are not effective for intermediate- and long-term regulation of BP because they are "reset" at a higher level in 1–2 days.

Q.12. What is hypertension and what are its causes and complications?

Classification of hypertension

The disease is grouped into the following two main categories:

1. *Essential hypertension:* About 90–95% of hypertensives belong to this category in which the cause of the high pressure is not known—although obesity, high salt intake, alcohol ingestion, heredity and mental makeup (tense, irritable and overambitious individuals; the type I personality) are believed to play a role.
2. *Secondary hypertension:* The remaining 5–10% of hypertensives belongs to this group in which the cause of high BP is known. Secondary hypertension which is curable should always be considered in patients under age of 30 years or those who develop hypertension after age of 55 years. Its common causes are:
   a. Renal diseases.
   b. Coarctation of aorta
   c. Endocrine diseases: Pheochromocytoma (catecholamine-secreting) tumor of adrenal medulla (hyperaldosteronism) and Cushing syndrome (hyperthyroidism).
   d. Toxemias of pregnancy.

Malignant hypertension

In some patients, the BP, especially the DP, is accelerated and rises to very high levels within a short time (DP above 120 mm Hg is a medical emergency). If untreated, the patient may die within 1–2 years.

Complications of hypertension

Hypertension has been called a "silent killer". It may go unnoticed and undiagnosed for years when permanent damage has already occurred in vital organs. The common causes of death are myocardial infarction (*heart attack*), hemorrhage or occlusion of a blood vessel in the brain (*brain attack*) and renal failure. Hemorrhages in the retina may cause blindness.

Q.13. What is hypotension and what are its effects?

Hypotension or low BP is hardly if ever considered a disease or a cause of alarm in otherwise healthy individuals. However, the BP may show low readings under certain conditions:

1. **Sudden fall in blood pressure:** This may be due to myocardial infarction, acute loss of large amounts of blood, severe diarrhea and vomiting and excessive intake of diuretics. The person may go into a state of shock.
2. **Postural hypotension:** When the SBP falls by 20 mm Hg or more on sudden standing from supine position (*See* Fig. 3.2.5), it is called postural hypotension. It is usually due to autonomic insufficiency as a result of diabetic polyneuropathy or during treatment with sympatholytic drugs in hypertension. Rising from bed after prolonged illness may also cause fall in BP.
3. *Chronic primary hypotension:* It is seen in some elderly persons, but its cause is not known.

> **NOTE**
> The BP readings are seldom identical in the two arms. It has been suggested that both arms be used, preferably the right arm and then the left arm.

OBSERVATION AND RESULT

Tabulate your results as shown here.
For report, express your result as: **SBP/DBP mm Hg**

Record of systemic arterial blood pressure				
A. *Palpatory method (mm Hg)*				
First reading				
Second reading				
Third reading				
B. *Auscultatory method (mm Hg)*				
	Systolic pressure	Diastolic pressure	Mean arterial pressure	Pulse pressure
First reading				
Second reading				
Third reading				
Final reading				

INTERPRETATION

....
....
....
....
....

STUDY NOTES

Date ....

CHAPTER 3.3

Effect of Posture on Blood Pressure and Heart Rate

AIM

To study the effect of posture on blood pressure.

INTRODUCTION

1. Gravity affects the fluid distribution in man. As the person changes the position from lying to sitting and then to standing, the blood is redistributed to regions below heart toward the splanchnic, pelvic and leg vasculature.
2. This results in decreased venous return causing fall in BP; unchecked this can lead to loss of consciousness and ultimately death.
3. There are physiological adaptations in human cardiovascular system to counteract the effect of gravity on the circulatory system under postural changes, such as in standing, sitting and lying down position.

BLOOD PRESSURE AND HEART RATE RESPONSES AFTER CHANGE IN POSTURE

The effect of changes in posture on BP and HR depends on whether these are recorded immediately after sitting or standing from supine position or after prolonged standing. Prolonged standing, poses an additional problem because of increased capillary hydrostatic pressure which causes fluid to be filtered out into the tissues that leads to further decrease in venous return. There is also increased catecholamine release and renin-angiotensin aldosterone system (RAAS) activation to restore the BP during prolonged standing (*See* Flowchart 3.3.1).

APPARATUS

1. Sphygmomanometer
2. Stethoscope
3. Watch.

PROCEDURE

1. Allow the subject to rest and relax for at least 5 minutes in the supine position before recording the BP. Record the HR (pulse rate) and BP. Disconnect the cuff from the BP apparatus but do not untie the cuff from the arm.
2. Ask the subject to sit up and immediately record the BP and HR. Repeat the determinations after 1 minute, 2 minutes and 5 minutes.
3. Ask the subject to lie down again and rest for a few minutes. Then record the BP and HR. Now ask him to suddenly stand up and record the BP and HR immediately. Repeat the determinations after 1 minute, 2 minutes and 5 minutes.
4. Record your observations below.

PRECAUTIONS

1. The subject should relax for at least 5 minutes before recording BP and pulse rate in the supine position.
2. Record the BP in the arm, with the cuff wrapped around it, at the level of the heart.
3. Do not remove the cuff in between the estimations but leave it in position by disconnecting the connection between the cuff and the mercury reservoir. (Aneroid BP apparatus is preferred nowadays).

Flowchart 3.3.1: Compensatory mechanism on immediate sitting/standing from supine position.

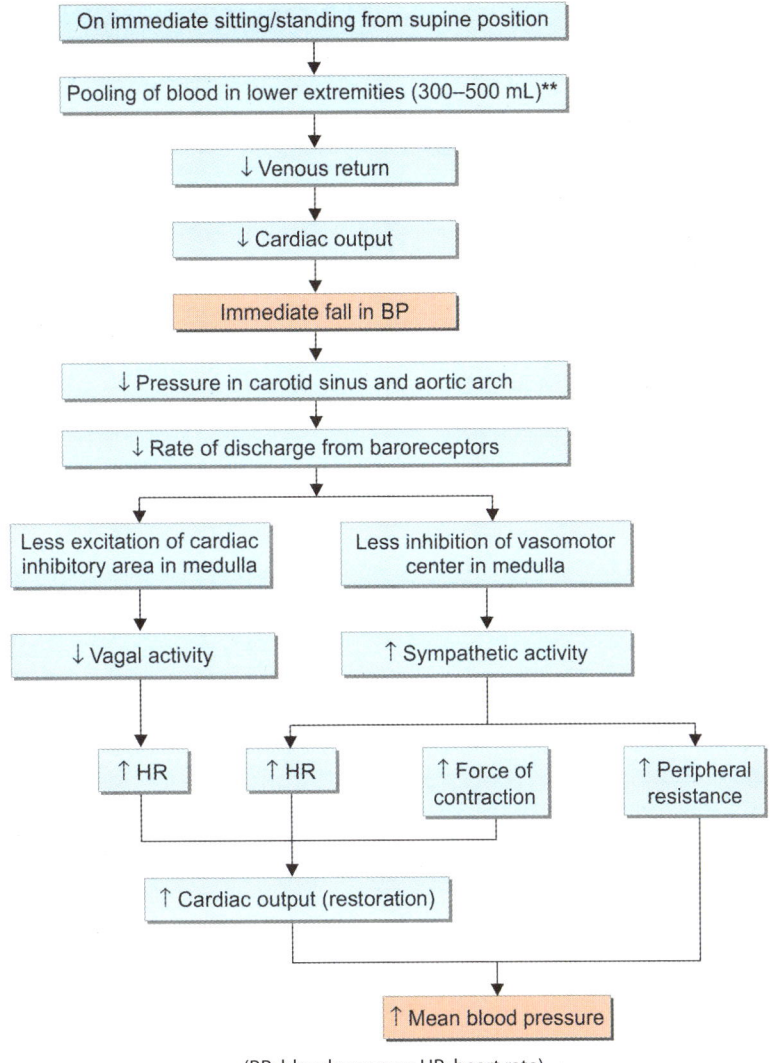

(BP: blood pressure; HR: heart rate)

**In standing position, BP changes are more marked as compared to that in sitting position, because of greater pooling (300–500 mL) of blood in lower extremities. HR increases in sitting and standing position as compared to that in supine position because of decreased vagal tone.

4. Record the heart rate and BP as soon as possible after a change in posture within 30 seconds (preferably within 10-15 seconds) because the changes in BP are rapid and short lasting.

PHYSIOCLINICAL SIGNIFICANCE

1. Effect of change in posture on BP and HR helps to assess the *integrity of the autonomic nervous system (ANS)*.
2. The consequences of prolonged standing are commonly seen in sentries, soldiers and traffic policemen. They are, therefore, advised to tense their leg muscles and walk around from time to time (to promote venous return by the *muscle pump*). They also wear "wrappings" (tight strips of thick cloth) around their legs.
3. Through this practical, we can come to know if the person is having postural hypotension or not.
   a. In some individuals, within 3 minutes of sudden standing there is a significant fall in BP (fall in systolic pressure of more than 20 mm Hg or fall in diastolic pressure of more than 10 mm Hg), which results in fainting. This is called *postural or orthostatic hypotension* (orthostatic = upright posture of the body; hypo = less + tension = pressure).
   b. Symptoms are: Lightheadedness, weakness, blurred vision and syncope.
   c. Seen in the following conditions:
      - Dehydration, blood loss.
      - Antihypertensive medication

Section 3: Human Experiments

- Old age (because of decreased baroreceptor sensitivity).
- Autonomic neuropathy (diabetes and syphilis).
- Primary autonomic failure.

Objective Structured Practical Examination

Aim: To record the effect of sudden standing from sitting position on the BP of the patient provided.

Procedural steps: See text above.

Checklist:
1. Explain the procedure to the patient and check the BP apparatus and stethoscope.
2. Record the BP by the palpatory and auscultatory methods. Note the heart rate.
3. Without removing the cuff, asks the patient to stand up quickly without support.
4. Record the blood pressure within 30 seconds.
5. Note the heart rate.

QUESTIONS

- Q.1. Why should BP be recorded within 30 seconds of change of body posture?
- Q.2. What is vasovagal syncope?
- Q.3. What is postural hypotension?
- Q.4. Discuss the physioclinical significance of this practical.

OBSERVATION AND RESULT

Compare heart rate, systolic blood pressure, diastolic blood pressure, pulse pressure and mean arterial pressure in lying, sitting and standing position. Enter the readings below.

Blood pressure and heart rate responses after change in posture.

Posture		HR	SBP	DBP	PP	MAP
Lying						
Sitting	Immediately					
	After 1 minute					
	After 2 minutes					
	After 5 minutes					
Standing	Immediately					
	After 1 minute					
	After 2 minutes					
	After 5 minutes					

(DBP: diastolic blood pressure; HR: heart rate; MAP: mean arterial pressure; PP: pulse pressure; SBP: systolic blood pressure)

INTERPRETATION

....

....

....

....

....

STUDY NOTES

CHAPTER 3.4

Effect of Exercise on Blood Pressure and Heart Rate

AIM

To record the effect of moderate exercise on blood pressure and heart rate.

INTRODUCTION

The effect of exercise on blood pressure (BP) and heart rate (HR) depends on the following:
1. **Intensity of exercise:** According to the WHO grading, exercise can be divided into mild, moderate, heavy and severe (Table 3.4.1).
2. **Type of exercise:** The exercise can be primarily isotonic or isometric (Table 3.4.2)

Effect of isotonic exercise: The arterial blood pressure starts to rise with the onset of exercise and the increase in BP roughly parallels the severity of exercise performed.

Table 3.4.2: Types of muscular exercise.

Isotonic exercise	Isometric exercise
Exercise in which there is a change in muscle length, e.g. walking, jogging and running	Exercise in which there is no change in muscle length, e.g. pushing against the wall
Systolic blood pressure (SBP) rises only moderately, whereas diastolic blood pressure (DBP) varies as explained below.	Within a few seconds of the onset of exercise, SBP and DBP rise sharply
Cardiac output increases markedly due to increase in HR and stroke volume	Stroke volume changes relatively little
Blood flow to exercising muscle increases	Blood flow to steadily contracting muscle is decreased, as a result of compression of their blood vessel

Table 3.4.1: World Health Organization (WHO) grading of exercise.

Grade	Level	Heart rate (beats/min)	O_2 consumption (L/min)	Relative load index (RLI) (% of maximum O_2 consumption)	METs
I	Mild	<100	0.4–0.8	<25	<3
II	Moderate	100–125	0.8–1.6	25–50	3.1–4.5
III	Heavy	125–150	1.6–2.4	51–75	4.6–7
IV	Severe	>150	>2.4	>75	>7

VO_2 max is the maximum oxygen consumption.
Metabolic equivalent of task (METs) is the oxygen consumption in multiples of basal oxygen consumption.
RLI (relative load index) is the oxygen consumption as a percentage of VO_2 maximum.

SBP and mean BP both increase in mild, moderate and severe exercise. There is a continuous increase in the cardiac output (CO) with increase in severity of exercise. DBP remains unchanged in mild exercise or it may fall slightly during moderate exercise.

During severe exercise, the DBP may increase slightly as sympathetic vasoconstrictor activity supersedes the vasodilator influence on the cutaneous blood vessels.

> **NOTE**
> Training of an individual results in lower basal HR (because of higher vagal tone and a lower sympathetic tone), lower submaximal HR with exercise, increased stroke volume and lower peripheral resistance than they had before training. During exercise, the maximal HR of a trained individual is same as that in an untrained person, but it is attained at a higher level of exercise.

APPARATUS

1. Sphygmomanometer
2. Stethoscope
3. Harvard/Master step.

PROCEDURE (EFFECT OF MODERATE ISOTONIC EXERCISE)

1. Make the subject comfortable and record the BP and the pulse rate of the given subject after 5 minutes of rest.
2. Ask the subject to perform any of these exercises: **spot running** with the thighs brought up to the horizontal alternately, for 3–5 minutes; **hopping** on each foot for 3 minutes raising the feet 12–15 inches off the ground; **climbing up and down the stairs**; **jogging, Master's two step test** (Fig. 3.4.1) or **Harvard step test**.

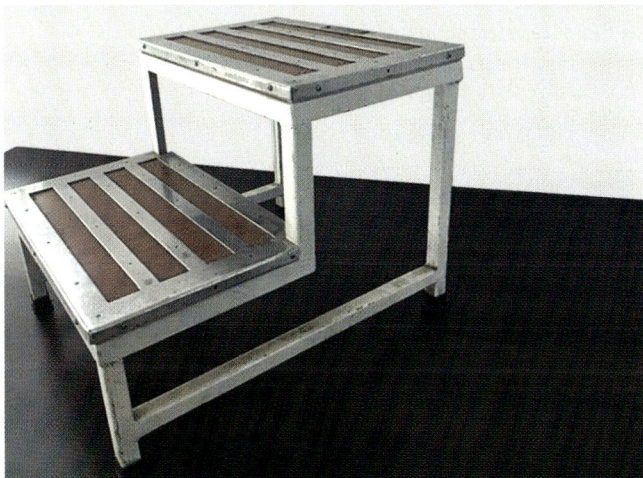

Fig. 3.4.1: Two-step exercise test.

> **NOTE**
> - **Harvard** step is a single level bench, 20 inches or 50 cm. in height is used. A stepping rate of 30 per minute is adjusted with the help of a metronome.
> - **Master's** two step test utilizes a two-step bench (22.5 cm per step). The stepping rate is determined from tables based on weight and age. The speed of climbing up and down should be kept constant by using a metronome.

3. Record the pulse rate and BP immediately, 2, 4, 6, 8 and 10 minutes after exercise.
4. Calculate pulse pressure, mean pressure and compare the pre- and postexercise values.

> **NOTE**
> Graded exercise can also be performed on a bicycle ergometer or treadmill.

PHYSIOCLINICAL SIGNIFICANCE

The effects of regular exercise on health are well-known.

There is a marked improvement of cardiovascular function, especially endurance. The basal heart rate decreases due to increased vagal tone. The stroke volume increases due to increased cardiac muscle mass (hypertrophy). A trained athlete achieves the target CO mainly by increasing stroke volume, while in an untrained individual, CO increases chiefly by increase in HR.

- The respiratory benefits include increased breathing capacity and maximal O_2 extraction.
- The size of skeletal muscles increases along with work capacity.
- Exercise also promotes better mental functions. The "feel good" effect can work as a powerful treatment for depression.

Long-term Benefits

Experts say that if you do moderate exercise, say, brisk walking for 30–40 minutes most days of the week, you can cut down the risks of heart attacks and strokes, hypertension, diabetes mellitus, arthritis, etc. This exercise regimen, combined with dietary and lifestyle changes raises the "good" high-density lipoprotein (HDL) cholesterol, while lowering the "bad" low-density lipoprotein (LDL) cholesterol.

PRECAUTIONS

1. The recording of HR and BP before and after exercise should be recorded in the same posture.
2. The sphygmomanometer cuff should be disconnected from the tubing while exercising.

3. If during exercise the subject feels discomfort, fatigue and pain in the legs, breathlessness, giddiness and suffocation tell him/her to discontinue the exercise.

> **NOTE**
> Blood pressure returns to normal within 5–7 minutes of termination of moderate exercise whereas the HR takes a longer time to return to normal.

Objective Structured Practical Examination

Aim: To record the effect of exercise on the BP of the subject provided.
Procedural steps: See text above.
Checklist:
1. Explain the procedure to the subject and check the BP apparatus and stethoscope. (Y/N)
2. Record the BP by the palpatory and auscultatory methods. Note the heart rate. (Y/N)
3. Without removing the cuff, ask the subject to do exercise. (Y/N)
4. Record the BP and HR following exercise at appropriate intervals. (Y/N).

QUESTIONS

Q.1. What is the WHO criteria of grading the exercise based on HR?

Q.2. What are the different types of classification of exercises?
1. **Based on metabolic consideration: Aerobic and anaerobic exercise**
   Aerobic exercises are those that primarily rely on oxygen to supply energy. These include jogging, cycling, spot running, rebounding (running in place on a mini trampoline), swimming, skipping rope, etc.
   Anaerobic exercise is short-lasting, high-intensity activity, where your body's demand for oxygen exceeds the oxygen supply available. **Therefore, the energy is supplied mainly by anaerobic mechanisms.**
2. **Based on muscle shortening and lengthening:**
   Isotonic exercises are those where muscle tension remains the same while the length of the muscle changes during contraction. The two types of isotonic contractions are **concentric isotonic** where a muscle shortens and produces movement (e.g. flexion of elbow) and **eccentric isotonic** where a muscle gradually lengthens while continuing to contract (e.g. gradually lowering a weight held in the hand such as in weight lifting).
   In **isometric exercises,** the tension in the muscle increases during contraction without a change in muscle length.

Q.3. What are the effects of muscular exercise on cardiovascular system?
1. **Effects of acute isotonic exercise**
   a. *Heart rate:* There is a quick rise in HR, the increase depending on the severity of exercise. The maximum HR achieved in young persons may be 180–200 beats/min. In older persons, it may increase to 150–160 beats/min.
   b. *Cardiac output:* There is an increase in HR and CO, the latter may increase to 25 L/min or even more. This is due to generalized sympathetic excitation.
   c. *Systolic blood pressure:* The increased rate and force of heart causes a prompt rise of SBP.
   d. *Diastolic blood pressure:* The diastolic blood pressure may remain the same, increase a little or even decrease somewhat, i.e. it is affected to a much less degree.
   e. *Muscle blood flow:* As a result of local metabolites in the contracting muscles (increased CO, K^+, H^+, adenosine, increased osmolality and decreased pO_2) and activity of sympathetic vasodilator nerve supply to the exercising muscles, there is vasodilatation. This increases the blood flow to the working muscles.
2. **Effects of long-term isotonic exercise**
   See physioclinical significance above.

Q.4. What are the benefits of regular exercise?

Q.5. What is steady state exercise?
A steady state exercise is that muscular activity where oxygen consumption increases upon exercise onset to attain a steady level, which can be maintained for a long period of time. In this state, the energy requirement for the working muscles are matched by the oxygen supply available. It is reached at about 4–5 minutes after moderate exercise.

OBSERVATION AND RESULT

Record your observation in the table below.

	HR	SBP	DBP	PP	MAP
Before exercise					
Immediately after exercise					
Two minutes after exercise					
Four minutes after exercise					
Six minutes after exercise					
Eight minutes after exercise					
Ten minutes after exercise					

HR returned to resting level after ……………… minutes
BP returned to resting level after ……………… minutes

(DBP: diastolic blood pressure; HR: heart rate; MAP: mean arterial pressure; PP: pulse pressure; SBP: systolic blood pressure)

INTERPRETATION

……………………………………………………………………………
……………………………………………………………………………
……………………………………………………………………………
……………………………………………………………………………
……………………………………………………………………………

STUDY NOTES

Date ....

CHAPTER 3.5

Recording and Interpretation of an Electrocardiogram

AIM

To record an electrocardiogram (ECG).

INTRODUCTION

Electrocardiogram (ECG/EKG) is a graphic representation of the electrical activity associated with heart beat. **Electrocardiography** is the method of recording an electrocardiogram. The machine that records an ECG is called the **electrocardiograph.** Since the body is a good volume conductor, the electrical activity spreads from the heart to the body surface from where, after suitable amplification, it can be graphically recorded as the ECG. Thus, the ECG recorded at the body surface represents the algebraic summation of activity of individual cardiac muscle cells, i.e. **the algebraic summation of action potential of the individual cardiac muscle cells**.

APPARATUS

1. Electrograph (ECG machine)
2. Electrodes
3. Electrode jelly
4. Electrocardiogram paper

1. **The electrocardiogram machine (Fig. 3.5.1):** The **electrocardiograph** works on the household current AC—230 V or on battery and has a very **sensitive galvanometer**. The potentials picked up from the surface of the body are suitably **amplified** before flowing through the galvanometer. **The ECG machine can have single channel/3 channel/6 channel or 12 channel recording facility**. **The recording** facility consists of an electrically heated stylus that inscribes on a chemically treated/wax coated paper.

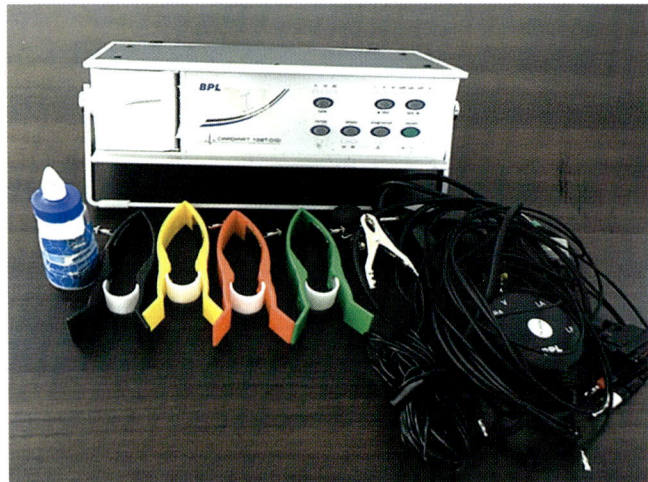

Fig. 3.5.1: Electrocardiogram (ECG) machine (single channel recording).

The control panel of the machine has the following main components:
- **Mains switch:** The on/off switch controls the power supply. A filter cuts off unwanted 50 Hz interference.
- **Calibration/sensitivity switch:** A commonly used sensitivity is 1 mV/10 mm, so that a calibration signal of 1 mV causes a pen deflection of 10 mm.

- **Centering knob:** The baseline control knob is used for bringing the pen to the center of the paper. This knob is not required in modern machines.
- **Lead selector switch:** It permits selection of various unipolar or bipolar electrodes.

2. **Electrodes:** The electrodes for the limbs are flat metal plates which are kept in position by rubber straps or plastic clamps. The chest electrode is a metal cup which is kept in position by "suction" produced by a rubber bulb.

3. **The electrode jelly** is a paste that contains fine sand and glass particles. When it is rubbed on the skin it caused mild erythema, thereby reducing the skin resistance and enhancing the conduction of electric current. Cable lead wires connect the subject to the machine.

4. **Electrocardiogram paper:** The ECG paper
   - Is thermosensitive, wax coated/chemically treated standard graph paper.
   - Divided into 1 × 1 mm squares.
   - The horizontal axis represents time. Each small square on this axis = 0.04 second.
   - The vertical axis denotes the voltage. On this axis 10 mm =1 mV.
   - Since the machine is capped at the standard speed of 25 mm/s normally so the machine covers a distance of 1,500 mm horizontally in 1 minute (25 × 60).
   - In normal ECG, the HR = 1,500 mm/distance between two consecutive R waves in millimeter
   - When RR interval is irregular, i.e. not uniform, the number of QRS complexes counted in 5 s are multiplied by 12 to determine the average HR.

Electrocardiographic leads: The paired electrodes applied to the surface of the body along with wires connected to the machine completing the electric circuit constitute an ECG lead. There are 12 conventional leads which are used to record an ECG.

> **NOTE**
> There are ten electrodes ("4" electrodes on the limbs and "6" electrodes on the chest) that are put on the surface of the body to record a 12 lead ECG.

CLASSIFICATION OF ELECTROCARDIOGRAPHIC LEADS

The classification of electrocardiographic leads is described in **Flowchart 3.5.1**.

The leads are classified as unipolar/bipolar leads depending upon whether ECG is recorded using one exploring/active electrode (**unipolar**) or two exploring electrodes (**bipolar**). In **unipolar lead**, the active electrode acts as the positive pole and the other electrode (indifferent electrode) is kept at zero potential. **Precordial** (chest) leads and **augmented leads** (aVR, aVL and aVF) are unipolar leads. In **bipolar leads**, one electrode forms the positive pole and the other acts as a negative pole.

Bipolar limb leads/standard limb leads or "classical" limb leads I, II and III

These were the earliest leads to be used (Willem Einthoven of Leyden, 1860-1927). These leads measure the potential using two active electrodes placed on any two limbs and represent the algebraic sum of the potentials of two constituent active (electrodes) leads. The two shoulders and the point where the left thigh joins the torso form the Einthoven triangle (Fig. 3.5.2) as described here. Since the potentials at these points are the same as at the wrists and left ankle, the limb electrodes can be attached at these locations, as they are more convenient to use. The right leg (RL) is used as a ground electrode to reduce the electrical interference. There are three bipolar limb leads:

Flowchart 3.5.1: Classification of electrocardiogram (ECG) leads.

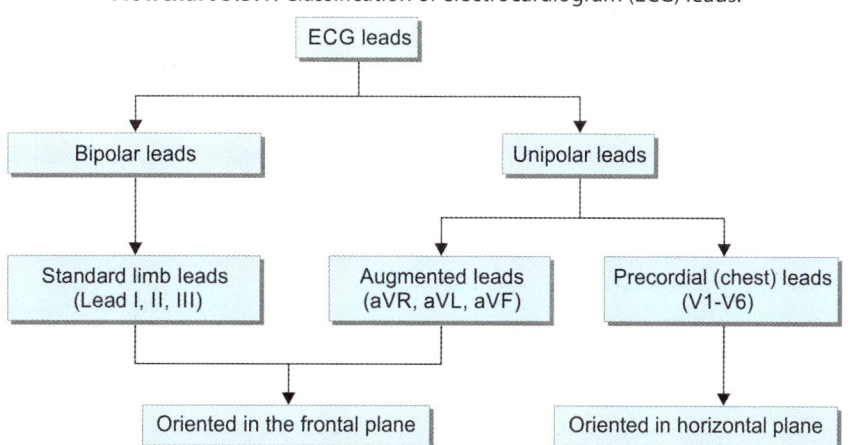

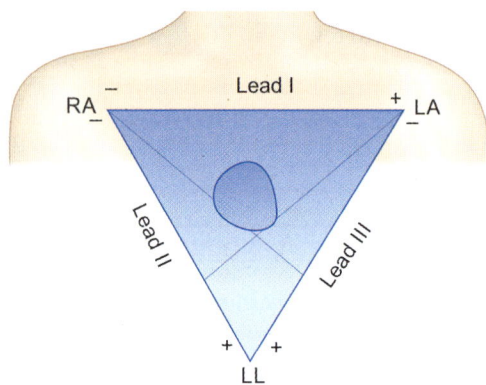

Fig. 3.5.2: The Einthoven's triangle.
[LA: left arm; LL: left leg (left foot); RA: right arm]

1. **Lead I:** It records the potential at the left arm (LA) minus the potential at the right arm (RA) or LA-RA (LA positive).
2. **Lead II:** It is the potential at the left leg (LL) minus the potential at RA or LL-RA (LL positive).
3. **Lead III:** This leads records the potential at the LL minus the potential at the LA or LL-LA (LL positive).

Einthoven's Triangle

As pointed out earlier (Fig. 3.5.2) the two shoulders and the point where left thigh joins the torso form the apices of an equilateral triangle—the Einthoven triangle—that surrounds the heart. The heart is thus placed approximately in the center of a volume conductor. Lines that bisect each side of the triangle (i.e. at the zero axis of each side, where the potential is zero at all times), meet the center of the triangle at the heart.

Einthoven's Law

The Einthoven law states that the sum of the potentials recorded in leads I and III will equal the potential in Lead II:

$$I + III = II$$

In other words, if the potentials of any two of the three limb leads are known at any instant, the third can be obtained mathematically just by summing the first two.

Unipolar Leads

These leads record the potential from a single region of the body (limbs or chest). In unipolar recording one electrode, the indifferent electrode, is kept at zero potential by connecting the three limb electrodes (right arm, left arm and left foot) to a common central terminal through 5000 Ω resistance in the machine where the currents from the 3 limbs neutralize each other. In a volume conductor, the sum of potentials at the points of an equilateral triangle with a current source in the center is zero at all times. Since, the 3 limbs are considered as the linear conductors connected to the points of equilateral triangle, the potentials recorded in these three limbs will be more or less the same. When the electrodes put on the 3 limbs are connected to a common central terminal, the sum of the three potentials is also zero. The insertion of high resistance (5,000 Ω) ensures zero potential in the eventuality if the sum of potentials from the three limbs does not become zero. This is how the indifferent electrode is kept at zero potential. The other electrode in unipolar recording is an exploring electrode that is put **on a limb** or **on the chest**. Thus, there are three such limb leads and a number of chest leads:

1. **Unipolar limb leads:** Any of the limb electrodes can be used to record cardiac potentials in comparison to the indifferent electrode kept at zero potential. Thus, there are three limb leads, each denoted by the letter V (vector)—(1) VR, (2) VL and (3) VF (left foot).
2. **Augmented limb leads:** Since the recorded voltages are small, disconnecting one lead from the common terminal increases the potential difference by 50%. Thus, the augmented limb leads are:
   - **aVR** = Between RA and (LA + LL)
   - **aVL** = Between LA and (RA + LL), and
   - **aVF** = Between LL and (RA + LA).

   The disconnection of a lead is automatically done in the ECG machine.
3. **Unipolar chest (precordial) leads:** These leads record the potentials from the anterior surface of the heart, from the right side to the left side of the chest in relation to the indifferent electrode (RA + LA + LL).

   The standardized sites for the unipolar chest leads are as follows (Fig. 3.5.3):
   - **V1** is in the fourth intercostal space (ICS), just to the right of the sternum.
   - **V2** is in the fourth ICS, just to the left of the sternum.
   - **V3** is halfway between V2 and V4.
   - **V4** is at the midclavicular line in the fifth ICS.
   - **V5** is in the anterior axillary line at the same level as V4 in the fifth ICS.
   - **V6** is in the midaxillary line in the fifth ICS.

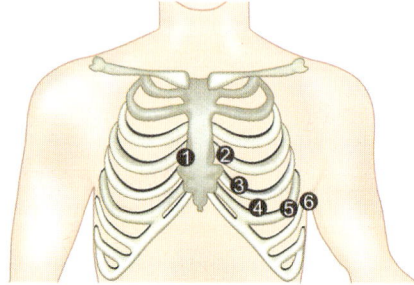

Fig. 3.5.3: Diagram to show the placing of unipolar precordial (chest) leads for recording electrocardiogram (ECG).

The 12-lead ECG is used to gain information about the orientation of the heart, size of its chambers and general direction of activation in the myocardium during any interval. It is also used to evaluate arrhythmias, conduction abnormalities, electrolytes disturbances, drug effects and location, extent and progress of myocardial ischemia and infarction.

PHYSIOLOGICAL BASIS OF ELECTROCARDIOGRAM

The wave of depolarization that spreads through the heart during each cardiac cycle has vector properties defined by its direction and magnitude. The net direction of the wave changes continuously during each cycle which causes changes in the deflections of the ECG. The size of the deflections is a function of muscle mass, while the direction of the waves depends on direction of depolarization. The electrical field of the heart decreases algebraically with the distance from the center. With distances greater than 15 cm from the heart, this decrement in the intensity of electric field is very small. Therefore, the electrodes when placed at a distance greater than 15 cm from the heart will record the same potential irrespective of the distance.

If the wave of depolarization spreads toward the positive electrode of a lead, the deflection is positive (upward). If it spreads toward the negative electrode, the deflection is negative (downward).

The ECG deflection produced by the atria (P wave) is smaller than that produced by the ventricular muscle (QRS) **(Fig. 3.5.4)**. The ventricular depolarization vector has two components:

1. **Septal vector:** It represents septal depolarization and is directed transversely from left to right through the lower third of the interventricular septum.
2. **Ventricular vector**: This represents the activation of the walls of left and right ventricles. It is directed from endocardium to epicardium and since the left ventricular muscle depolarization is dominant, the resultant direction is from right to left.

The various components of a normal electrocardiogram are shown in Fig. 3.5.5 and Table 3.5.1.

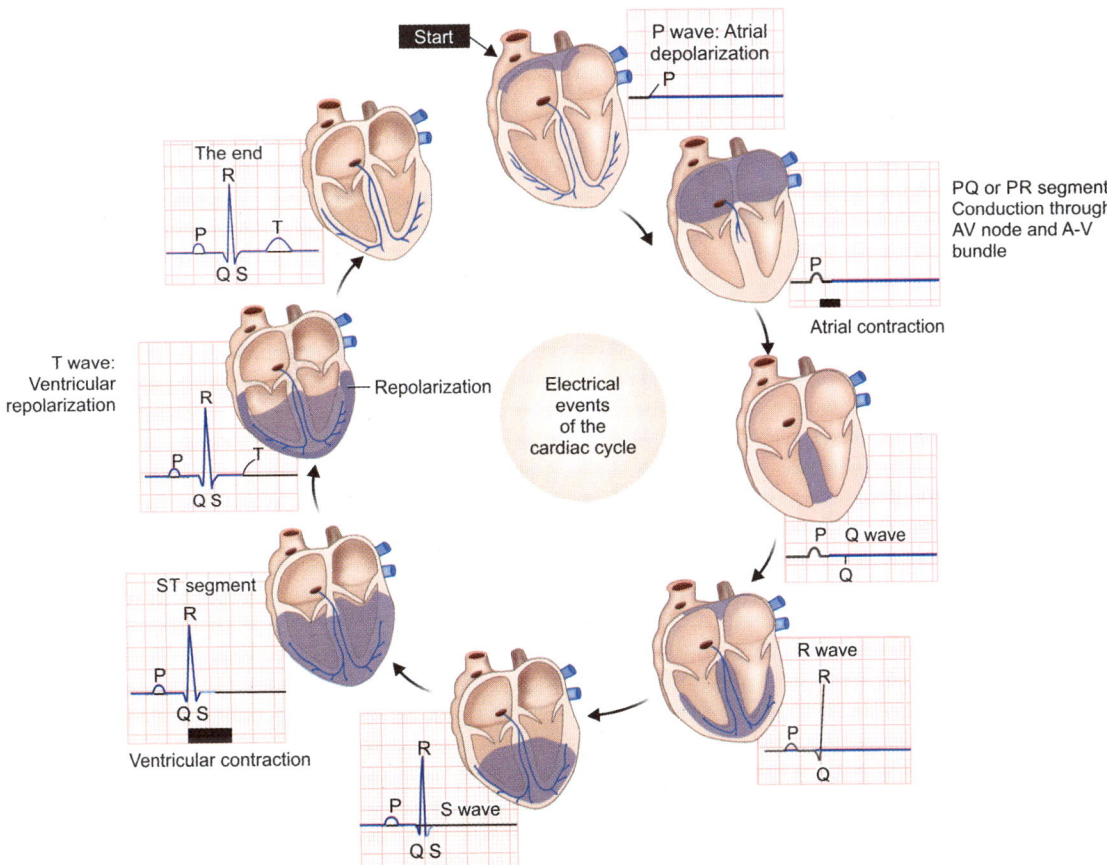

Fig. 3.5.4: Electrical events of cardiac cycle.

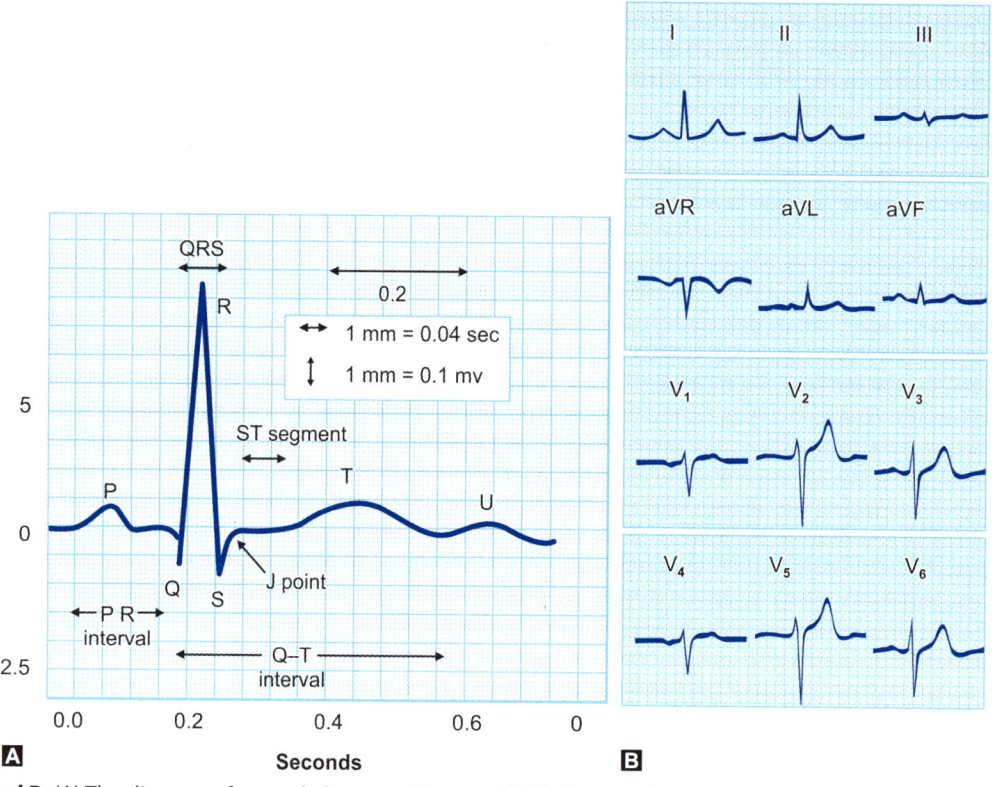

Figs. 3.5.5A and B: (A) The diagram of normal electrocardiogram (ECG) showing the various waves, segments, times and voltages; (B) The normal sequence of PQRS and T wave in an actual 12-channel ECG record; leads I, II, III, aVR, aVL, aVF, V1, V2, V3, V4, V5 and V6.

Table 3.5.1: Electrocardiogram components.			
Components of ECG	**Duration and amplitude**	**Cause**	**Remarks**
P wave	Duration: 0.08–0.10 sec Amplitude: Not greater than 2.5 mm (Lead II)	Atrial depolarization	Duration >0.10 sec—left atrial enlargement Amplitude >2.5 mm—right atrial enlargement
QRS complex	Duration: 0.08–0.10 sec	Ventricular depolarization	Duration >0.10 sec may represent a bundle branch block
T wave		Represents ventricular repolarization	
U wave		Slow repolarization of papillary muscles	
PR segment	Isoelectric	Extends from the end of P wave to the start of QRS complex	
PR interval	Isoelectric Duration: 0.12–0.20 sec Average: 0.18	Beginning of P wave to the start of QRS complex It includes the conduction delay in the AV node	It shortens as heart rate increases
QT interval	QT interval: 0.39 sec at a heart rate of 60/min Duration QTc: 0.35–0.43 sec	Onset of Q wave to end of T wave Represents ventricular depolarization + repolarization and corresponds to the duration of electrical systole	Shortens with tachycardia and lengthens with bradycardia so it must be corrected for the effect of the associated heart rate (QTc)
ST segment	Isoelectric	Extends from the J point to the onset of T wave	
ST interval		End of S wave to the end of T wave	

> **NOTE**
> **J point:** The J point occurs at the end of QRS complex. At this point, the entire ventricular muscle is depolarized. Normally, the J point is on the isoelectric line but it is displaced up or down by the current of injury resulting from myocardial ischemia or infarction.

Why is T wave of repolarization positive?
Normally, it is in the same direction as the QRS complex because repolarization follows a path that is opposite to that of depolarization, i.e. it occurs from epicardium to endocardium (one of the reasons for this is that the endocardial areas have a longer period of contraction and are thus slow to repolarize). *A vulnerable period* occurs during the down slope of T wave when the ventricle is partially repolarized and the cardiac muscle fibers are in a state of relative refractoriness. An ectopic stimulus in the ventricles due to myocardial damage may bring on extrasystoles or fibrillation.

Cardiac Vector or Cardiac Axis

- In electrophysiology, a **vector** represents both the magnitude and direction of the potential generated by the current flow. A vector is represented by an arrow. The arrow is directed from negative to the positive direction. The length of the arrow represents the voltage of the potential. The average vector of all of the instantaneous vectors is called the **mean vector**. The **direction** of the **mean vector** is called the **mean electrical axis**.
- **Cardiac vector:** The magnitude and direction of the electromotive force generated in the heart represents the cardiac vector. The direction of the mean cardiac vector is called the **mean cardiac axis**.
- The QRS complex, which represents ventricular depolarization, is used for the determination of the electrical heart axis.
- The term, electrical heart axis, usually refers to the electrical axis in the frontal plane as measured by the limb leads.

The mean frontal axis is the sum of all the ventricular depolarization forces. The average direction of the flow of current is called **the electrical axis of the heart** (the mean QRS axis) lies between −30° and +110° and averages around 59°.

Calculation of Mean Electrical Axis of the Heart (The Mean QRS Axis)

- This is generally calculated from leads I and III (any two of the limb leads can be used in reality).
- Net QRS amplitudes are calculated in millimeter in the two leads by subtracting any negative peak deflections (usually the negative peaks of the Q and S waves) from the R wave peak.
- The two values so obtained are then plotted in the appropriate polarity direction along the respective lines (leads I and III here) in the hexaxial system (Fig. 3.5.6).
- The two perpendiculars are drawn from those two points until they intersect.
- A line is then drawn from the center of the hexaxial system to the point where the two perpendiculars intersect with each other.
- This line represents the mean QRS vector in the heart at that moment in time (Fig. 3.5.6A).

The **mean QRS axis lies between −30° and +110°**.
- **Right axis deviation** is said to be present if the calculated axis falls to the right of +110°. In right axis deviation, the QRS waves in these leads point toward each other.
- **Left axis deviation** is when they point in opposite direction. In left axis deviation, the calculated axis falls to the left of −30°. If QRS complex is primarily positive in these two leads, the axis is normal.

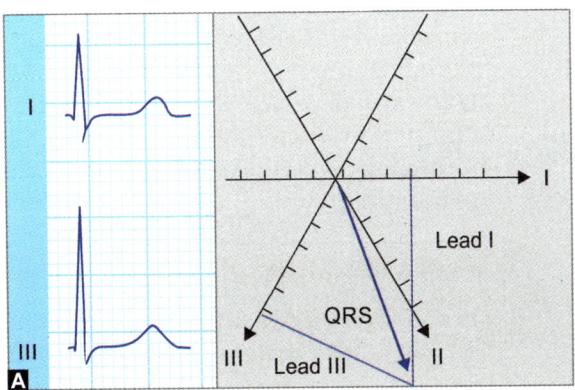 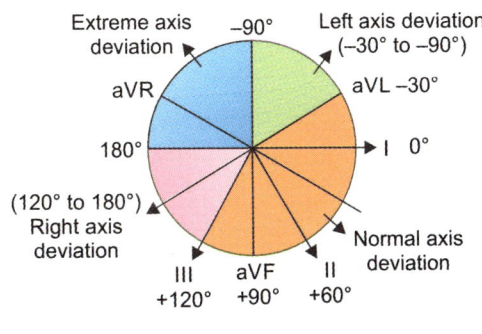

Figs. 3.5.6A and B: (A) Calculation of cardiac vector; (B) Hexaxial system (Cabrera system).

Because the orientation of each lead to the depolarization is different, the **direction and magnitude of deflections** of ECG are different—still the **sequence of deflections**—P wave, QRS complex and T wave is identical.

PROCEDURE

1. Ask the patient to lie down supine on the bed and be comfortable and relaxed. Check that the ECG machine is properly earthed. Rub small amounts of electrolyte jelly on the fronts of wrists and just above the ankles.
2. Apply the limb electrodes firmly on these points and fix them in place with plastic clamps. Fix the lead wires, identified with the letters—RA, LA, LL and RL electrodes. Connect the connector cable to the machine.
3. Switch on the machine and "center" the stylus (pen); run the paper and using the CAL (calibration), push the button 2–3 times and adjust the pen deflection to 10 mm.
4. Using the lead selector switch, record 4–6 ECG complexes in the standard order—leads I, II, III, aVR, aVL and aVF—in this order (Figs. 3.5.5A and B).
5. Stop the machine and apply the electrode jelly on the chest positions for V1-V6. Using the chest electrodes, record the ECG from these positions one after the other.
6. Tear off the paper from the machine and label the various leads. Note down the name of the person and date.

NOTE
Color coding of limb leads (red—RA, yellow—LA, black—RL and green—LL). Color coding of chest leads (white/red—V1, white/yellow—V2, white/green—V3, white/brown—V4, white/black—V5 and white/violet—V6).

NOTE
In modern machines, there are three modes of recording, i.e. manual mode, auto mode and analysis mode. Under manual mode the operator can choose which lead group needs to be recorded and determine the record length. Under auto mode, the leads switch and calibrate automatically while recording. In analysis mode, the machine will sample the ECG for a prefixed time (1–3 minutes) and analyze all the waveforms of lead II for R-R analysis.

PRECAUTIONS

1. The patient must be completely relaxed and comfortably supported. Explain the procedure to him. This will alleviate his anxiety and help in smooth recording.
2. Electrocardiogram should be recorded in the supine position. Hair should be parted or shaved.
3. Electrocardiogram machine should be properly earthed.
4. Electrode jelly should be rubbed properly to ensure good conduction of current.
5. There should be good contact between the electrodes and the skin. Poor contact may result instability of the baseline.
6. Ensure that RL is properly grounded.
7. Ask the subject to remove any magnetic or metallic articles which interferes at the time of recording.
8. Ensure that the ECG machine is properly calibrated (with respect to sensitivity, speed and number of complexes recorded per lead) before recording the ECG.
9. Ensure the sequential recording of ECG machine with respect to sequence of leads. Recording should be done in a proper sequence. I, II, III, aVR, aVL, aVF and V1-V6 in manual mode.

RECORDING OF ELECTROCARDIOGRAM ON STUDENT PHYSIOGRAPH

The student physiograph with ECG coupler can be used for recording ECG. Calibration of sensitivity, centering of pen, connecting subject to five-pin junction box through patient cable and the latter to the coupler are required for recording ECG.

SYSTEMATIC ANALYSIS OF ELECTROCARDIOGRAM

1. **Heart rate:** It can be determined by any of the following two methods:
   a. By dividing 1,500 by the number of small squares between two successive R waves (1,500 small squares represent 1 min). For example, number of small squares between two R waves = 21
   Heart rate = 1,500/21 = 70 beats/min.
   b. By dividing 60 by the RR interval in seconds. For example, number of small squares between two R waves = 20
   RR interval = 20 × 0.4 = 0.80
   Heart rate = 60/0.80 = 75 beats/min.
2. **Rhythm:** In normal sinus rhythm, P waves precede each QRS complex. Atrial, junctional and ventricular arrhythmias are detected by in-hospital and ambulatory ECG monitoring.
3. **Mean cardiac vector:** Evaluation of the frontal plane QRS axis provides the information.
4. **Morphology of various waves, intervals and segments are** carefully studied.

CLINICAL APPLICATIONS OF ELECTROCARDIOGRAM

Electrocardiogram provides useful information in:
1. Diagnosis and prognostic information in ischemic heart disease [coronary artery disease (CAD)] such as angina, heart attack (acute CAD).

2. Detection of cardiac arrhythmias—both atrial and ventricular.
3. Different types of heart block. For example, in complete heart block, diseases of AV node or bundle of His which is the only pathway from atria to ventricles, there is complete dissociation between atria and ventricles. The HR may be 15–20 beats/min and serious emergency may arise with prolonged periods of asystole. Due to cerebral cortical ischemia (Stokes–Adams syndrome), there is dizziness or "faints". It is in such cases that artificial pacemakers are implanted.
4. Hypertrophy of atria and ventricles.
5. Electrical activity resulting from general metabolic and electrolyte changes.

SPECIAL USES OF ELECTROCARDIOGRAM

1. **In-hospital electrocardiogram monitoring:** Cardiac arrest or severe arrhythmia patients who are shifted to the hospital need special care.
2. **Ambulatory electrocardiogram monitoring (Holter):** Patients with episodic palpitation and dizziness or unstable angina, are given a Holter monitor to wear for 24 h. Analysis of the recorded tape often identifies the cause of the condition.
3. **Exercise electrocardiogram:** The ECG recorded during exercise [treadmill test (TMT)], as per Bruce protocol in otherwise normal. Arrhythmias and ST segment changes are more likely to be detected during TMT.

SOME COMMON ABNORMALITIES OF ELECTROCARDIOGRAM

These include abnormalities of HR (tachycardia and bradycardia), new rhythm centers (e.g. extrasystoles), axis deviation, ischemic cardiac conditions and various types of heart block.

QUESTIONS

- Q.1. What is ECG and what is its basis?
- Q.2. What is meant by the term lead?
- Q.3. What do the lines on ECG paper indicate?
- Q.4. What are the different waves recorded in normal ECG and what do they represent?
- Q.5. Which wave represents atrial repolarization?
- Q.6. What is complete heart block? Is this condition compatible with life?
- Q.7. What is the function of electrode connected to the right leg?
- Q.8. How do you calculate the HR and mean QRS axis from an ECG record?
- Q.9. Where is the indifferent electrode in your recording setup?
- Q.10. Why 12 ECG leads are employed?
    The heart is a three-dimensional organ, so its electrical activity must be studied in three dimensions. Each lead views the heart at a unique angle, increasing its sensitivity to a particular region of the heart at the expense of the others. In simple terms, each lead looks at the heart from a different perspective and therefore, employment of 12 leads enables to record the electrical activity of the heart in FRONTAL and HORIZONTAL plane thus making a correct and more accurate detection of pathology possible.

OBSERVATION AND RESULT

Enter your observations in relation to heart rate, P wave, QRS complex, PR interval, QT interval, ST segment and mean QRS axis.

Heart rate	Wave form	Duration	Amplitude
P wave			
QRS complex			
PR interval			
QT interval			
ST segment			
Mean QRS axis			

INTERPRETATION

....
....
....
....
....

STUDY NOTES

CHAPTER 3.6

Cardiac Efficiency Tests

CARDIAC EFFICIENCY TESTS (EXERCISE TOLERANCE TESTS)

The response of the cardiovascular system to standardized exercise (**"exercise tolerance test"**, also called **"stress testing"**) is the single and the best test for assessing the efficiency of the heart.

During exercise, there is a progressive increase in the heart rate (HR) and blood pressure (BP). However, after the exercise is over, these values return to the pre-exercise levels during the next few minutes.

In a trained person, there is a greater increase in the HR and BP than in an untrained individual. During exercise, these values take a longer time to return to basal levels. This forms the basis of exercise tolerance tests.

The response to physical exercise depends on the cardiac reserve (i.e. efficiency of the heart), muscle power, training, motivation and the state of nutrition. Therefore, the cardiac efficiency tests can also be used to test physical fitness in an individual.

Caution: This is a test for physical fitness and should not be used in patients.

- **Record the basal pulse rate,** then ask the subject to hop 20 times on each foot, raising the shoulders 6 inches at each step.

    If the heart is healthy, there should be little disturbance of breathing and the pulse rate should not increase by more than 10–20 beats per minute and should return to pre-exercise level in about a minute.

    Record these timings in your workbook.
- **Harvard step test.**

Protocol: Record the basal pulse rate. Then ask the subject to alternately step up and down, lifting each foot about 20 inches (16 inches in females) off the ground, at a rate of 30 per minute for a period of 5 minutes [Alternately, the subject may step up and down a 50 cm bench (40 cm in females), at a frequency of 30 times/min for 5 minutes]. Stop the test if the subject feels breathless and exhausted and is unable to continue the test.

Count the pulse rate 1 minute after the end of the exercise.

The pulse rate is inversely proportional to the degree of cardiac efficiency. To obtain an approximate idea of the cardiac efficiency index, count the pulse rate at the following intervals:

- Between 1 and 1½ minutes = .../min (**a**)
- Between 2 and 2½ minutes = .../min (**b**)
- Between 3 and 3½ minutes = .../min (**c**)
- Time after which the pulse rate returns to basal levels = ... minutes

CARDIAC EFFICIENCY INDEX

$$\frac{\text{Duration of exercise in seconds (300)}}{a + b + c} \times 100$$

In normal individuals, the cardiac efficiency index is nearly 100%, but is more in sports persons.

Efficiency Index

Over 90%: excellent.
81–90%: good.

55–80%: average.
Below 55%: poor.

Master's step test: Master's step test employed in the past was a two-step wooden bench, each step being 9 inches high. The subject steps on and off the steps 12 times a minute and the pulse rate is noted. The time of recovery is about 5 minutes (the test also used to be repeated with stepping rates of 18 and 24 times a minute).

QUESTIONS

Q.1. How is physical exercise graded?
For the WHO grading of muscular exercise, according to heart rate and relative load index (RLI; i.e. percentage of maximum O_2 utilization) refer to Table 3.4.1.

Q.2. What is the purpose of the exercise tolerance tests?
Purpose of exercise tolerance tests: The exercise tolerance tests are the best tests for determining the efficiency of the heart as a pumping organ. These tests take the place of cardiac output (CO) measurements which cannot be made with ease in most clinical settings.

Q.3. What is meant by the term "cardiac reserve"?
Cardiac reserve: The cardiac reserve is the difference between the basal CO of an individual and the maximum CO that can be achieved in that person. It can also be expressed as cardiac reserve percent. For example, basal cardiac output = 5 liters/min; maximum achievable output = 25 liters/min. Thus, cardiac reserve percent = $[(25 - 5) \times 100]/25 = 80\%$.

Q.4. Name some other cardiac efficiency tests.
Treadmill test (TMT): A very sophisticated "stress test" employed these days is the one using a treadmill or a bicycle ergometer. The individual is subjected to standardized incremental increase in external workload, according to a definite protocol (Bruce protocol), while the person's 12-lead ECG, arm blood pressure and symptoms are continuously monitored by a physician present throughout the test. The performance is usually symptom-limited and the test is discontinued as soon as there is evidence of chest discomfort, severe dyspnea, dizziness, fatigue, ST-segment depression of more than 2 mm, a fall in systolic pressure exceeding 15 mm Hg or development of ventricular tachyarrhythmia.

The test is also done in cases of coronary artery disease to assess the degree of cardiac disability. The test can be enhanced by IV radioisotope (thallium 201) to assess regional myocardial perfusion by means of gamma camera. Radioisotope angiography using technetium 99 can also be employed to measure various parameters of ventricular performance.

> **NOTE**
> It may be noted that exercise testing can neither at present definitely exclude the presence of coronary artery disease, nor it is absolutely specific in predicting its presence.

STUDY NOTES

UNIT 2: RESPIRATORY SYSTEM

Date ....

CHAPTER 3.7

Stethography

AIM

To study respiratory movements by stethography and to see the effect of various maneuvers on it.

INTRODUCTION

Stethography is the process of recording respiratory movements with the help of a stethograph. The inspiratory and expiratory movements of the chest cause a change in the air pressure in the corrugated rubber tube of the stethograph. These respiratory movements are recorded on a moving drum.

PRINCIPLE

Corrugation of the tube keeps the mean radius unchanged during stretching. Thus during inspiration when the corrugated rubber tube is stretched, the length increases but the mean radius remains the same. This results in increase of its volume. Since the tube is airtight the pressure falls because of increase in volume leading to a fall in pressure inside the tube. This is transmitted to the tambour where the higher atmospheric pressure pushes the diaphragm and the writing lever downward. Thus, the downstroke of the lever is inspiration, while upstroke is expiration.

APPARATUS

1. **Stethograph:** It consists of a corrugated rubber tubing about 60 cm long and 3–4 cm in diameter. It has a hook and chain device for tying it across the chest wall. One end of the stethograph is closed, while the other end is connected via pressure rubber tubing to the Marey's tambour. This arrangement makes the corrugated tube airtight (Fig. 3.7.1).
2. **Marey's or Brodie's tambour:** This is a metallic cup or a small flat saucer with a rubber diaphragm stretched over its top. A light metal capillary writing lever is mounted on a small metal disk that rests on the diaphragm. The pressure variations in the rubber tube are thus transmitted accurately on to the rubber diaphragm. A rubber tube attached to an outlet connects the tambour to the stethograph.
3. Kymograph
4. Stop watch
5. Time marker

PROCEDURE

1. Ask the subject to sit on a stool with her/his back to the recording apparatus and ask the subject to relax and breathe normally. Tie the stethograph around the subject's chest at a level where respiratory movements are maximum (usually midchest at 4th-5th intercostal space below the nipples).
2. Slightly stretch the stethograph so that respiratory movements can cause adequate pressure changes within the stethograph.
3. Mount the tambour on the stand and connect the stethograph to it. Bring the writing point in contact with the drum surface at a tangent.

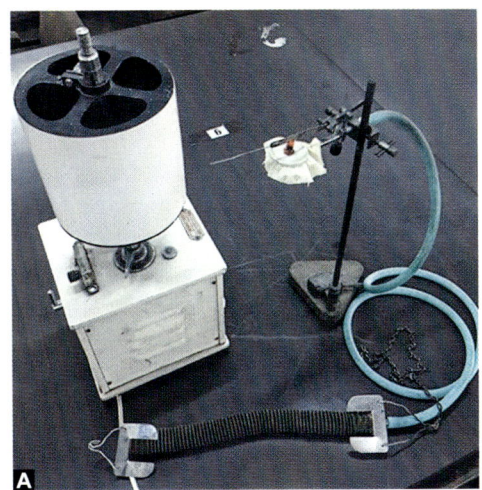
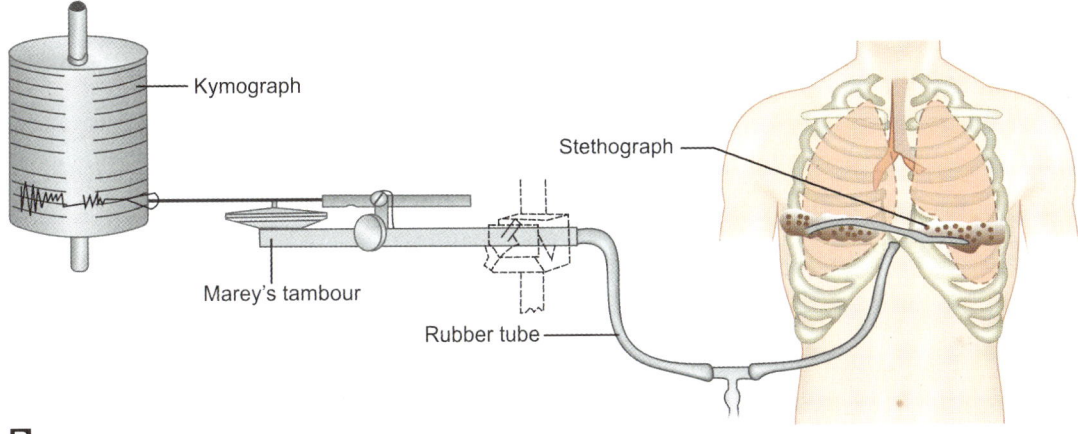

Figs. 3.7.1A and B: Stethography.

4. **Recording the respiratory movements:** Set the kymograph at a **slow speed of 2.5 mm/sec** and record a few normal respiratory movements and note the following:
   a. Rate of respiration
   b. Relative duration of inspiration and expiration
   c. Presence or absence of a gap between one inspiration and the next expiration and between one expiration and the next inspiration.
5. **Effect of deglutition (swallowing):** Ask the subject to take a mouthful of water and hold it in the mouth for a while. After a few normal respiratory movements are recorded, ask to swallow the water in one go. Note that there is a temporary stoppage of breathing and the condition is called **"deglutition apnea"** (apnea = temporary stoppage of respiration) (Fig. 3.7.2).
6. **Effect of breath holding:** Ask the subject to sit quietly and breathe normally for few minutes. Then ask the subject to hold his breath as long as possible in the following conditions and note the duration of breath holding time (BHT) in each conditions:
   - At the end of quiet expiration
   - At the end of maximum expiration
   - At the end of quiet inspiration
   - At the end of maximum inspiration
   - After voluntary hyperventilation.

> **NOTE**
> **"Breaking point":** The point at which the subject can no longer voluntarily hold his breath is called as the breaking point. It is due to increased arterial pCO_2 and decreased arterial pO_2.

   a. **Effect of voluntary hyperventilation:** Record few normal respiratory movements. Stop the drum and ask the subject to breathe deeply and rapidly for 1-2 minutes and then wait for the normal breathing to resume on its own. The tracing usually shows a short period of apnea or decreased breathing after stoppage of hyperventilation.

Section 3: Human Experiments

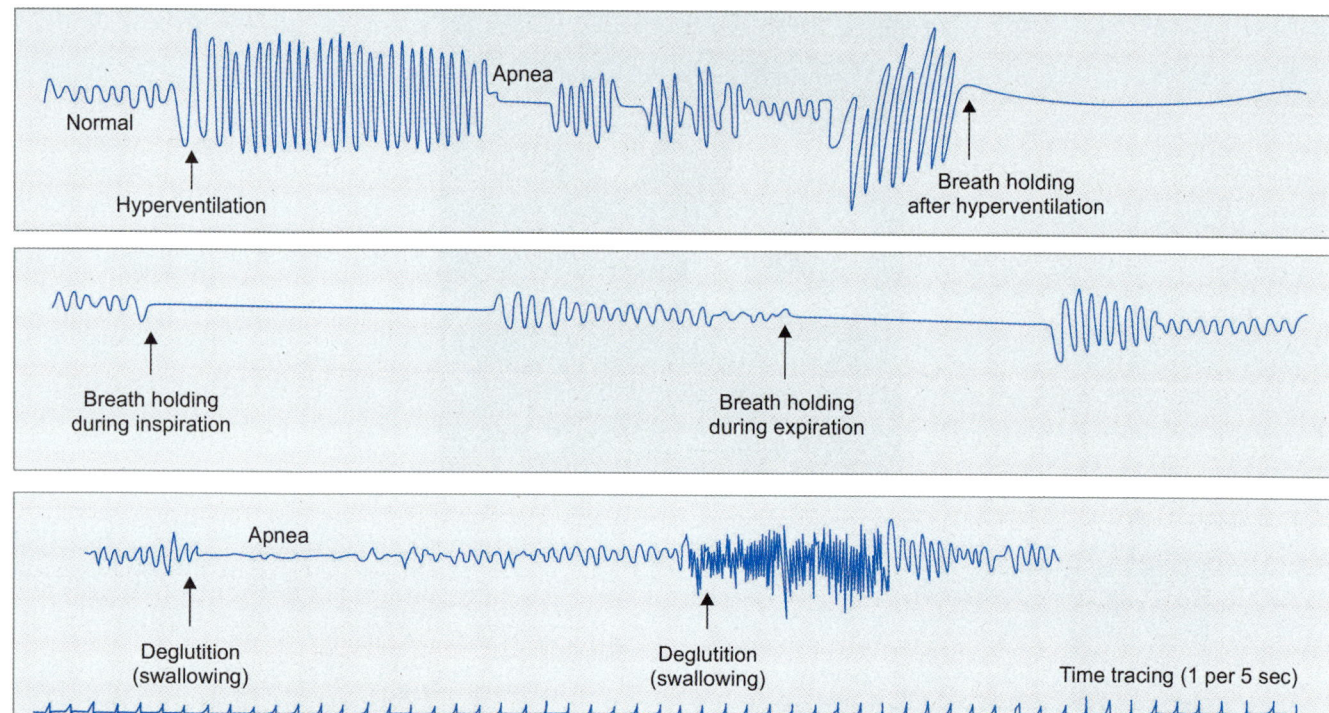

Fig. 3.7.2: Stethography recording.

b. **Effect of exercise:** Stop the drum and disconnect the stethograph from the tambour. Then ask the subject to do "running in place" or "spot running", bringing the thighs to horizontal position alternately for 3–4 minutes. Reconnect the stethograph to the tambour and record the effect of exercise. Also record the time taken for respiration to return to resting levels.

c. Record a 5 second time interval below the graph obtained, keeping the kymograph speed unchanged. Indicate various events with arrows. Remove the graph and fix it in the usual manner (Fig. 3.7.2).

7. **Effect of modified respiratory movements:** Record the effect of **coughing, sneezing, talking** on respiratory movements giving a 2–3 minutes interval between each act.

PRECAUTIONS

1. The stethograph applied to the chest should not be too tight or too loose.
2. Do not let the subject look at the tracings being obtained.
3. Do not allow the subject to hyperventilate for more than 2 minutes.
4. Record a few normal movements before each maneuver.

Objective Structured Practical Examination

Aim: To record the respiratory movements of the subject provided.
Procedural steps: See text above.
Checklist:
1. Check out the apparatus. (Y/N)
2. Seat the subject on a stool with his back to the recording apparatus. Tell him to relax and explain the procedure. (Y/N)
3. Tie the stethograph firmly around his midchest and connect it to the tambour. (Y/N)
4. Set the kymograph at slow speed (1.2 mm/sec) and record a few respiratory movements. (Y/N)
5. Using a signal marker, record the time tracing below the graph. (Y/N)

QUESTIONS

Q.1. What is the working principle of stethograph?
Q.2. Why should the subject not look at the tracings being obtained?
Respiratory movements are easily affected by our becoming aware of them—their rate, depth, rhythm, etc. If the subject looks at the record being obtained, he/she will become conscious (aware) of it so that the movements are bound to change and not represent the true effects of various maneuvers.

Q.3. What is deglutition apnea? Describe its mechanism and physiological significance.

This term refers to a **temporary stoppage** of breathing when we swallow food or fluids. It is a reflex phenomenon and occurs automatically when we swallow. This stops the breathing **at any point of inspiration or expiration**.

Physiological significance of deglutition apnea: The stoppage of breathing and closure of glottis prevents the entry of food or fluid into the upper respiratory passages, which would cause aspiration pneumonia or other complications.

Q.4. What is "breaking point" and what is its cause?

The point at which the subject can no longer voluntarily hold his breath is called breaking point. It is due to increased arterial pCO_2 and decreased arterial pO_2.

Q.5. How can breath-holding time be prolonged?

The breath-holding time can be increased by:
1. Hyperventilating before holding the breath (This will decrease the arterial pCO_2 and raise pO_2 a little)
2. Breathing 100% oxygen before breath-holding
3. Psychological factors: Motivation increases the breath-holding time.

Q.6. Define hyperventilation and what are its effect on the respiratory system?

Hyperventilation refers to increased volume of air moving into and out of the lungs per unit time—whether due to increase in rate, depth or both. It can result from:
1. Voluntary effort
2. Exercise
3. **Chemical stimuli:** High pCO_2, low pO_2 or increased H$^+$ ion concentration resulting from lung and heart diseases can increase the ventilation.

Effects of voluntary hyperventilation: Hyperventilation for 1–2 minutes leads to a short period of apnea followed by a few breaths till normal rhythm is restored.

Harmful effects of hyperventilation: Though a single bout of hyperventilation may have no ill effects, chronic hyperventilation as seen in neurotic subjects may produce certain ill effects.

- The arterial pCO_2 may fall from the normal level of 40 mm Hg to 15–20 mm Hg. This degree of hypocapnia produces vasoconstriction of cerebral blood vessels. The cerebral ischemia causes dizziness, lightheadedness, etc.
- Constriction of retinal blood vessels may cause blurring of vision.
- A more serious effect of chronic hyperventilation and associated hypocapnia is alkalosis which causes precipitation of ionic calcium. If the serum calcium is already low, an attack of tetany may be precipitated. As a result, there are extensive tetanic spasms of the skeletal muscles especially in limbs and larynx.

Q.7. What is the cause of increased ventilation during exercise?

A variety of factors are involved in increasing the ventilation during exercise.
1. **Psychic stimuli:** Ventilation often increases in anticipation of the exercise, i.e. before the exercise has started. Soon after the start of exercise and before blood pCO_2, pO_2 and H$^+$ ions have time to change, there is a sudden and large increase in ventilation (mainly due to increase in depth).
2. **Impulses from motor cerebral cortex:** As the motor cortex sends impulses via corticospinal tracts to the motor neurons of active muscles, it also sends via collaterals of the tracts, excitatory impulses to the respiratory center (as it does to vasomotor center).
3. **Impulses from proprioceptors:** Body movements especially those of the limbs stimulate the proprioceptors (stretch receptors) in the active muscles, tendons, ligaments, joints, etc. These excitatory impulses are also relayed to the respiratory center (it is important to note that even passive movements of the limbs increase the ventilation).
4. **Chemical stimuli:** Increased ventilation removes the excess of CO_2 produced without any significant change in arterial pO_2 and pCO_2 especially in trained athletes. In fact, the pO_2 may be higher and pCO_2 lower than the normal. Thus, low pO_2 and high pCO_2 cannot explain respiratory stimulation during exercise. Sometimes, the neural signals may be too weak to stimulate the respiratory center; it is then that the chemical stimuli play a role.
5. **Other factors:** Increased body temperature, increased blood K$^+$, lactic acidosis, hypoxia in exercising muscles stimulating the sensory nerve endings, fluctuations in blood gases.

Q.8. What is periodic breathing?

Periodic breathing is a disturbance of respiratory control where periods of apnea alternate with periods of increased respiration. This waxing and waning of breathing begins with shallow breaths which gradually increase in depth, each phase lasting 20–30 seconds. This is called **Cheyne–Stokes breathing**. Various irregular forms, such as **Biot's breathing**, Kussmaul's breathing, sleep apnea syndrome, etc. are also seen. It is generally a sign of brain damage, increased intracranial pressure, congestive heart failure, uremia, etc.

Q.9. Why cannot a person hold his/her breath for periods longer than a minute or so? What is the cause of breaking point?

The normal level of CO_2 in the body (arterial pCO_2 of 40 mm Hg) is just sufficient to maintain a resting ventilation of 6–8 L/min. This degree of ventilation is enough to supply adequate amounts of O_2 to the tissues at rest. Any increase in ventilation by high pCO_2 (or low pO_2) or other stimuli shows that the "ventilatory drive" has increased (i.e. the medullary respiratory center has been stimulated). On the other hand, the cerebral cortex can temporarily allow voluntary breath-holding and thus oppose the ventilatory drive.

Thus, two opposing factors are operating during breath-holding: **Ventilatory drive** and **voluntary stoppage of breathing**. Since the ability to hold breath remains unchanged in a normal person, "breaking point", i.e. the point when a breath has to be taken is reached when the ventilatory drive is so strong that it overcomes the desire to continue to hold breath (It is interesting to note that the world record for breath-holding is 5 min 13 sec). It is also obvious that a person cannot commit suicide by holding breath because breathing will begin even if that person losses consciousness.

Section 3: Human Experiments

> **NOTE**
> Usually, the breaking point is reached when the arterial (and alveolar) pCO_2 increases from the normal 40 mm Hg to about 60 mm Hg and the pO_2 falls from the normal 100 mm Hg to about 50 mm Hg.

Q.10. What is the effect of prolonged hyperventilation on breath-holding time?

Hyperventilation washes out CO_2 from the body so that both pCO_2 and H^+ ion concentration decrease. At the same time, there is some increase in pO_2. Therefore, it will take some more time for these chemical stimuli to increase the ventilatory drive so that it reaches the breaking point.

Q.11. What are the factors that increase and decrease the BHT?

The normal BHT after a deep inspiration may vary from 40 seconds to over a minute. It can be increased by practicing breathing exercises as part of yoga training. Breathing pure O_2 before holding breath delays the breaking point. Hyperventilation increases BHT as described above. Reflex or mechanical factors also affect BHT. Psychological factors, such as motivation (e.g. telling the subject that his performance is improving, increases the BHT).

Breath-holding time decreases in many diseases, e.g. chronic bronchitis, emphysema, congestive heart failure and so on.

OBSERVATION AND RESULT

Record and analyze the results under the following headings:

1. Normal respiration:
   a. Rate of respiration

   ....
   ....

   b. Duration of inspiration and expiration

   ....
   ....

2. Effect of deglutition

   ....
   ....

3. Effect of breath-holding:

Breath-holding time after		Readings (in sec)
a.	Quiet inspiration	
b.	Quiet expiration	
c.	Deep inspiration	
d.	Deep expiration	
e.	Voluntary hyperventilation	

4. Effect of voluntary hyperventilation

   ....
   ....

5. Effect of exercise

   ....
   ....

6. Effect of modified respiratory movement:
   a. Coughing

   ....
   ....

   b. Sneezing

   ....
   ....

   c. Talking

   ....
   ....

INTERPRETATION

....
....
....
....
....

STUDY NOTES

CHAPTER 3.8

Spirometry: Lung Volumes and Capacities

AIM

Determination of lung volumes and capacities.

INTRODUCTION

Pulmonary function tests (PFTs) are noninvasive tests that show how well the lungs are working. These tests help the physician to make a physiological assessment of lung function rather than a pathological diagnosis which the physician has in most cases already arrived at during clinical examination.

CLASSIFICATION OF PULMONARY FUNCTION TESTS

The PFTs are employed to assess the three basic processes involved in the supply of O_2 to and removal of CO_2 from the body—***ventilation, diffusion*** and ***perfusion of lungs***. Thus, they can be classified on the basis of these tests:
1. Tests of ventilatory function
2. Tests to assess gas exchange function
3. Tests to assess the perfusion of lungs.

Tests of Ventilatory Function

Assessment of ventilatory function can be accomplished by:
1. Measurement of lung volumes and capacities
2. Measurement of dead space
3. Measurement of compliance
4. Measurement of airway resistance.

Measurement of Lung Volumes and Capacities

Lung Volumes

The term lung volumes refer to the nonoverlapping subdivisions or fractions of the total lung air while the term capacities refer to the combination of two or more lung volume. It may either be **static** or **dynamic** depending on whether or not time factor has been taken into consideration.
1. **Static lung volumes and capacities:** These measurements are those where time factor is not taken into consideration. They are expressed in milliliters or liters and include:
   a. **Static Lung Volumes (Table 3.8.1)**
      - **Tidal volume:** It is the amount of air inspired or expired with each normal breath (tidal respiration).
      - **Inspiratory reserve volume:** It is the extra volume of air that can be inspired over and above the normal (resting, quiet) tidal volume (i.e. from the spontaneous end-inspiratory point), with maximum effort.
      - **Expiratory reserve volume:** It is the extra amount of air that can be expelled from lungs by forceful effort after normal expiration, i.e. over and above the normal tidal expiration.
      - **Residual volume:** It is the amount of air that remains behind in the lungs after a maximum voluntary expiration.
   b. **Static lung capacities (Table 3.8.2)**
      - Vital capacity (VC)

Table 3.8.1: Static lung volumes.

Static volumes	Definition	Normal volume	Importance	Factors affecting
Tidal volume (TV)	Resting volume	500 mL	Normal breathing rate calculation	Restrictive and obstructive disorders
Inspiratory reserve volume (IRV)	Volume inspired above the TV	2.5–3.2 L	Reserve for exercise	Restrictive and obstructive disorders
Expiratory reserve volume (ERV)	Volume expired after TV	1,000–1,200 mL		
Residual volume (RV)	Air in lungs after maximal expiration	1,200 mL	• Maintains gas exchange • Prevents collapse	↑ In emphysema, old age ↓ In fibrosis

Table 3.8.2: Static lung capacities.

Static capacities	Definition	Normal value	Importance	Factors affecting
Inspiratory capacity (IC)	TV + IRV	2.5–3.7 L	Exercise reserve	Strength of muscles
Vital capacity (VC)	TV + IRV + ERV	4.8 L in males 3.2 L in females	Important index of pulmonary function	Strength, age, size, posture, diseases
Functional residual capacity (FRC)	RV + ERV	2.3–2.5 L	Same as RV	Same as RV
Total lung capacity	VC + RV or IC + FRC	6 L	Reserve for gas exchange	Age, lung diseases

- **Inspiratory capacity (IC):** It is the maximum amount of air that a person can breathe in with maximum effort starting from the normal end-expiratory point. [IRV (2,500 mL) + TV (500 mL) = 3,000 mL].
- **Functional residual capacity (FRC):** This is the amount of air remaining in the lungs at the end of a normal (quiet) expiration. It cannot be determined directly by spirometry. Normal value is 2.3–3.3 L (30–35 mL/kg body weight). Determination of functional residual capacity:
  - *Nitrogen washout method*
  - *Helium dilution method*
- **Total lung capacity (TLC):** It is the volume of air that is present in the lungs at the end of a deepest possible inspiration.

NOTE
- All static volumes are measured by spirometer except residual volume, functional residual capacity and total lung capacity.
- All values have to be changed to standard temperature and pressure, dry (STPD) for comparison by using "gas equation".
- **Functional residual capacity** is determined **by nitrogen wash-out method** or **helium dilution method** and then residual volume and total lung capacity are calculated.

2. **Dynamic lung volumes and capacities:** These measurements are those where time factor is taken into account, that is, they are time-dependent. They are expressed in milliliters or liters per second or per minute and include:

a. **Dynamic lung volumes and capacities**
- **Minute ventilation/Pulmonary ventilation (MV/PV):** It is the volume of air inspired or expired per minute. It equals the tidal volume multiplied by respiratory rate [TV (500) × RR (12) = 6 L/min].
- **Alveolar ventilation:** Out of a tidal volume of 500 mL, 150 mL air remains in the upper respiratory passages up to respiratory bronchioles (anatomical dead space), while only 350 mL reaches the respiratory zone (respiratory bronchioles, alveolar ducts and alveoli) for exchange of gases. Thus, alveolar ventilation would be
  = (500 – 150 = 350) × 12 = 4.2 L/min.
- **Maximum voluntary ventilation (Maximum ventilation volume) (MVV):** It is the amount of air which can be moved into or out of the lungs with maximum effort during 1 minute. It was formerly called **maximum breathing capacity (MBC)**, the MVV amounts to 80–170 L/min (average 120 L/min). The subject breathes quickly and deeply for 15 seconds and MVV is calculated for 1 minute (This means that pulmonary ventilation of 6–8 L/min can be increased by 15–20 times with maximum effort, though for short periods). MVV is profoundly reduced in patients with emphysema, airway obstruction and very poor respiratory muscle strength.
- **Timed vital capacity/Forced vital capacity (FVC):** It is the largest volume of air a person can

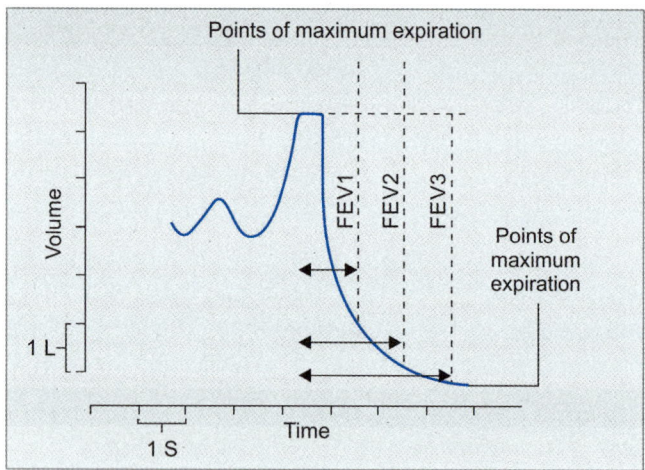

Fig. 3.8.1: Components of timed vital capacity.

expel from the lungs with maximum effort after first filling the lungs fully by a deepest possible inspiration. It amounts to 3.5–5.5 L.

Components of TVC/FVC (Fig. 3.8.1): The volume of expired air can be timed by recording the FVC on a spirograph moving at a known speed. From the graph so obtained the FVC can be divided into the following components:

- **Forced expiratory volume during 1 second (FEV1):** Volume of air expired during the 1 second of FVC. It is the most commonly used screening test for airway diseases. FEV1 is actually a flow rate. FEV1% is the percentage of VC expired in 1 second. FEV1% = FEV1/FVC × 100 (Normally FEV1% = about 80% of FVC). The FEV1 recorded is a dynamic capacity. In a normal person, a single forced expiration takes about 3 seconds and the tracing thus obtained is called an **"expiratory spirogram"**. Figure 3.8.2 shows such a tracing where the fractions of FVC are: 80% in 1 second (FEV1), 95% in 2 seconds and 98% in 3 seconds. The FEV1 is called the **"first expiratory volume at 1 second (FEV1)"** or **"forced expiratory volume in 1 second"**.
- **Forced expiratory volume in 2 seconds (FEV2):** It represents the volume of air expired in first 2 seconds of an FVC, FEV2% is about 90% of FVC under normal condition.
- **Forced expiratory volume in 3 seconds (FEV3):** It represents the volume of air expired in first 3 seconds of an FVC, FEV3% is 98–100% of FVC under normal condition.

Physioclinical significance of timed vital capacity: FEV1 and the ratio FEV1/FVC help in differentiating between two major patterns of abnormal ventilation—**obstructive** and **restrictive** lung diseases.

- **Obstructive pattern:** Patients with obstructive lung disease (bronchial asthma) have relatively low expiratory flow rate throughout expiration as a result of high airway resistance therefore, their **FEV1% is abnormally low.** The main feature is a **decrease in PEFR, FEV1, FEV1/FVC and MMEFR are all reduced (Figs. 3.8.2 and 3.8.3).** Over many years more and more air tends to remain in the lungs which increase TLC and RV (Fig. 3.8.3).
- **Restrictive pattern:** Patients with restrictive lung disease (kyphoscoliosis, ankylosing and spondylitis) have a reduced FVC but are able

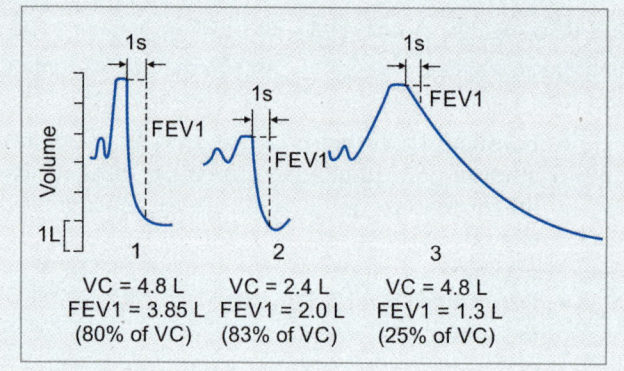

Figs. 3.8.2: The expiratory spirogram: Forced expiratory volume in 1 second (FEV1) component of timed vital capacity. 1. Normal patient; 2. Patient with restrictive lung disease; and 3. Patient with obstructive lung disease.
(VC: vital capacity)

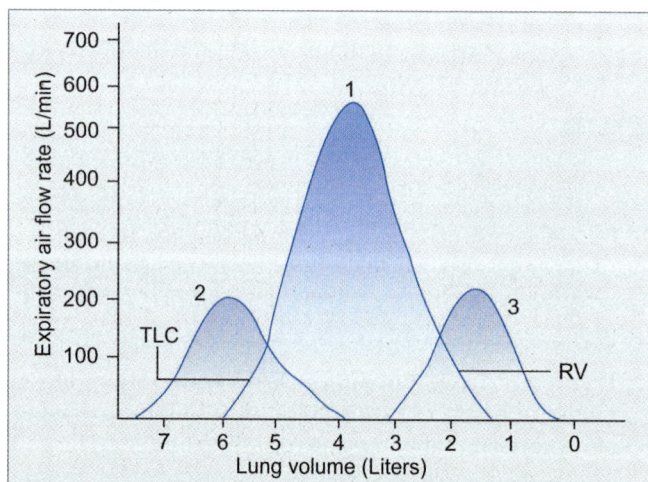

Fig. 3.8.3: Maximum expiratory flow volume curve. 1. Normal, 2. Chronic obstructive lung disease, 3. Restrictive lung disease.
(RV: residual volume; TLC: total lung capacity).

to achieve relatively high flow rates; therefore, their FEV1% exceeds 80%. The main feature is reduced lung volume (mainly TLC and RV), which may be due to *interstitial lung disease (ILD)* or *chest wall deformity* that reduce the air in the lungs. There is no obstruction to the outflow of air. **FEV1 is normal though FVC is low and FEV1/FVC may be normal or slightly increased as shown in Figure 3.8.2 and Table 3.8.3.**

- **Maximum expiratory flow-volume curve (MEFVC) (Fig. 3.8.3):** It represents outflow of air from lungs during a forceful expiration after a deep inspiration. The curve starts at a TLC of about 6.0 L, quickly reaches a peak of 550 L/min and then falls gradually to a residual volume of 1,100 mL. The decline in expiratory flow rate is due to compression of airways by the increasing intrathoracic pressure due to compression of chest by the forced expiration.
- **Forced expiratory flow during 25–75% of expiration (FEF 25–75%):** It is the mean expiratory flow rate during middle 50% of FVC.

Table 3.8.3: Obstructive and restrictive pattern of lung diseases.

Interpretation	FVC	FEV1	FEV1/FVC% (Tiffeneau index)
Healthy person	Normal (>80%)	Normal (>80%)	Normal (>0.7)
Airway obstruction	Low/normal	Low	Low
Restrictive	Low	Low/normal	Normal/increased (>0.7)
Mixed	Low	Low	Low

Normal value: 300 L/min. In addition to FVC and FEV1, the average expiratory flow rate during the middle 50% of FVC also called **"maximal mid-expiratory flow rate" (MMEFR; or FEF 25–75%)** can also be calculated (Fig. 3.8.4). A horizontal line drawn from 25% (t) and a vertical line from the 75% mark (V) will denote FEF 25–75%. This indicates the patency of smaller airways.

- Figure 3.8.4 also shows that in the middle 50% of FVC, 2.0 liters of air is expired in 0.5 second (t). This is also known as **mid-expiratory time (MET)**.
- **Pulmonary reserve (PR) or breathing reserve:** PR refers to the maximum amount of the air above the pulmonary ventilation that can be inspired or expired in 1 minute. It equals maximum ventilation volume minus pulmonary ventilation (minute ventilation), i.e. PR = MVV – PV/min.
- Pulmonary reserve is usually expressed as percentage of MVV and is known as percentage pulmonary reserve or **dyspneic index (DI)**, i.e. DI = (MVV – PV)/MVV × 100.
  - Normal values of DI or % PR range from 70–95% with an average of 75%.
  - Dyspnea is usually present when the value of DI becomes less than 60%.

Most of the lung volumes and capacities can be measured using a **recording spirometer**.

Spirometry

Spirometry is a simple and useful technique for assessing the ventilatory functions of the lungs. It refers to the recording of volume changes during various clearly defined breathing maneuvers. There are two types of spirometers:
1. Recording spirometer
2. Computerized spirometer with display

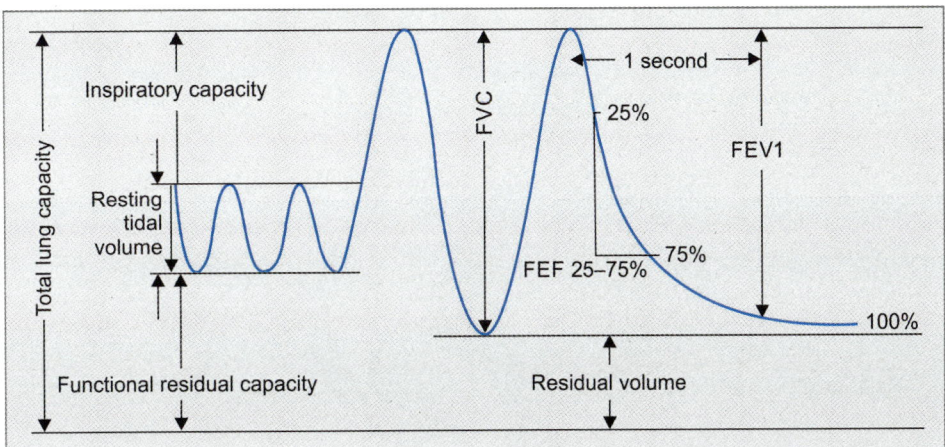

Fig. 3.8.4: Calculation of FEF 25–75% from forced expiratory spirogram.
(FVC: forced vital capacity)

Section 3: Human Experiments

1. **Recording Spirometer** (Figs. 3.8.5 to 3.8.7)
   The **recording spirometer,** which is electrically driven, is used to provide a graphic record (called **spirogram**) of various lung volumes and capacities. It consists of:
   a. *Double-walled cylindrical chamber:* It contains water between its two walls to maintain an airtight seal. A 9-L lightweight metal "gas bell" dips into the water from above and floats in it. A chain attached to the top of the bell passes over a frictionless pulley and carries **a counter-weight and a pen writer**. As the volume of air increases and decreases, the writing point moves down and up on the surface of the paper that passes under it. This provides a continuous record of the displacement of air in the bell with each inspiration and expiration.
   b. *Soda lime tower:* It is fitted within the spirometer and removes (absorbs) CO_2 from the expired air so that one can continue to breathe into and out of the spirometer (color change of soda lime from white to pink indicates that is near the point of exhaustion).
   c. *Kymograph:* There is an on/off switch and a pilot lamp on the front of the apparatus. The paper assembly carries **mm graph paper** calibrated for both **volume**

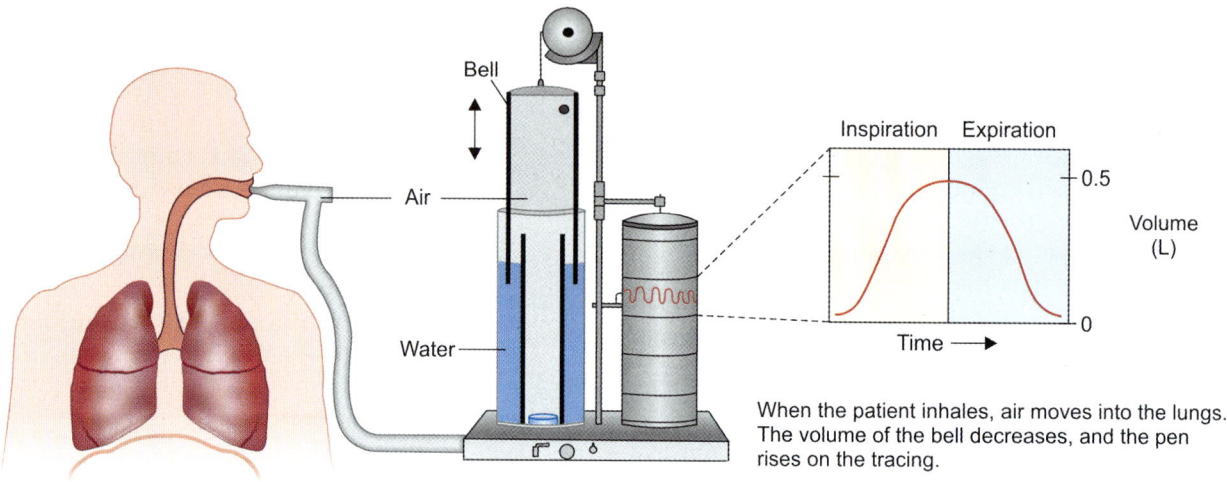

Fig. 3.8.5: Working of spirometer.

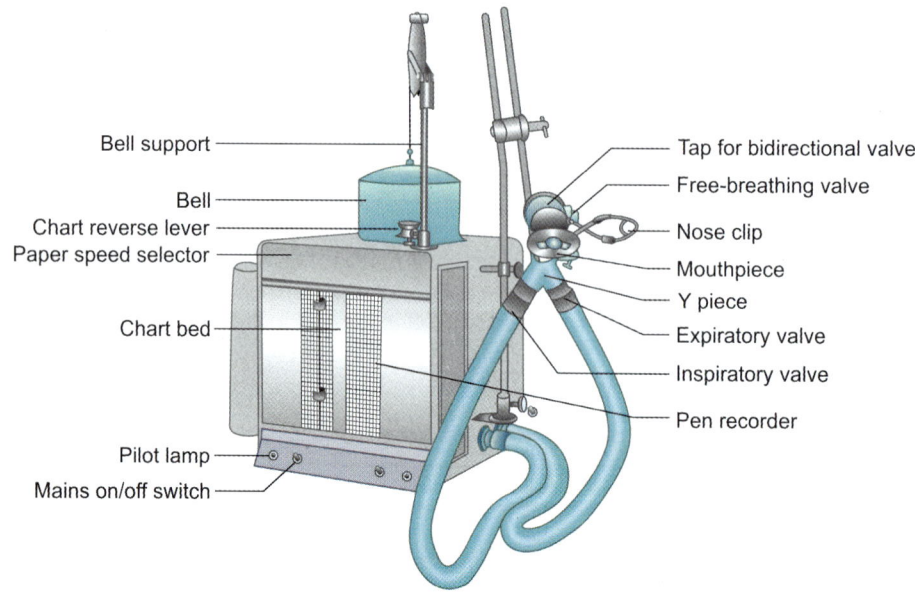

Fig. 3.8.6: Parts of spirometer.

Chapter 3.8: Spirometry: Lung Volumes and Capacities

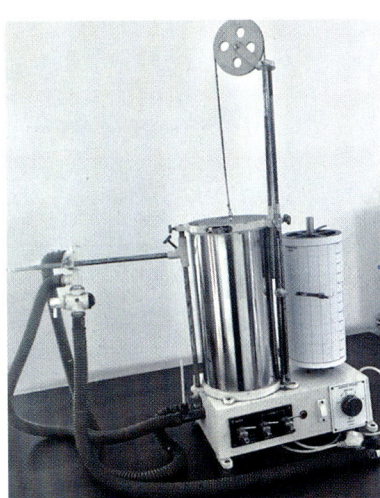

Fig. 3.8.7: Recording spirometer (Actual photograph).

of air and time. The paper speed selector has three markings:
- 60 mm/min speed is for normal recordings.
- 1,200 mm/min is for recording timed vital capacity.
- The "zero" mark is for "neutral" position of the kymograph at which the paper does not move.

d. *Chart paper:* A slot on the side of the unit allows exit of recorded paper.
It is calibrated for time along the X-axis, where 1 mm = 1 sec at the slower speed and 20 mm = 1 sec at the faster speed.
The calibration along Y-axis is for volume where **1 mm on paper represents 30 mL.**

e. *Breathing assembly:* The breathing assembly has a mouthpiece which is connected to the spirometer via a Y piece by two rubber-canvas corrugated tubes, one carrying a unidirectional valve for inspiring air from the bell and the other carries a unidirectional valve for expiring air into the atmosphere. The third component of the assembly is a free-breathing valve which has a directional tap. The tap can be turned to permit a person either to breathe room air or air from the spirometer bell (Fig. 3.8.6).

f. **Inlet** for filling the gas bell with oxygen or any other gas.

g. A *tap* for draining water out of the apparatus.

h. A *chart reverse knob* can rewind the recorded chart paper by turning the knob clockwise.

i. A *nose clip* is provided for closing the nostrils during recording.

Procedure

1. Fill three-fourths of the space between the two walls of the chamber with water. Dip the gas bell from above into the water. Connect the valve to the atmosphere and wash and fill the gas bell with fresh room air by slowly raising and lowering it 3–4 times.
2. Seat the subject facing the spirometer and instruct her/him about the procedures that will be carried out. Insert the mouthpiece between the teeth and lips and apply nose clip on the nostrils. Tell the subject to breathe through the mouth for about a minute to familiarize her/him with mouth breathing.
3. Connect the subject to the spirometer and allow her/him to breathe quietly for a short time. Then start the kymograph at the speed of 60 mm/min and record the excursions of the pen writer for about a minute.

> **NOTE**
> Upstrokes are for inspiration and downstrokes are for expiration.

4. The record of tidal breathing will be used for calculating the rate of respiration, tidal volume (TV) and minute ventilation (minute volume; MV).
5. To record IRV (Fig. 3.8.8), ask the subject to breathe in as deeply as possible after a quiet inspiration. IRV + TV will give IC. Record a few tidal breaths.
6. To record ERV, ask the subject to breathe out as forcefully as possible after a quiet expiration.
7. To record MVV (MBC) ask the subject to breathe quickly and deeply for 15 seconds. Convert the heights of all the excursions of the pen writer in 15 seconds into volume per minute to obtain MVV.
8. To record forced vital capacity (FVC) and timed vital capacity (FEV1), quickly change the kymograph speed to 1,200 mm/min and ask the subject to first take a deep breath and then expel the air from the lungs as forcefully and as quickly as possible (as for VC). Take 3 readings at intervals of about 2 minutes.

Precautions

1. Subject should not be facing the recording spirometer during the recording.
2. All lung volume and capacities are measured from end that is expiratory position.
3. Look for the color of soda lime (change of color from white to pink indicates that is near the point of exhaustion).

2. Computerized Spirometer

Nowadays portable computerized spirometers with graphic display are used for the pulmonary functions tests. These are quick and easy to use and are accurate as well (Fig. 3.8.9). The spirometric data can be seen and printed too.

Peak expiratory flow rate (PEFR): It is the maximum or peak rate (or velocity), in liters per minute with which air is expelled with maximum force after a deep inspiration.
Normal range = 350–600 L/min.

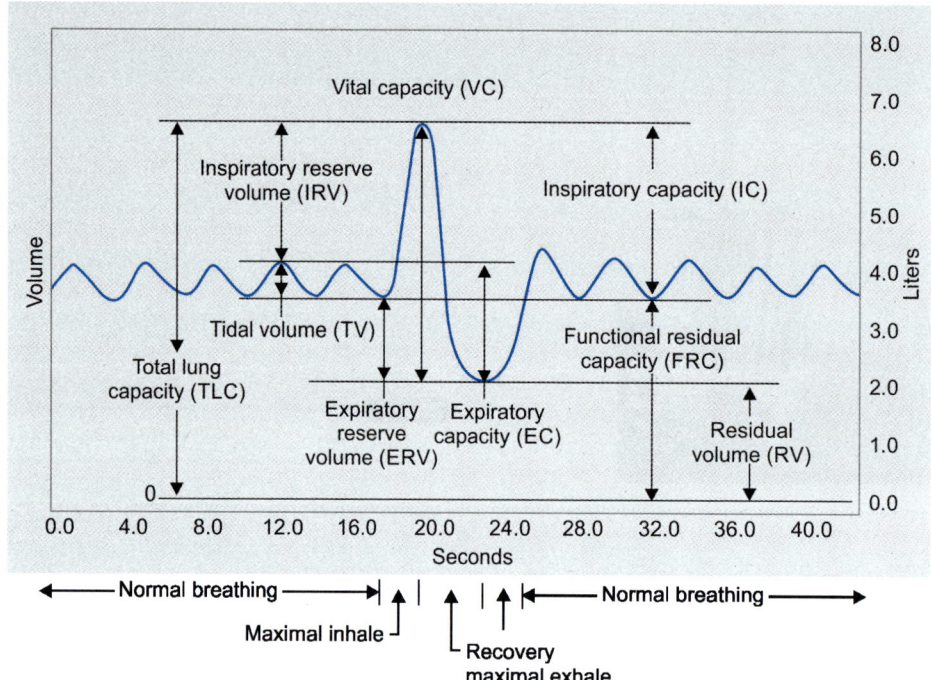

Fig. 3.8.8: Lung volumes and capacities (normal spirogram).

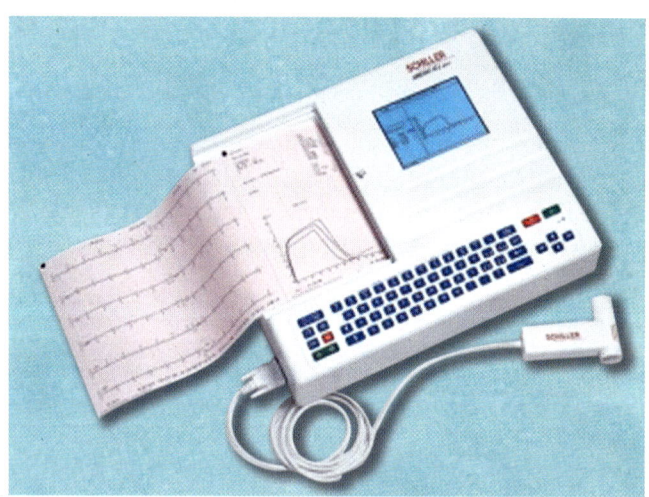

Fig. 3.8.9: Computerized spirometer.

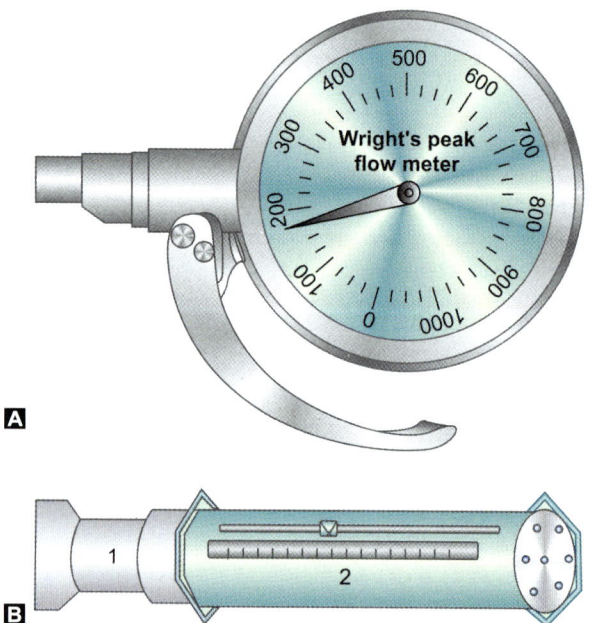

Figs. 3.8.10A and B: (A) Wright's peak flow meter. It directly measures expiratory flow rate; (B) Mini Wright's peak flow meter. 1. Mouthpiece, 2. Calibrated scale with marker.

The Wright's peak flow meter is a simple device for the measurement of the PEFR. A mini version is available which can be carried in one's pocket for bedside use (Figs. 3.8.10A and B). The flow meter is a short cylinder made of plastic material. An indicator (pointer) moves in a slot alongside a scale with numbers on it which indicates liters/minute. There is a handle provided near the mouthpiece. The end, opposite the mouthpiece, has holes in it for allowing air to exit from the apparatus.

Procedure

1. Ask the subject to hold the peak flow meter by its handle making sure that the fingers are clear of the scale and the

slot and are not obstructing the holes at the end of the apparatus.
2. Tell the subject to take a deep breath, place the mouthpiece firmly between the teeth and lips and then to blow out with a short sharp blast. Note the reading on the scale. Bring the indicator back to zero by pressing the button located near the mouthpiece.
3. Take six readings at intervals of 1 minute and select the maximum value for report.

Precautions
1. Subject should be instructed to blow out rapidly, completely and forcefully into the mouthpiece.
2. There should be no leakage from the mouthpiece.

Measurement of Dead Space

Dead space air is the portion of minute ventilation that does not take part in the exchange of gases. Normally, it is constituted by the air present in the conducting zone of respiratory passages *(anatomical dead space)*, but in some diseases may additionally include also poorly perfused alveoli *(physiological dead space)*. Anatomical dead space can be measured by **single breath N_2 curve**.

Measurement of Compliance

Compliance (C) expresses the distensibility (expansibility) of the lungs and chest wall. Compliance is defined as the change in lung volume (ΔV) per unit change in transpulmonary pressure (ΔP) where transpulmonary pressure is the difference in the pressure between the alveolar pressure and pleural pressure.

$$C = \Delta V/\Delta P$$

1. Total respiratory compliance or combined compliance of lungs and chest wall, i.e. lungs inside the thoracic cavity. Normal value of total respiratory compliance is 0.13 L/cm H_2O.
2. Pulmonary compliance, i.e. of lungs only (lungs outside the chest wall). Normal value of compliance for the lungs alone is 0.22 L/cm H_2O.

Measurement of Total Compliance

Total respiratory compliance (combined compliance of chest wall and lungs) can be measured by the pressure–volume curve of respiratory system. Pressure–volume curve of the respiratory system can be obtained in living subjects by using a spirometer.

Measurement of Airway Resistance

Airway resistance is one of the fundamental features of the respiratory system. Total airway resistance (Raw) the driving pressure is the pressure difference between the mouth (P_{mouth}) and the alveoli (P_A).

$$Raw = \frac{P_{mouth} - P_A}{V}$$

Normal value in healthy adults = 1–3 cm of H_2O/L per second.

Flow-volume Loop

In contrast to the spirogram which displays airflow (in L), over time (in sec), the flow-volume loop displays airflow (in L/sec) as it relates to lung volume (in L) during maximal inspiration from complete exhalation (residual volume) and during maximum expiration from complete inhalation (TLC). A normal, nonpathological F/V loop will descend in a straight or a convex line from top (PEF) to bottom (FVC) (Fig. 3.8.11).

Tests of Gas Exchange Functions

1. **Tests of diffusion:** Pulmonary diffusion refers to the transfer of gases across the alveoli to the capillary blood across the respiratory membrane. Diffusion capacity is defined as the volume of any gas that diffuses across the alveolar-capillary membrane per minute per mm Hg difference of pressure across the membrane.

   Diffusion capacity: As it is technically difficult to measure the diffusing capacity of lungs for O_2 directly, CO is used instead. The diffusion capacity measured for CO at rest is about 17 mL/min/mm Hg.

   Since the diffusing coefficient for O_2 is 1.23 times that for CO, the diffusing capacity for O_2 is = 17 × 1.23 = 21 mL/min/mm Hg.

2. **Estimation of arterial pO_2, pCO_2, pH:** Also known as ABG (arterial blood gas) test. This test measures oxygen

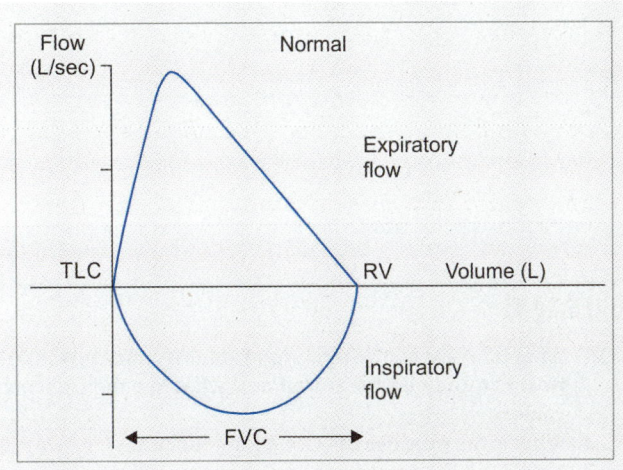

Fig. 3.8.11: Normal flow-volume loop.
(TLC: total lung capacity; RV: residual volume; FVC: forced vital capacity)

and carbon dioxide levels along with pH of the arterial blood.

Tests for Perfusion Functions

Special methods (e.g. lung scan and catheterization) are employed to determine blood flow through different zones of the lungs. The ventilation/perfusion balance can also be determined.

Special Techniques

Some of these tests are the following:
1. **Plain X-ray chest and screening** for evidence of lung disease
2. **Determination of pulmonary vascular pressures** by catheterization
3. **Computerized axial tomography** (CAT, CT scan)
4. **Magnetic resonance imaging** (MRI)
5. **Bronchoscopy**
6. **Lung scan**
7. **Ventilation scan**
8. **Computerized multifunctional spirometers.**

PHYSIOCLINICAL SIGNIFICANCE OF PULMONARY FUNCTION TESTS

1. To assess the normal functioning of the lungs.
2. To evaluate the physical fitness and effects of physical training.
3. To reach a diagnosis when a patient complains of dyspnea (breathlessness) and to assess the degree of disability.
4. To follow the progress of lung disease and the effectiveness of treatment.
5. To assess respiratory status before anesthesia and cardiothoracic surgery especially if a lung is to be removed.
6. To determine the incidence of respiratory dysfunction in the community and workers in hazardous industries.
7. To obtain medicolegal information and opinion in certain situations, e.g. claim for lung damage in a hazardous occupation.

QUESTIONS

Q.1. What is meant by the terms lung volumes and capacities? How can they be measured and what are their normal values?
Q.2. What is the purpose of testing lung functions?
Q.3. Name the lung volumes and capacities that cannot be measured on a spirometer.
Q.4. What is the difference between minute ventilation and maximum voluntary ventilation?
Q.5. What is timed vital capacity (FEV1) and what is its clinical importance?
Q.6. What is peak (expiratory) flow rate and what is its significance?
The peak expiratory flow rate (PEFR): The peak expiratory rate is the maximum flow rate or peak flow rate of air, during a single forced expiration. This estimation is useful in distinguishing reversible (e.g. asthma) from irreversible (e.g. emphysema) diseases. The peak flow meter which measures PEFR is of special value in cases of asthma where the effectiveness of treatment with a bronchodilator can be quickly evaluated.
Q.7. What is the physiological significance of functional residual capacity (FRC)?
Functional residual capacity (FRC), the air that remains in the lungs at the end of a normal (quiet) expiration is important for the gas exchange function of the lungs. The FRC amounts to about 2,200 mL, half of which is residual volume which cannot be expired into the spirometer.

Of the 500 mL of tidal volume (fresh air), 150 mL remains in the dead space, while only 350 mL reaches the depths of the lungs. There, it is added to the large amount of 2,000–2,500 mL of FRC. This causes dilution of the gases and a steady gas exchange throughout the respiratory cycle. The steady exchange prevents sudden changes in arterial pO_2 and pCO_2 which would make the control of breathing extremely difficult. The FRC is increased when lungs are overinflated with air as in old age, emphysema (due to loss of elasticity), asthma, etc.
Q.8. Name the precautions that must be observed during spirometric recording?
Q.9. What is breathing reserve and what is its clinical importance?

OBSERVATION AND RESULT

Sl. No.	Parameters	Values
1.	TV (mL)	
2.	IRV (mL)	
3.	IC (mL)	
4.	ERV (mL)	
5.	VC (mL)	
6.	FEV1	
7.	$FEF_{25-75\%}$	
8.	MVV (L/min)	
9.	PEFR	

INTERPRETATION

....
....
....
....
....

STUDY NOTES

CHAPTER 3.9

Vitalography and Effect of Posture on Vital Capacity

VITAL CAPACITY

Vital capacity (VC) is the maximum volume of air that can be expired after a maximal inspiration. It is computed as VC = TV + IRV + ERV*. VC is 4.8 L in males and 3.2 L in females. It is the most commonly performed pulmonary function test. It can be **measured** as:
1. Slow vital capacity
2. Forced vital capacity

1. **Slow Vital Capacity (SVC):** It is the volume of air expired (after maximum inspiration) during a slowly performed maximum expiratory effort.
2. **Forced vital capacity (FVC):** It is the largest volume of air, a person can expel from the lungs with maximum effort after first filling the lungs fully by a deepest possible inspiration. It amounts to 3.5–5.5 L. When FVC is timed it is known as **timed vital capacity (TVC).**

NOTE
SVC is more than FVC in patients with airway obstruction.

Measurement of Vital Capacity

Vital capacity is a simple and useful measurement for assessing the ventilatory functions of the lungs in health and disease. VC can be measured by:
1. Simple spirometer
2. Recording spirometer
3. Computerized spirometer

1. **Simple spirometer (student spirometer** also called a **vitalograph):** It is a common low-cost instrument (metallic or a bellows type), used in colleges, hospitals, sports facilities and gymnasia (Figs. 3.9.1A and B).
2. **Recording spirometer:** It is a sophisticated, electrically driven, recording system used in respiratory physiology laboratories, hospitals, etc. It provides a graphic record of various lung volumes and capacities.

VITALOGRAPHY

The procedure of recording the vital capacity with the help of a vitalograph is called as vitalography.

Apparatus
1. Vitalograph
2. Nose clip
3. Mouthpiece

Vitalograph
- It consists of a double-walled metal **cylindrical chamber** having an outer container filled with water in which a light metal gas bell of 6 L capacity floats.
- The **bell (or float)** is attached on its upper surface to a chain which passes over a graduated frictionless pulley.
- The **pulley** bears a spring-mounted indicator needle that moves with the pulley and indicates the volume of air present in the bell.
- The bell is counterpoised by a weight (counterweight) attached to the other end of the chain (Fig. 3.9.2). This weight allows a smooth up and down movement of the bell.

---
*TV: tidal volume; IRV: inspiratory reserve volume; ERV: expiratory reserve volume.

Chapter 3.9: Vitalography and Effect of Posture on Vital Capacity

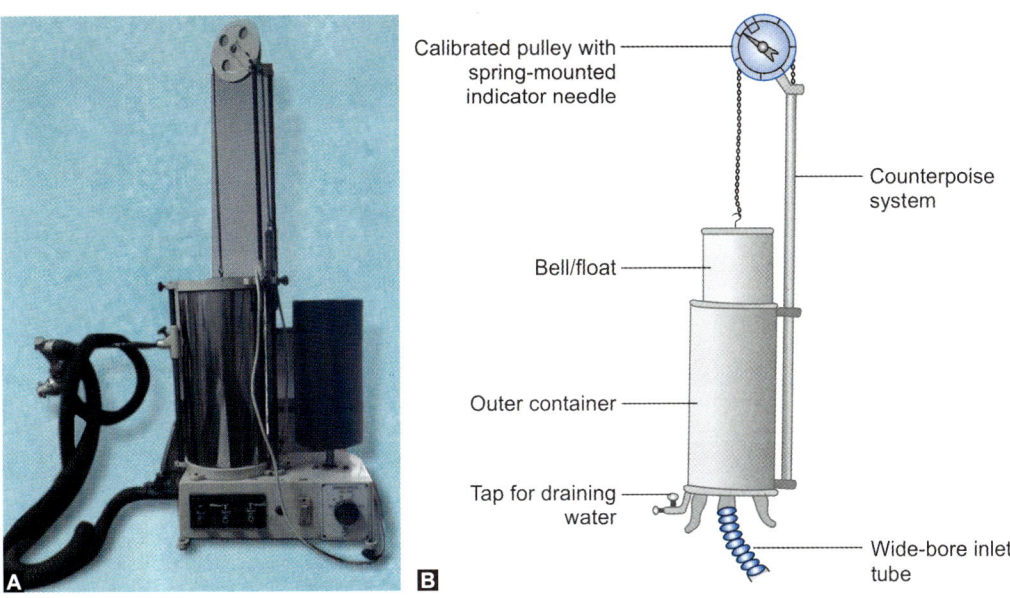

Figs. 3.9.1A and B: Vitalograph.

- The inlet tube through which air moves into or out of the bell is a corrugated canvas-rubber tubing bearing a **mouthpiece** (this tube is attached to a metal pipe fitted at the bottom of the apparatus, the upper end of which lies above the level of water in the outer container). When air is blown into the inlet tube, it raises the bell, the water acting as an **airtight seal**.

> **NOTE**
> One can record not only VC with this apparatus but also a few lung volumes and capacities, though only approximately. Their accurate recording is done on the recording spirometer.

Procedure

1. Bring the bell to its lowest position by gently pushing it down. Adjust the pointer needle to zero which indicates that the bell is completely empty.
2. Ask the patient to stand comfortably, facing the vitalograph so that she/he can see the movement of the bell.
3. Tell the subject to breathe normally (quietly) for a minute or so. Now direct the subject to inspire as deeply and as completely as possible to fill the lungs.
4. Keeping the nostrils closed with a nose clip and the mouthpiece held firmly between the lips, tell the subject to expel all the air that he/she can maximally into the vitalograph. The bell moves up and the pointer on the pulley indicates the volume of expired air.
5. Take two more readings at intervals of 2–3 minutes in the standing position as before.
6. **Effect of posture on vital capacity:** Ask the subject to sit comfortably on a stool and record the VC three times as before at intervals of 2–3 minutes.
7. Then ask the subject to lie down on the couch in supine position and record the VC three times.

> **NOTE**
> The maximum of three readings should be considered for each posture.

PRECAUTIONS

1. The arrow mark of the scale should be adjusted to zero each time before taking the recording.
2. A minimum of three attempts should be made in all posture.
3. The maximum of the three should be taken as the final reading.
4. The time interval between each attempt should be minimum of 2–3 minutes.

PHYSIOCLINICAL SIGNIFICANCE

The VC is an effort-based measurement therefore it indicates the strength of the respiratory muscles. The VC is frequently determined clinically as an index of lung function and provides useful information about abnormal ventilation due to airway obstruction, fibrosis of the lungs, mechanical interference with chest expansion and compression, strength of respiratory muscles and so on. However, it cannot help in differentiating between obstructive and restrictive lung diseases, where timed VC is of greater help.

Section 3: Human Experiments

Objective Structured Practical Examination–I

Aim: Determine vital capacity by using a vitalograph.
Procedural steps: See text above.
Checklist:
1. Adjust the vitalograph reading to zero and check for any leak in the apparatus.
2. Ask the subject to stand comfortably facing away from the vitalograph.
3. Give instruction to the subject to put in maximum effort in during the recording.
4. Instruct the subject to repeat the procedure three times and record the best reading.

Objective Structured Practical Examination–II

Aim: Effect of posture on vital capacity.
Procedural steps: See text above.
Checklist:
1. Adjust the vitalograph reading to zero.
2. Instruct the subject to lie down supine on a couch.
3. Give instructions to the subject to exhale forcefully and maximally after a deep inspiration and record the reading.
4. Ask the subject to repeat the procedure in sitting and standing position.
5. Compare all the readings and report.

QUESTIONS

Q.1. What is the normal vital capacity? Can it be predicted?
The normal VC varies between 3.2 L to 4.8 L, the value being 20% lower in females. In general, the VCs (and other volumes and capacities) are larger in males, taller persons and in younger adults. Thus, since the VC depends on age, sex, body build, occupation, etc. various formulae have been introduced to predict VC in an individual. Various disorders may then be diagnosed by comparing the actual (determined) values with the predicted normal values for one's age, sex, height, etc. The VC is high in athletes, swimmers, divers, etc. but is low in persons who have sedentary habits.

Q.2. How will you check for the leak in the system?
Let the vitalograph bell float on water in the inner cylinder. While obstructing the corrugated rubber tube to prevent any leakage of air, apply pressure from above. If there is a leak in the system the bell will begin to move down.

Q.3. What is the clinical importance of determination of vital capacity?

Q.4. Why do we take maximum of three reading to obtain the best result?
This is done as vitalography is an effort dependent procedure.

Q.5. What is two-stage vital capacity?
Two-stage vital capacity is defined as the sum of inspiratory capacity (IC) and ERV measured separately with the help of a vitalograph.

Q.6. Describe the effect of posture on vital capacity?
The VC is maximum in the standing position, less in the sitting position and least in the supine position. This effect of posture is due to the following factors:
1. In the sitting and supine positions, the muscles of respiration (both primary and accessory) cannot be employed as forcefully and effectively for the expansion and compression of lungs and chest.
2. In the supine position, the abdominal viscera push the diaphragm up and interfere with its movements. The mobility of the chest is also reduced by the contact of the back with the bed.
3. There is accumulation of more blood in the blood vessels of the lungs (especially veins) in the supine position. This decreases the total lung capacity and hence the VC.

Q.7. Name the factors that affect vital capacity.
The factors affecting VC are:
1. **Physiological factors:**
   a. *Size and development of the subject:* Males have larger chests, greater body surface area (BSA) and greater muscle power.
      VC in males—2.6 L/m^2 BSA; Females—2.1 L/m^2 BSA
   b. *Age:* It is lower in children. VC decreases in old age due to loss of elasticity of lungs and weaker compressing forces.
   c. *Strength of respiratory muscles:* VC increases in swimmers and divers.
   d. *Posture:* VC is maximum in the standing position, less in the sitting position and least in the supine position.
   e. *Pregnancy:* Decreases VC.
2. **Pathological factors:** Diseases like lung congestion, diseases of lungs and chest wall and accumulation of fluid in the abdominal cavity (ascites) decreases the VC.

OBSERVATION AND RESULT

All the readings should be taken in standing, supine and sitting positions.

Record your observations as indicated below:

Vital capacity (Readings in mL)				
Position	1st	2nd	3rd	Maximum value
a. Standing				
b. Sitting				
c. Supine				

INTERPRETATION

....
....
....
....
....

STUDY NOTES

Date ....

CHAPTER 3.10

Cardiopulmonary Resuscitation

INTRODUCTION

Cardiopulmonary resuscitation (CPR) is a first aid, but life-saving, emergency procedure and must be started without losing a second.

Cardiopulmonary arrest is said to have occurred when there is a sudden stoppage of heart or breathing or both. It is an extreme emergency that threatens life. Consciousness is lost within 10–15 seconds of stoppage of oxygen supply to the brain and some brain damage occurs in 5–6 minutes. Circulatory arrest for more than 10–15 minutes causes permanent damage to the brain.

Important: Artificial respiration (AR) alone may be needed if breathing has stopped suddenly though the heart is still beating (as it happens in many cases). However, if breathing is not restarted within 3–4 minutes, the heart will also stop. In this case, both AR and external cardiac compression will be required.

> **NOTE**
> The survival rates of out-of-hospital cardiopulmonary arrest (say due to a heart attack on a roadside or in a building) are sadly very low. The main reason is ignorance of the value of CPR in saving lives, but even in trained health personnel and bystanders, there is unwillingness to provide CPR for fear of catching acquired immunodeficiency syndrome (AIDS), hepatitis or tuberculosis through mouth-to-mouth respiration. Also, when professionals do CPR, it is often not done well.

It is for this reason that medical/dental and other lifesciences students must be seriously trained in this life-saving procedure.

AIM OF CARDIOPULMONARY RESUSCITATION

The aim of CPR is to "artificially" push oxygen-containing blood to the brain and other vital organs (when the heart and lungs fail to do this vital job), till the heart and lungs regain their normal function or the victim is shifted to the hospital.

GENERAL PLAN FOR CARDIOPULMONARY RESUSCITATION

Management of a case of cardiopulmonary arrest involves two phases:
1. **Phase I: Emergency measures—basic life support (BLS)**
   The management sequence of BLS
   Initially the sequence of management in order of importance was **ABC**, i.e.
   A: Airways
   B: Breathing
   C: Circulation.
   According to the new guidelines of CPR, this order has been changed to—**CAB,** i.e.
   - **Circulation:** Re-establish circulation if there is insufficient heart beat or if the heart has stopped.
   - **Airway:** Establish an airway or maintain it if it is open.

- **Breathing:** Provide artificial ventilation if breathing has stopped.

> **NOTE**
> These procedures must be performed in that order.

- **C—Circulate:** Give external cardiac massage. Alternate 30 cardiac compressions with two quick lung inflations. Continuous compressions at the rate of 100–120/min.
  If unconscious, but breathing and pulse are present:
- **A—Airway:** Tilt the head back with a hand under the neck to maintain an open airway.
  If not breathing:
- **B—Breathe:** Give mouth-to-mouth respiration (or mouth-to-nose). Inflate lungs 14–16 times/min to provide adequate oxygen supply.
  Maintain head tilt to avoid flaccid tongue from falling back into pharynx.
  Feel carotid pulse.
  If pulse present, continue lung inflations. **If pulse absent (death-like appearance, fixed, dilated pupils).**

2. Phase II: Definitive treatment—advanced cardiac life support
   This phase of treatment is carried out in the hospital and includes:
   D: Drugs (adrenaline, intravenous sodium bicarbonate for acidosis, etc.)
   E: Electrocardiogram (ECG) monitoring
   F: Fibrillation treatment with a defibrillator, lidocaine or procaine
   G: Gauging and restoration of normal breathing and circulation
   H: Hypothermia
   I: Management of the patient in the intensive care unit (ICU) of the hospital.

CAUSES OF CARDIOPULMONARY ARREST

Acute Conditions

1. Drowning
2. Hanging
3. Electric shock
4. Massive, acute myocardial infarction (MI) leading to cardiac standstill (asystole) or fibrillation
5. Inhalation of poisonous gases (e.g. carbon monoxide)
6. Overdose or sensitivity to an anesthetic agent, poisoning with narcotics and drugs (accidental or suicidal) (e.g. barbiturates, opium, etc.), acids and other chemicals
7. Head injuries
8. Obstruction of respiratory passages by inhalation of a foreign body (e.g. a fishbone)
9. Anaphylactic shock.

Chronic Conditions

1. Poliomyelitis
2. Diphtheria
3. Ascending paralysis
4. Obstruction of air passages by a tumor of pharynx, larynx, etc.

SIGNS AND SYMPTOMS OF CARDIOPULMONARY ARREST

1. The victim is unconscious, lips, face, earlobes, fingers and toes are blue and there is death-like appearance.
2. The skin is pale, cold and moist and the pupils are dilated and fixed, i.e. nonresponsive to light (these features are due to sympathetic stimulation).
3. **Absent or weak arterial pulse:** The carotid artery must be palpated because the radial pulse may be too weak to be felt.
4. **Absence of heart sounds:** Put your ear on the chest of the victim and try to confirm presence or absence of heart sounds.
5. **Breathing is absent:** There is no movement of the chest or the alae nasi (nostrils). There is no air coming out of the nose or mouth.
6. Blood pressure is not recordable.

What to Do Immediately:
Confirm the diagnosis: Unconsciousness, absent carotid artery pulse. Note what time is it. One person should be in-charge.

1. **Assess:**
   a. **Thump the chest** (if there is no carotid pulse). This may stop fibrillation. Recheck pulse. If absent, start CPR.
   b. Make sure you are in a safe place. Trying CPR on the road may risk your life as well.
   First establish unresponsiveness:
   a. Determine the responsiveness of the victim by tapping him/her on the shoulder and asking "Are you all right?"
   b. Check carotid pulse and breathing to make sure that the heart and breathing have really stopped, because if the heart is still beating, there will be enough muscle tone so that external cardiac massage may cause fracture of the ribs.
2. **Start CPR routine** after confirming cardiopulmonary arrest and find out if a bystander can help.

Section 3: Human Experiments

3. **Ask a bystander to phone the hospital emergency** for an ambulance because you do not have time to do so yourself. If no one is available, continue CPR till the victim is revived.

> **NOTE**
> CPR is never demonstrated on a normal waking person for the same reason. Demonstration dummies are available for CPR training.

What Not to Do:
1. Do not delay resuscitation; immediate intervention is required after establishing unresponsiveness.
2. The victim must not be made to sit or stand. No pillow should be placed under the head or neck, as this will bend the head and close the trachea.
3. The feet and legs should be raised by placing a pillow, etc. under the hips/legs. This will help promote venous return to the heart.
4. Nothing should be given by mouth to a semiconscious or unconscious individual for fear of aspiration of the fluid into the lungs.
5. There should be no crowding around the victim.

ARTIFICIAL RESPIRATION (PULMONARY RESUSCITATION)

Artificial respiration (AR; assisted ventilation) may be given by **manual methods, mouth-to-mouth method** (sometimes called **"kiss of life"** or **"rescue breath"**) **or** by **mechanical methods.**

> **NOTE**
> Though mouth-to-mouth respiration has been found to be the best general first aid procedure, but which method to use in a given case will depend on the cause of cardiopulmonary arrest. For example, in a case of drowning or near drowning, face injuries, fracture of jaw and chemical burns on lips and in the mouth, it may not be possible to give mouth-to-mouth respiration. In such cases, International Red Cross recommends Holger Nielsen method.

Manual Methods

The old prone or supine position methods: Schafer's prone position, back pressure, Sylvester's supine position arm lift and Thomson's hip-lift chest pressure methods are no longer employed since they rely on compressing the thorax to cause expiration and then allowing lungs to expand passively. The Holger Nielsen method described here is used when mouth-to-mouth respiration is not possible.

Holger Nielsen Method (Back-pressure Arm-lift Method)

1. Place the victim, face downward (Figs. 3.10.1A to D) on a hard surface with the arms bent and the head turned to one side and resting on the hands.
2. Kneel down on one knee at the victim's head with the opposite foot placed near the elbow.
3. Place your hands with fingers widespread on the victim's back just below the scapulae. Now rock forward with the arms held straight at the elbows until your arms are vertical and pressing down on the back. This compresses the chest and produces expiration.
4. Slide your hands sideways and outward on to the victim's arms just above the elbows. Now rock backward, lifting the victim's elbows until some resistance is felt at her/his shoulders. This movement expands the thorax, decreasing the intrathoracic pressure and causing inspiration.
5. Repeat this cycle of compression and expansion (that lasts for about 3 seconds each) for about 12 times a minute.

Mouth-to-mouth Respiration (Rescue Breath; Exhaled-air Ventilation)

Mouth-to-mouth respiration (Figs. 3.10.2A to C) has proved to be superior to all the manual methods in all age groups. Comparative studies have proved it to be the only technique capable of producing satisfactory ventilation.

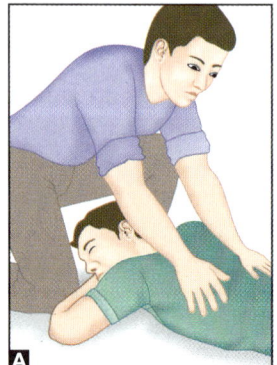 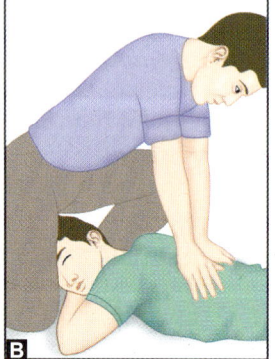 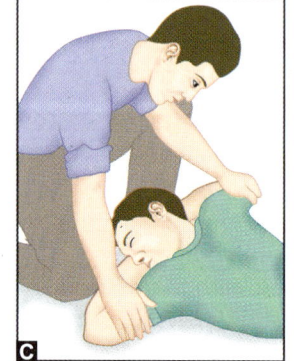 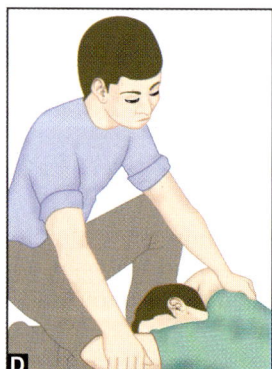

Figs. 3.10.1A to D: Holger Nielsen (back-pressure arm-lift, BPAL) method of artificial respiration. (A and B) Back pressure; (C and D) Arm lift.

Chapter 3.10: Cardiopulmonary Resuscitation

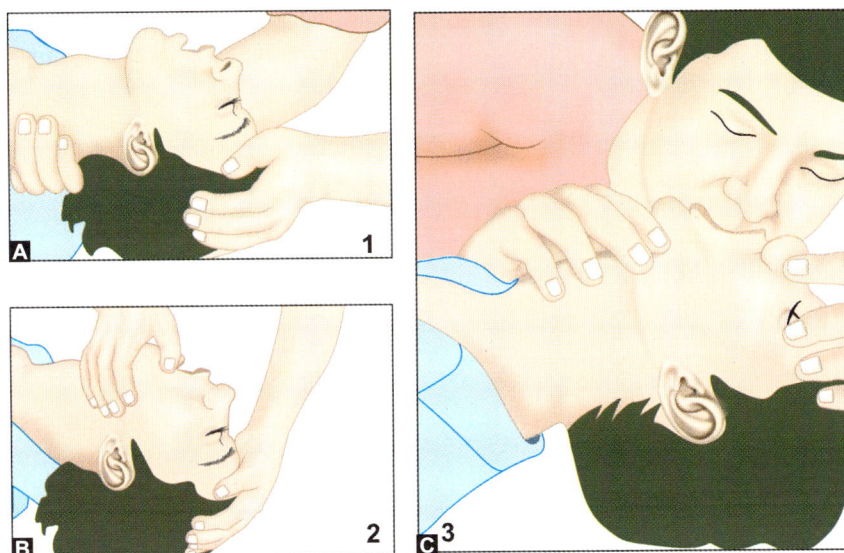

Figs. 3.10.2A to C: Mouth-to-mouth respiration. (A) Tilting the head back; (B) Lifting the chin and angle of law; and (C) Clamping the nostrils and blowing air into victim's lungs.

Advantages and Disadvantages of Mouth-to-mouth Respiration

The method is simple, safe and easy to perform, even by a layman with minimum instruction. Above all, it does not require any apparatus. The only disadvantage is that the victim's flaccid (toneless) tongue tends to fall back into the pharynx and thus obstruct the airway. However, this can be avoided by extending the neck and turning the head slightly to one side.

Procedure

1. Place the victim on his/her back on firm ground and loosen the clothing around the neck, chest and waist.
2. Remove any mucus, food, saliva or any foreign material (e.g. grass, dentures, etc.) from the mouth and nose with your fingers wrapped in a handkerchief.
3. Open the airway by tilting the head back. Kneel by the right side of the victim. Place your right hand under the neck and lift it while keeping a pressure on the forehead with the heel of the other hand (Figs. 3.10.2A to C) (the extension of the neck lifts the flaccid tongue from the back of the throat). Using your right thumb and fingers, lift the chin and angle of the jaw upward and forward. This simple procedure keeps the airway open.
4. Clamp the nostrils with your left thumb and fingers, take a deep breath, apply your mouth firmly on the victim's mouth (or nose if the pharynx cannot be cleared) and blow a liter of air into the victim's lungs, watching the expansion of the chest at the same time (remember, the expired air contains 15% oxygen).
5. Remove your mouth, turn your head to one side and take another deep breath as the elastic recoil of the chest causes expiration. You may feel and hear the expiratory airflow from the victim's mouth and nose.
6. **Repeat the cycle of** blowing out—turning the head—breathing in—about 14–16 times a minute till spontaneous breathing returns or the victim is shifted to the hospital.
7. **Important:** Feel the carotid pulse. If after 6–8 lung inflations, there is no improvement in the color of the victim, suspect cardiac arrest and start external cardiac massage as well.

> **NOTE**
> If the airway is clear, only a moderate resistance will be felt when you exhale air into the victim's lungs.

Mechanical Respirators

Mechanical ventilation is employed when AR has to be given for long periods, e.g. during chronic respiratory failure. Airtight metallic or plastic devices are placed around the chest and negative pressure is applied at intervals; this draws air into the lungs. The elastic recoil of the lungs and chest causes expiration.

Alternate positive and negative pressures are also employed.

1. **Drinker's tank respirator (also called the "iron lung"):** It is an iron chamber in which the patient is placed with the head kept outside, an airtight collar sealing the body inside. The pressure in the chamber is alternately raised

(2–3 cm water) for expiration and lowered (–10 cm to –14 cm H_2O) for inspiration by means of a pump.

2. **Sahlin's jacket model, Bragg–Paul pulsator**: These employ elastic chest jackets in which pressure can be increased and decreased at intervals.
3. **Eve's rocking method**: The victim is laid on a stretcher or a plank and the shoulders and ankles are fastened to it. A rhythmic rocking up and down like a see-saw causes the abdominal viscera to push up against the diaphragm (expiration) or pull it down (inspiration).

> **NOTE**
> In operation theaters and critical care units, the acute respiratory failure patients are intubated (an endotracheal tube put in the trachea via the mouth) and pulses of air or a mixture of gases are delivered through an Ambu bag/machine. It is common to maintain positive end-expiratory pressure (PEEP) to help in expansion of the lungs.

EXTERNAL CARDIAC MASSAGE (CARDIAC RESUSCITATION)

Rationale

One may doubt the efficacy of external cardiac massage in causing blood to circulate when the heart has stopped or fibrillating. However, there are two reasons for believing that cardiac output and coronary perfusion can be partially maintained by CPR:

1. When the heart stops suddenly, the pulmonary veins, left heart and the arteries are full of oxygenated blood. Cardiac massage causes this blood to start flowing.
2. Since the heart is situated between two rigid structures—sternum in front and vertebrae behind— pressure (compression) applied on the chest in front of it squeezes it, thus producing a mechanical systole. The right and left ventricular pressures exceed the pulmonary and aortic pressures which cause a forward flow of blood. When the pressure is released, it causes diastolic filling of the ventricles due to the pressure gradient between the large peripheral veins and intrathoracic structures—especially the thin-walled right ventricle.

Procedure

1. Lay the victim on a firm surface. Kneel beside him and place the heel of your left hand (fingers extended and not touching the chest) on the junction of upper two-thirds and lower one-third of the sternum. Place the heel of the other hand over the first parallel to it (Figs. 3.10.3A and B).
2. Keeping the elbows straight, bend forward and depress the sternum toward the spine by 4–5 cm at a rate of 80–90/min. The movement should be at the shoulders so that the force can be transmitted through the hands to the chest.

   Cardiopulmonary resuscitation:
   - One person CPR cycle is 30 compressions to 2 breaths.
   - Two persons CPR cycle is 30 compressions to 2 breaths.
     (Alternate 30 cardiac compressions with two quick lung inflations)
   - Two person CPR for child and infant is 15 compressions to 2 breaths.

> **NOTE**
> If the CPR is being given correctly, you will quickly see an improvement in skin color of the victim; pupils will return to normal size and neck pulsations will be visible and heart sounds will be heard.

In Infants

Press the sternum with two fingers of a hand or with a thumb with the fingers supporting the back of the infant. Compress by 2–3 cm and maintain cardiac compressions at a rate of 100–110/min.

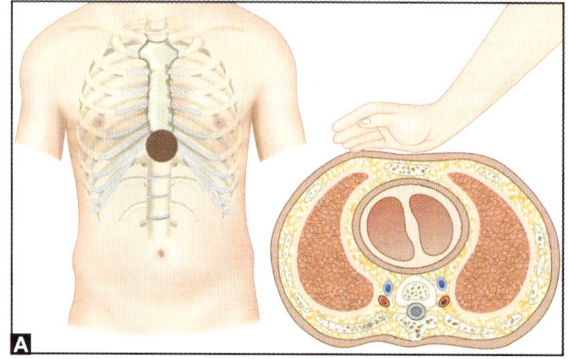 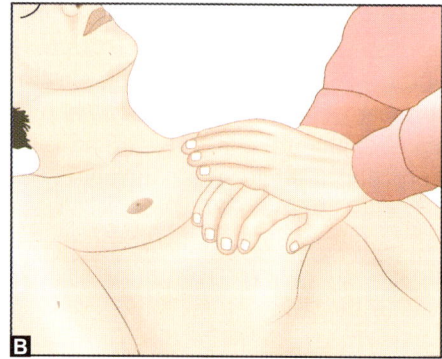

Figs. 3.10.3A and B: External cardiac massage (cardiac resuscitation). (A) The black circle over the region of the heart shows the area where compression should be applied and (B) The position of hands for chest compression. The victim must be placed on a firm surface.

INTERNAL OR OPEN CARDIAC MASSAGE

This procedure is employed in hospitals. The chest is opened in the left intercostal space in the midclavicular line; a hand is inserted into the thorax and the heart is compressed against the chest wall. There is a transdiaphragmatic approach as well.

CARDIOPULMONARY RESUSCITATION FOR ONESELF

What to do when one gets an attack of MI when alone. Coughing very vigorously and repeatedly can save life. A breath and a forceful cough, repeated every 3 seconds, without let up till help arrives or the heart is felt to be beating normally.

REASONS FOR FAILURE OF CARDIOPULMONARY RESUSCITATION

In every case you must try your best to get the heart and lungs functioning again. However, in some cases, all efforts at CPR may fail. It may be that:
- The injury to the heart is very severe or
- Acid-base disturbances (lactic acidemia) and electrolyte imbalance do not allow the heart rate and rhythm to be restored.

VENTRICULAR FIBRILLATION

Ventricular fibrillation (VF) is the most common cause of cardiac arrest because a fibrillating (trembling) heart cannot act as an effective pump. It is most frequently caused by acute MI as a result of which an "ectopic" irritable focus starts to discharge action potentials (APs) in a fast and irregular manner. The heart responds to these APs and goes into fibrillation. If VF is not stopped within 2–3 minutes, it almost always leads to death. The specific treatment includes:

1. **Electroshock defibrillation (cardioversion):** While a weak AC current (as in accidental shock or in death penalty) causes VF and death, a strong, high voltage current applied to the chest via large, flat electrodes, can stop fibrillation. All APs stop and the heart remains quiescent for 4–5 seconds after which it starts to beat at the normal rate and rhythm. The shock may have to be repeated a couple of times.
2. **Intravenous injection of 100 mL of 8% sodium bicarbonate** is used to neutralize lactic acidemia.
3. Intravenous injection of 5–10 mL of 1% calcium chloride.
4. Intravenous or intracardiac injection of 0.5 mL of 1:1000 adrenaline often revives the heart.

HEIMLICH MANEUVER (ABDOMINAL THRUST) FOR INHALATION OF FOREIGN BODY

This procedure can be life-saving when a person begins to choke on something he/she is eating (e.g. a fishbone) or in a child who puts something in his mouth and inadvertently "inhales" it, e.g. coin, marble, etc.

> **IMPORTANT**
> Choking must not be confused with an attack of MI. A person who chokes on something cannot speak but only make gestures, while a heart attack victim can (and, of course, choking is likely to occur while eating. Therefore, ask, can you speak?).

Procedure

1. Stand behind the person, place your clenched fist below his epigastrium (between the costal margin and the umbilicus) and grasp this fist with the other hand.
2. Now give a sudden upward and inward thrust. It is important that the thrust is applied to the upper abdomen and not to the thorax.
3. The sudden thrust pushes the diaphragm up so that the forceful blast of air from the lungs carries the foreign body out of the respiratory passages. The maneuver may be repeated until the foreign object is expelled.

> **IMPORTANT**
> In many cases of choking, the respiratory passage is not completely blocked (though there may be laryngeal spasm), so that if the person breathes quietly and without panic, enough air may reach the lungs to keep him alive until he is shifted to the hospital.
> If you happen to choke on something, when alone, position yourself over the high back of a chair or some other suitable furniture and thrust your abdomen suddenly and forcefully against it. Repeat if necessary.

Emergency Procedure in Children

Bend the head of the victim forward and downward so that it is lower than the chest. Then, with the heel of a hand, give a few blows on the child's back between the scapulae till the offending object is expelled.

Note that the head must be kept lower than the chest, otherwise the foreign object is likely to be pushed further down into the lungs rather than upward.

QUESTIONS

Q.1. Name the indications for cardiopulmonary resuscitation.
Cardiopulmonary resuscitation is a first aid measure and is indicated when there is a sudden stoppage of breathing or heart or both.

Q.2. What are the causes and signs of cardiopulmonary arrest?

Q.3. Name the advantages and disadvantages of mouth-to-mouth respiration.

Q.4. How will you handle a case of drowning?
1. As soon as the victim is brought out of the water, check carotid pulse and breathing. If both present but unconscious, press on lower abdomen to expel water from stomach, if any. Then place the victim in "recovery position", i.e. partial supine position, head turned to one side, left arm under left thigh, right arm above the head and right leg bent.
2. If the pulse is present, but the victim is not breathing—start mouth-to-mouth breathing or Holger Nielsen method of AR.
3. If both pulse and breaching are absent—start CPR till the victim recovers or is shifted to the hospital.

Q.5. How does defibrillation help in ventricular fibrillation?
A strong, high voltage AC current applied to the chest can stop a fibrillating heart. However, within a few seconds, normal heart beat usually returns.

Q.6. What is Heimlich maneuver?
It is an emergency procedure to clear the upper respiratory passages after a foreign body has been accidentally inhaled.

STUDY NOTES

Teacher's Signature

CHAPTER 3.11

Basal Metabolic Rate

AIM

To measure the basal metabolic rate (BMR) of the subject.

INTRODUCTION

The total heat production or energy expenditure of the body is the sum of the energy required to carry out various body functions. The lowest level of energy production is called the basal metabolism. The measurement of the heat production under basal conditions is called as **BMR**. It is measured as kcal/h/m² body surface area (BSA).

Basal conditions essential for measuring BMR:
1. Complete physical and mental rest
2. Postabsorptive state, i.e. after 12–16 hours from the last meal
3. Comfortable ambient temperature: 20–25°C.
4. Test is carried out in awake stage in recumbent position.

The BMR can be estimated with sufficient accuracy merely by measuring the oxygen consumption of the subject for 6 minutes under basal conditions.

Normal values for adults:
- Males: 40 kcal/h/m² BSA
- Females: 37 kcal/h/m² BSA.

BMR is considered within normal limits if the values are between ± 10% of the normal values.

MEASUREMENT OF BASAL METABOLISM

Oxygen consumption can be measured by:

- **Open circuit method:** Collection of expired air in Douglas bag and analyzing it for carbon dioxide and oxygen. The difference in the composition of the atmospheric air and the expired air when computed for the total expired indicates total oxygen consumption.
- **Closed circuit breathing:** Most commonly used method for measuring BMR clinically. The indirect principle is employed whereby oxygen consumption if the subject is measured and is then translated into terms of heat production.

PROCEDURE

1. The subject is made to sit on a stool, relaxing close to the spirometer which has been filled with 100% oxygen.
2. A nasal clip is fixed on the nose of the subject and he is asked to respire through the nose piece, valve with inlet open to the atmosphere, till he is relaxed and adapted to breathe through the mouthpiece.
3. Subject is connected to the spirometer and 6 minutes graph is recorded (Fig. 3.11.1).
4. Determine the mean value of oxygen utilization per minute (This is taken from the slope of oxygen utilization graph).
5. During rest the oxygen utilized for 6 minutes by the subject is corrected to Standard Temperature and Pressure, Dry (STPD) by multiplying with a factor after consulting the charts. As the subject had a mixed diet breakfast his respiratory quotient may be presumed to be 0.85. Therefore each liter of oxygen provides 4.83 calories.

Chapter 3.11: Basal Metabolic Rate

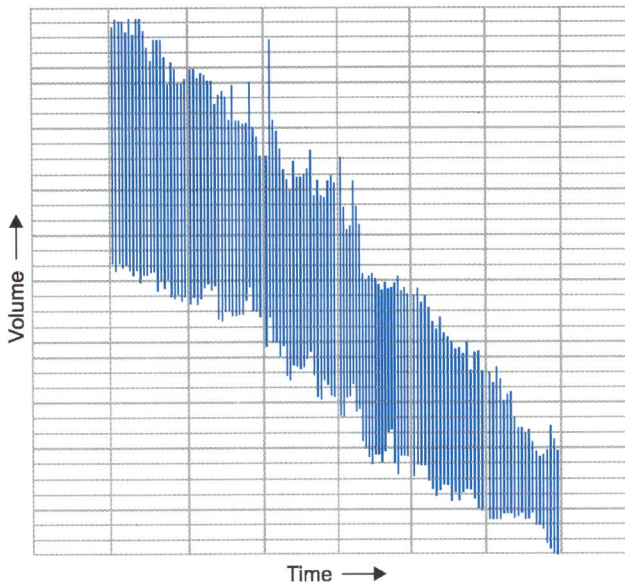

Fig. 3.11.1: Graph showing the respiratory movements for recording oxygen consumption on a spirometer.

6. Under basal conditions, the energy output will represent the basal metabolic rate. However, for this calculation, compare the energy output of the subject with that of the standard for the same age, sex (per sq m body surface area) and represent the result as percentage in ± above or below the expected value.
7. Surface area is calculated by using the "nomograms", taking into consideration the weight and height of the subject. Energy output per hr per sq m body surface area is then calculated.
8. Energy output of normal human being under basal conditions depends upon the age and sex of the person.
9. Experimental values obtained are compared with the standard value. The results are expressed as % variation ± from the normal.

CALCULATIONS

Calculation of oxygen consumption per minute

$$= \frac{\text{Initial level of } O_2 - \text{Final level of } O_2 \text{ (after 6 minutes)}}{6}$$

Oxygen utilization per hour (60 min) = Oxygen utilization in 6 min × 10 at BTPS (body temperature, ambient pressure, saturated with water vapour) = A

Oxygen utilization at STPD (B) = A × Correction factor (C)
= B × 4.82*

> **NOTE**
> *Caloric equivalent of 1 L of oxygen consumed per hour at STPD at a respiratory quotient (RQ) of 0.80 = 4.82 kcal). STPD is Standard Temperature and Pressure, dry; denoting a volume of dry gas at 32°F (0°C) and a pressure of 760 mm Hg.

Hence, BMR of the subject = (B × 4.82)/BSA in kcal/h/m²
Refer Appendix for BSA nomogram and Du Bois nomogram.

PHYSIOCLINICAL SIGNIFICANCE

1. For diagnosing various pathological conditions, e.g. hypothyroidism and hyperthyroidism.
2. To understand how different types of food affects the BMR which will help in prescribing an adequate diet.

QUESTIONS

Q.1. What is BMR?
Q.2. What is the normal value of BMR?
Q.3. What are the conditions necessary for the measurement of BMR?
Q.4. What are the factors that affect the BMR?

Factors that affect the BMR:

Factors that increase BMR:
- Higher lean body mass
- Greater height (more surface area)
- Younger age
- Elevated levels of thyroid hormone
- Stress, fever, illness
- Male gender
- Pregnancy and lactation
- Certain, drugs, such as stimulants, caffeine and tobacco.

Factors that decrease BMR:
- Lower lean body mass
- Lower height
- Older age
- Depressed levels of thyroid hormone
- Starvation or fasting
- Female gender.

Section 3: Human Experiments

STUDY NOTES

UNIT 3: SPECIAL SENSES

Date ....

CHAPTER 3.12

Perimetry

AIM

To map the peripheral field of vision with Priestley Smith perimeter.

INTRODUCTION

Field of vision: The part of the external world visible to one eye when a person fixes his gaze at one particular point is called the field of vision for that eye.

The visual field can be tested by **confrontation method** and **perimetry**. The process of mapping the monocular field of vision using a perimeter is called as **perimetry**. It is employed for the diagnosis of various lesions of the visual pathways, diagnosis of glaucoma and retinal lesions. The peripheral limits for the field of vision are largely determined by the margins of the orbit, nose and cheek.

Normal extent of field of vision using **5 mm of white object** for monocular vision:
1. Superior (Upward): 60° restricted by superior orbital margin
2. Temporal/Lateral (Outward): 100° restricted by lateral orbital margin
3. Inferior (Downward): 75° restricted by inferior orbital margin
4. Medial/Nasal (Inward): 60° restricted by the nose.

NOTE
The two visual fields, one for each eye, overlap in the medial part forming an area of **binocular vision.** In this area, the object is seen by both the eyes. Binocular vision enables in appreciating the depth and proportion of objects. For binocular vision, the field of vision extends more than 200° laterally and about 140° vertically. It is to be remembered that monocular field of vision is not a circle, but an irregular ovoid and the outer and inner parts of the field are unequally divided.

PRINCIPLE

One eye is covered while the other is fixed at the central fixation point of the perimeters. A small test object is moved towards this central point along different meridians. Along each meridian, the location where the test object **first** becomes visible, is plotted in degrees marked on the arc, away from the central point. This is repeated in at least 12 different meridians and plotted.

VISUAL PATHWAY

The **optic nerve** fibers from the nasal (medial) half of each retina cross to the opposite side in the **optic chiasma**, while fibers from the temporal (lateral) half of each retina remain on the same side. At the optic chiasma, fibers from the inner nasal half of each retina decussate. The **optic tract** formed by this decussation project to the:

Section 3: Human Experiments

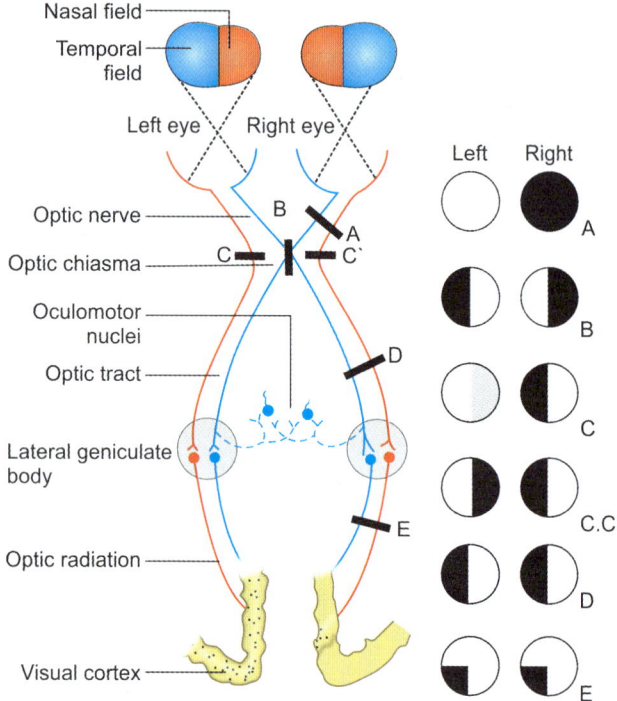

Fig. 3.12.1: Visual pathway. Lesions of the pathway at different locations produce defects in the fields of vision as shown on the right.

1. Pretectum of midbrain to synapse on the **Edinger-Westphal nucleus** (for light reflex).
2. Lateral geniculate body (LGB).

Fresh relays from LGB pass back in the geniculocalcarine tracts (**optic radiations**) which pass through the internal capsule where they lie behind the somatic sensory fibers to reach the **primary visual area (area 17 of Brodmann)** on the medial surface of the occipital lobe. **Areas 18 and 19** on the lateral surface are the **visual association areas** (Fig. 3.12.1).

Perimeter

Priestley Smith perimeter (Fig. 3.12.2), Lister perimeters (Fig. 3.12.3) and Student's perimeter (Fig. 3.12.4) (a simple hand perimeter) are the commonly used instruments for perimetry. These instruments accurately map the field of vision.

The Priestley Smith perimeter consists of the following parts:

1. **Stand:** A vertical stand on which a metal arc is fitted on a pivot, provides stability to the apparatus. A large black disk with a frame for holding the perimeter chart is provided on the back.
2. **Metal arc:**
   - A broad metal arc shaped like a half circle is mounted on the stand and can be rotated in any meridian around its central pivot.

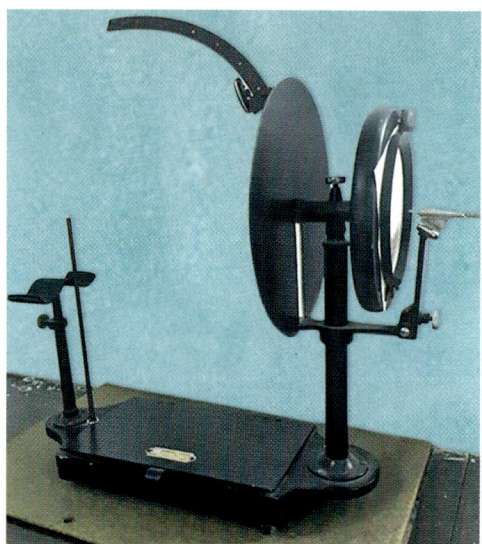

Fig. 3.12.2: Priestley Smith perimeter.

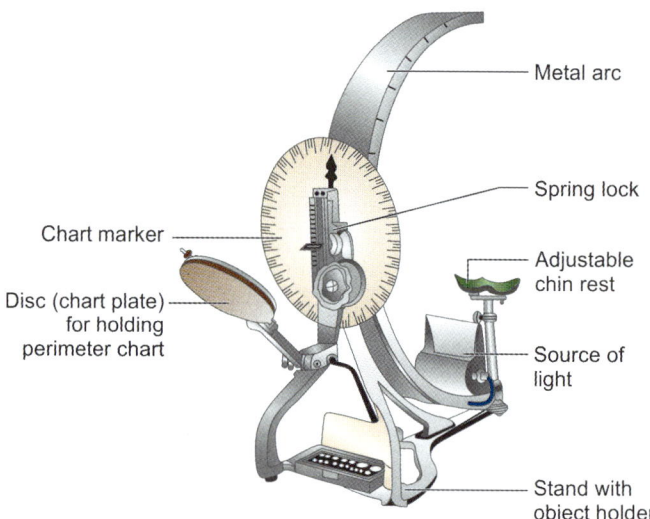

Fig. 3.12.3: Perimeter (Lister model).

- One half of the arc, the concavity of which is directed toward the subject, has a scale of 0°–90° marked on its convex surface. The "zero" mark is at the center and 90° at the periphery.

> **NOTE**
> In Lister's perimeter there is a source of light fitted at the end of the other limb and a small plane mirror is fixed in the center of the arc.

- There is a circular white spot of 5 mm diameter present at the point where the arc is pivoted on the vertical stand. This is the **fixation point** at which the subject is asked to fix his gaze, while the field of vision is being mapped.
- **Test objects** of various sizes and colors can be fitted in a carrier, which can be moved in a groove in the

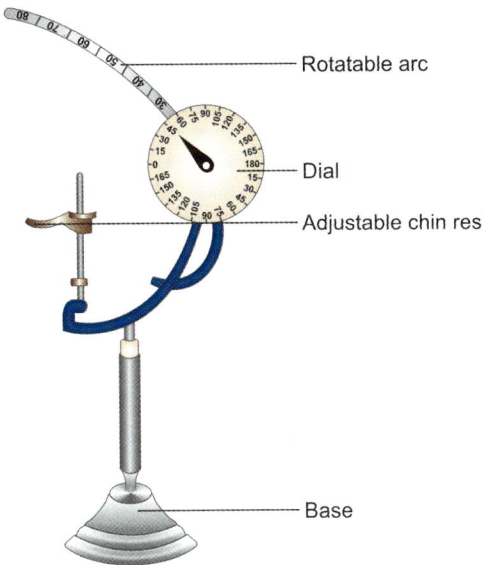

Fig. 3.12.4: Student's perimeter.

graduated limb of the arc from the periphery to its center.
- The radius of the arc, i.e. the distance between the test object and the eye varies between 250 mm and 330 mm in different types of perimeters. In Priestley perimeter, it is usually 330 mm.
3. **Chin rest:** An adjustable chin rest having two chin cups is provided to keep the head steady.

The chin of the subject rests on the **right cup when the left eye is to be tested and the left cup is used when the right eye is tested.**

4. **Scale and chart frame:** The chart frame or chart plate is meant to hold the chart paper in position. Priestley Smith model has a pin punch pointer moving on the fixation chart along the scale. It marks the distance in degrees from the central fixation point.
5. **Chart:**
   - The perimeter chart (**Figs. 3.12.5A and B**) on which the field of vision is to be plotted is divided by circles from 0° to 90° at an interval of 10°. Each circle or concentric line denotes a point of equal visual acuity. These concentric lines are called **isopters.**
   - The radii of the circles are marked at 15° intervals which indicate the **meridians**. In whatever meridian the arc is placed, all the points on it are equidistant from the eye.
   - There is a tightening screw to hold the arc in a particular meridian.
   - Both the isopters and the meridians are printed on the chart. The limits for the normal peripheral fields of vision for the two eyes and the blind spots are printed on the chart for comparison with the plotted fields of vision.
   - The **term "peripheral field" refers to the peripheral or outer limits of the field.**

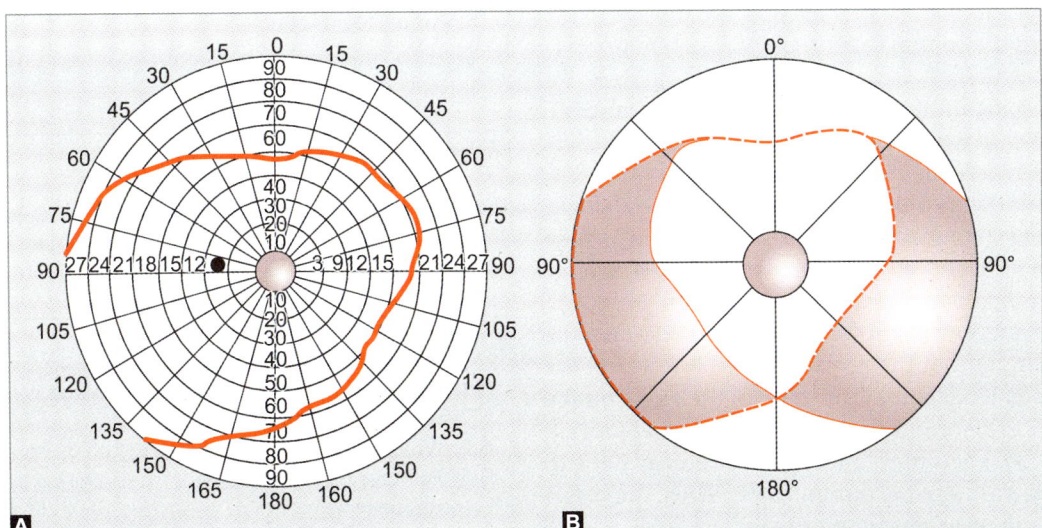

Figs. 3.12.5A and B: Perimeter chart: The fields of vision of both eyes are shown. Note that the binocular segments of the two eyes overlap and are seen by both eyes. The monocular segments of the two eye lie outside the binocular segments.

Student's Perimeter

In this model (Fig. 3.12.4), the inclination of the arc is read from a plastic dial fitted behind the mirror. When an object which is moved along the inside of the arc becomes visible. The angle it subtends at the fixation point (i.e. the mirror) in a given meridian can be read from the scale engraved on the outside of the arc. The readings—the meridian and the angle are then transferred to the corresponding points on the chart.

FACTORS AFFECTING VISUAL FIELD

1. **Visual acuity:** Obviously, the visual acuity should be sufficient to enable the subject to see the test object clearly.
2. **Size of object:** Though the visual field is better with a large object, a standard test object is used.
3. **Color of object:** The field is widest for white color and smaller for blue, red and green in that order.
4. **Brightness and contrast:** Adequate illumination affects the brightness and contrast of the object.

PROCEDURE

1. Place the perimeter on a table of suitable height and seat the subject in front of it. Fix a perimeter chart in the frame. Ask him to place his chin on the chin rest and adjust its height so that the tip of the detachable rod touches the lower eyelid and fix the chin rest in this position.
2. Ask the subject to fix his gaze on the fixation point and instruct the subject not to move his eye, but keep the gaze fixed at the central fixation point. Tell him to cover his left eye with his hand.
3. Position the arc on the zero meridian on the temporal side. Fix a 5 mm white object in the carrier and take it to the peripheral end of the arc. Instruct the subject to say "yes" as soon as the object comes into view. Now slowly move the object toward the center of the arc and as soon as the subject says "yes", strike the chart holder against the pin so that it punches a hole in the chart.
4. Rotate the arc downward (or upward) by 30°, take the object to the end of the arc and move it towards the center. When it becomes visible, mark the angle on the chart paper as before. Repeat the procedure after moving the arc by 30° each time until the arc returns back to the starting position, i.e. through 360°. Thus, the test is performed along at least 12 meridians.
5. **Mapping the blind spot:** To mark the **blind spot**, **position the arc at 100° meridian (i.e. 10° below the horizontal) on the temporal side.** Move the object from the periphery toward the center. The subject will continue to see the object up to about 20°, then it will disappear, but reappear once again after about 5°. Mark both the points on the chart; a small circle around these points will mark the **blind spot** which is **5–6° in diameter and situated about 15° lateral to the central fixation point**.
6. Plot the field of vision for the other eye in a similar manner.
7. Remove the chart from its holder and join all the pinholes with a pen to obtain the peripheral fields of vision for both the eyes. Note the area that is common to both eyes.
8. Examine the entire field of vision, in addition to mapping only the peripheral field of vision by bringing the test object right up to the fixation point at the center in all meridians and noting if the object disappears after appearing at the periphery of the field. This will reveal if there is any **scotoma** in any part of the field.

PRECAUTIONS

1. The subject should be instructed not to move the eye from the fixation point.
2. While testing for one eye, the other eye should be kept closed.
3. Adequate illumination should be provided.
4. If the subject wears glasses, these should be removed as they may restrict the field of vision. Contact lenses should not be removed.
5. Healthy eye should be tested first—to get an idea of the reliability of the subject's response and the extent of his normal visual field.
6. Ensure that the test object (especially the white test object) is clean.

PHYSIOCLINICAL SIGNIFICANCE

Perimetry is used:
1. For diagnosis of lesions in visual pathway.
2. Diagnosis of scotomas.

QUESTIONS

Q.1. What is meant by field of vision? What is the extent of a field of vision for normal eye?

Q.2. Which parts of the retina are tested by perimetry?
Perimetry tests most parts of the retina **except the macular region** which contains the fovea centralis. The fovea contains only the cones and is the region of most acute vision.

Q.3. What is physiological blind spot and what is its significance?
The **physiological blind spot** is also known as **physiological scotoma**. It corresponds with the optic disc which is the

region where the optic nerve leaves and the blood vessels enter the eye. The optic disc is 1.5 mm in diameter and is located 3 mm medial to and slightly above the posterior pole of the eye (the location of macula lutea). As there are no rods or cones in the optic disc, any image falling on it is not visible.

Q.4. Describe the visual pathway.
See Figure 3.12.1.

Q.5. What is bitemporal hemianopia and what is its cause?
Blindness in the temporal fields of vision of both eyes is called **bitemporal hemianopia**. A lesion of crossed fibers in the central part of optic chiasma, commonly due to a pituitary tumor causes this type of visual defect (*See* Fig. 3.12.1).

Q.6. What is binasal hemianopia and what is its cause?
Blindness in the nasal halves of fields of vision of both eyes is called **binasal hemianopia**. It occurs when the uncrossed optic nerve fibers in the lateral parts of optic chiasma are damaged. Usually, there is right or left nasal hemianopia as a result of a calcified internal carotid artery pressing on one or the other side of the chiasma (*See* Fig. 3.12.1).

Q.7. What is homonymous hemianopia?
Blindness in the temporal half of field of vision of one eye and the nasal field of the other eye is called **homonymous hemianopia**. A lesion of optic tract or optic radiation by tumors of parietal or temporal lobes produces this type of defect. A lesion on the right side will produce left homonymous hemianopia and a lesion on the left side will produce right homonymous hemianopia (homonymous, because right half of field of one eye and right half of field of the other eye is affected. If right half of field of one eye and left half of field of the other eye is affected, it is called **heteronymous hemianopia**, e.g. binasal or bitemporal hemianopias). Partial damage to optic radiation will produce superior (lower part of radiation involved) or inferior (upper part affected) **homonymous quadrantanopia** (*See* Fig. 3.12.1).

Q.8. What is stereoscopic vision?
The visual fields of the two eyes overlap, the portion common to both eyes having a diameter of 120°. The images of an object falling on the two maculae are slightly different from each other because of the separation of the two eyes. This is the basis of stereoscopic or binocular vision which is responsible for depth perception.

Q.9. What is a scotoma? What are the pathological causes of scotoma?
Generally, the term scotoma (plural, scotomata) is applied to a small area of blindness (except the physiological blind spot) lying within a visual field. It is important clinically to detect the presence of scotomata and to map their location. Causes of scotoma include glaucoma, vitamin B_{12} deficiency, demyelination of optic nerve, lesion in the visual cortex.

Q.10. Name other method of determining the field of vision.
The **confrontation test** can provide a rough estimate of the peripheral field of vision (*Refer* clinical examination of the optic nerve in Chapter 4.5).

Q.11. List the factors affecting the field of vision.

Section 3: Human Experiments

STUDY NOTES

Teacher's Signature

UNIT 4: NERVOUS SYSTEM

Date ....

CHAPTER 3.13

Reaction Time (Visual and Auditory)

AIM

To determine the reaction time to visual and auditory stimuli.

APPARATUS

1. Two tapping keys (K1, K2)
2. Signal marker
3. Short circuiting key
4. Bulb
5. Low voltage current (6V DC mains)
6. Kymograph with drum.

PRINCIPLE

Reaction time is defined as the time interval between the application of an adequate stimulus and the voluntary motor response to it.

It varies with the complexity of reflex and interrelated sensory pathways associated with the course of the impulse as it travels to the center. The reaction time can be decreased with practice and training. It can also be decreased by alertness and concentration. The reaction time is prolonged with advancing age, distraction and muscular weakness, etc.

PROCEDURE

Visual Reaction Time

1. Set up a circuit with two tapping keys (K1, K2), electromagnetic signal marker and a bulb connected in series to the 6V DC mains current source (Fig. 3.13.1).

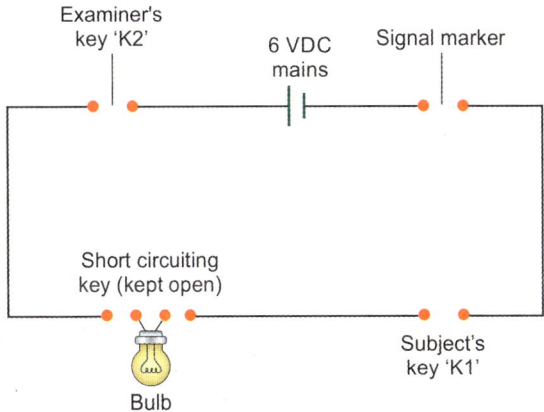

Fig. 3.13.1: Circuit diagram for visual reaction time.

2. Place the kymograph to record the movement of signal marker.
3. Without making any sound, the examiner gently press K2 to light the bulb.
4. Ask the subject to press the tapping key K1. Instruct the subject to be alert and to release the key the moment the bulb is lightened.
5. The event is marked on the drum with the signal marker as Event 1 (E1). The subject as instructed releases K2, which is marked on the drum as Event 2 (E2).
6. Take the time tracing using a tuning fork of 100 Hz and calculate the visual reaction time from the time interval between E1 and E2 (Fig. 3.13.2).

Auditory Reaction Time

1. Remove the bulb from the circuit.
2. Ask the examiner to press the tapping key K2 to produce the sound.

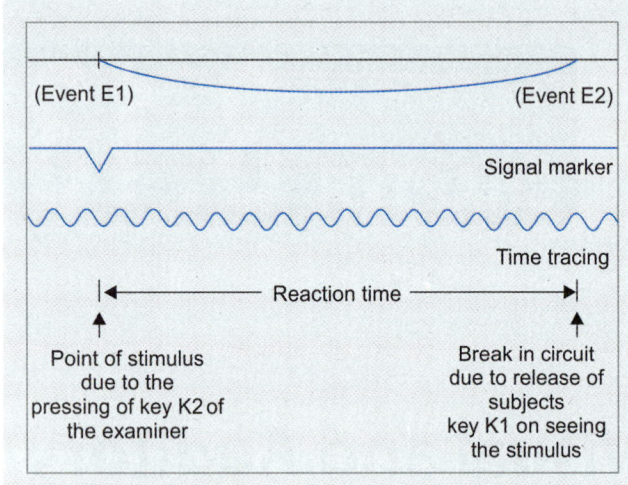

Fig. 3.13.2: Actual recording of the reaction time.

3. Ask the subject to press the tapping key K1. Instruct the subject to be alert and to release the key the moment he hears the tapping sound.
4. The event is marked on the drum with the signal marker as Event 1 (E1).
5. The subject is instructed to release K2, which is marked on the drum as Event 2 (E2).
6. Calculate the auditory reaction time from the time interval between E1 and E2.

PRECAUTIONS

1. The subject should be alert.
2. The subject should not be facing the examiner, as he should respond to the visual and auditory stimuli and not to the movement of the examiner's hand.
3. The examiner's key should be released without making any noise for the visual reaction time.

NORMAL VALUE

Visual reaction time: 200–400 ms
Auditory reaction time: 100–200 ms
Visual reaction time is more than the auditory reaction time because visual reaction time involves chemical changes in its occurrence, i.e. the conversion from a photon to a bioelectric stimuli takes *a lot* longer than the conversion from a pressure wave to bioelectric stimuli.

QUESTIONS

Q.1. Define reaction time.
Q.2. Which reaction time is longer, the visual or auditory? Explain why?
Q.3. What are the factors that affect the reaction time?

OBSERVATION AND RESULT

Take 3 readings and the best of three is taken as the final reading.

	Reading (in ms)			
	1st	2nd	3rd	Best of 3
1. Visual reaction				
2. Auditory reaction time				

INTERPRETATION

....
....
....
....
....

STUDY NOTES

CHAPTER 3.14

Electroencephalography

AIM

To demonstrate the recording of Electroencephalogram (EEG).

INTRODUCTION

The term **electroencephalogram (EEG)** denotes the record of electrical activity of brain obtained from the surface of the scalp. The procedure of recording EEG is called **electroencephalography**. The instrument which records **EEG** is called **electroencephalograph.** The term **electrocorticogram (ECoG)** is employed for recording the electrical activity recorded from the surface of the exposed brain. EEG records the electrical activity which arises without any obvious stimulation.

> **NOTE**
> **Evoked potentials** are the electrical potentials that are caused and recorded by the stimulation of sensory receptors or sensory nerve fibers.

APPARATUS

1. EEG machine
2. EEG jelly (paste)
3. EEG electrodes
4. Photostimulator.

PRINCIPLE

Gold-plated disks or shallow cups are placed on multiple analogous areas on the two sides of the scalp and simultaneous recordings are made from these areas for analysis and interpretation. The electrodes placed on the scalp record the electrical activity of the cerebral cortex. This **electrical activity arises because of the current flow in fluctuating dipoles on the dendrites of the cortical cells and cell bodies.**

FEATURES OF ELECTROENCEPHALOGRAM WAVES

Normally, all the recurring oscillations in potentials (EEG waves or brain waves) recorded from different areas of the scalp are more or less identical in waveform (shape), though their amplitude may differ slightly. The dominant rhythm of the waves is 8–13/sec and an amplitude of about 50 μV which is called the alpha rhythm. Depending on their frequency and amplitude which are inversely related, the following rhythms are described (Table 3.14.1).

Table 3.14.1: Rhythm of the electroencephalogram waves.

Rhythm	Frequency (Hz)	Voltage (μV)
Alpha (α)	8–14	50–100
Beta (β)	14–30	5–10
Theta (θ)	4–7	10
Delta (δ)	1–3.5	100

Alpha Rhythm (Berger Rhythm, 8–13/sec)

The alpha rhythm is the dominant rhythm of a normal EEG, especially from the parieto-occipital region. It is found in almost all normal, waking and relaxed adults with the eyes closed. It represents a resting state of cerebral activity, i.e. it is the rhythm of inattention.

The alpha rhythm is called a **synchronized EEG;** the synchronization is due to:
1. The synchronizing effect of neighboring, densely packed, parallel-arranged fibers (dendrites) in the cerebral cortex.
2. Rhythmic discharges from thalamus and possibly other subcortical structures.

Changes in Alpha Rhythm

Alpha rhythm is decreased in: Hypoglycemia, low body temperature, high arterial pCO_2, low levels of glucocorticoids, anesthesia and sleep.

Alpha rhythm is increased in: Hyperglycemia, rise in body temperature, low arterial pCO_2 and hyperventilation.

> **NOTE**
> Alpha rhythm, the rhythm of "inattention", is usually associated with a relaxed state of mind and a feeling of well-being. It can be promoted by "biofeedback" that is employed in the management of stress.

Desynchronization: Desynchronization or *arousal response* refers to the replacement of a rhythmic EEG pattern by irregular, low-voltage activity. The ascending reticular activating system (ARAS) is responsible for this desynchronization that follows any type of sensory stimulation, e.g. cutaneous, visual effort at mental arithmetic, etc.

Delta Rhythm

A rhythm slower than alpha rhythm, i.e. theta or delta rhythm does not usually occur in a normal waking individual (except in infants). However, the alpha rhythm is replaced by delta rhythm *in normal subjects during deep sleep.* The presence of delta rhythm during the waking state in adults may indicate the presence of organic brain disease.

Beta Rhythm

When the attention is focused on something alpha rhythm is replaced by beta rhythm.

Theta Rhythm

It may be seen in children where it is blocked by visual stimulation. It is often found over the parietal and temporal areas. These occur during sleep and deep meditation.

Electroencephalogram records may be:
1. **Unipolar:** A unipolar tracing records the potential difference between a sensitive scalp electrode and a indifferent or reference electrode placed at a distance away from the sensitive (or exploring) electrode.
2. **Bipolar:** A bipolar recording shows the fluctuations in potential between two sensitive electrodes placed on the scalp or on the exposed brain.
   a. **Electroencephalogram machine:** A variety of electroencephalographs having different numbers of recording channels (up to 32) are available. The number of channels is important because simultaneous recordings can be made from wide areas of the scalp (the number of electrodes is fixed). The potentials picked up by the electrodes are suitably modified and amplified before being fed to the recording unit. The machine has the following controls:
   - **Mains supply:** The ON/OFF power switch controls 220 volts AC, 50 Hz current supply. A 50 Hz filter excludes interference from the strong sources of AC current near the recording site. A wooden couch is used for the patient.
   - **Filters:** Special filters are provided to select desired frequencies and to modify the output of the amplifiers.
   - **Sensitivity control:** A commonly used sensitivity is 7 µV/mm so that a calibration signal of 50 µV causes a pen deflection of about 7 mm.
   - **Input selector switch:** Various combinations of electrode placements (montages)—unipolar, bipolar and unipolar plus bipolar can be selected by this control. Three montages—A, B and C are provided in this machine.
   - **Photic stimulation:** A stroboscopic lamp can give light flashes of desired frequency (usually 25/sec) and duration of stimulation (usually 5 sec).
   - **Hyperventilation time clock:** A time clock displays the duration of voluntary overbreathing (usually 3–4 minutes) during the EEG recording.
   b. **Electrodes:** The surface electrodes are shallow silver cups about 10 mm in diameter and have a central hole. Lead wires connect them to the electrode board. They are applied to the scalp with an electrode jelly which holds them in place and provides good mechanical and electrical contact with the skin. Cotton balls are placed over the electrodes to delay the drying of the conductive paste.
   c. **Electrode paste:** It is a bentonite paste prepared by thoroughly mixing 100 g of bentonite powder with 100 mL of normal saline and adding glycerin slowly.
   d. **Electrode or input board:** It connects the electrodes on the subject's head to the input selector switches of the machine. A diagram of the scalp showing various

electrode positions is printed on the board. There is a provision for checking any loose connections. There is a provision in the machine for minimizing skin to electrode impedance (resistance).

e. **Electrode placement:**
   The standard set of electrodes for adults consists of 22 electrodes including one ground electrode.
   - The international ***"10-20" (ten-twenty) system*** of electrode placement (Fig. 3.14.1A) uses the distances between **three bony landmarks** of the skull—**nasion** (bridge of nose), **inion** (occipital protuberance on the back of the head) and **preauricular point** (indentation just above the tragus cartilage) to generate a system of lines which run along and across the head and intersect at intervals of 10% or 20% of the distance between nasion to inion which is taken as 100%. This system is based on the proven relationships between the measured electrode site and underlying cortical structures and areas.
   - The electrodes are named with a letter and a subscript. The letter denotes the underlying region—frontopolar (F_p), frontal (F), central (C), parietal (P), occipital (O) and auricular (A).
   - The subscript is either the **letter "z" indicating zero or midline placement of electrodes while a number indicates the lateral placement** of electrodes (**odd numbers on the left side** and **even numbers on the right side**) on the head.
   - Thus, C_z is placed at 50% of the nasion-inion distance in the midsagittal plane, while C_3 and C_4 are 20% of this distance to the left and right of C_z.

f. **Electroencephalogram paper:** The paper transport system pulls the paper from a folded stack in a storage bin and moves it under the writing pens at the standard speed of 3 cm/sec (it can be increased or decreased). The paper has printed vertical lines at 3 cm intervals as shown in Figure 3.14.1.

g. **Pen recording system:** There are 21 recording pens, the lower most being for the time tracing. The pens are 120 mm in length to minimize arc distortion. The contact tension of the pens on the paper can be adjusted, if required, with cradle springs. A pen lift knob can lift the pens from the paper.

PROCEDURE

1. Records are taken simultaneously from multiple analogous areas of the scalp for at least 20-minute period.
2. No special preparation of the patient is required except that the scalp should not be oily. Ask the subject to lie down on the couch comfortably and relax.
3. Apply the reference electrodes on the earlobes and the ground electrode above the bridge of the nose. Place the sensitive electrodes on the scalp as per the "10-20" system. Connect them to the electrode board and check for any loose connections.
4. Sensitivity calibration. Calibrate the machine so that an input of 50 μV gives a pen deflection of 7 mm.
5. Ask the subject to close his eyes and make a test recording. Normally, alpha rhythm is recorded as shown in Figure 3.14.1B.
6. **Effect of opening the eyes:** Ask the subject to open his eyes. Note that the alpha rhythm is immediately replaced by desynchronization, i.e. by fast, irregular activity. Ask the subject to close his eyes, the alpha rhythm reappears.
7. **Photic stimulation:** As the record is running, deliver light flashes at a rate of 25/sec for 5 seconds, first with eyes closed, then with eyes open. Normally, there may be no change, but in abnormal cases (e.g. epilepsy), delta rhythm may appear. In some cases, even an attack of epilepsy may be precipitated (A flickering television is known to result in an attack of epilepsy).
8. **Effect of hyperventilation:** Ask the subject to breathe deeply and quickly for 3 minutes. Normally, the frequency of alpha waves decreases by low pCO_2 and the record may show theta or even delta rhythm. In epilepsy, an attack may be precipitated along with abnormal patterns.

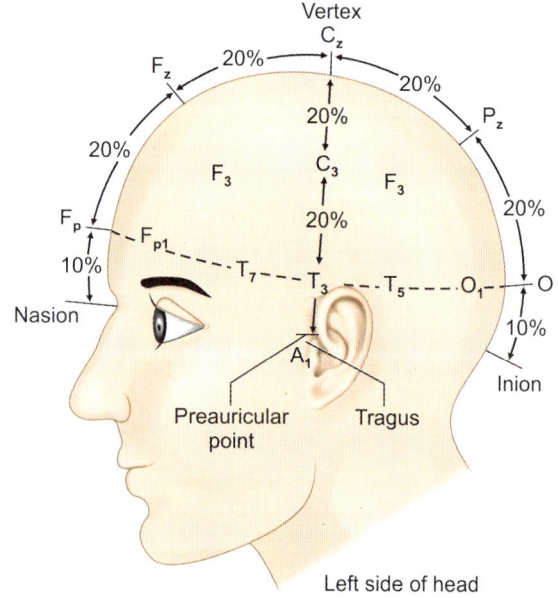

A

Fig. 3.14.1A

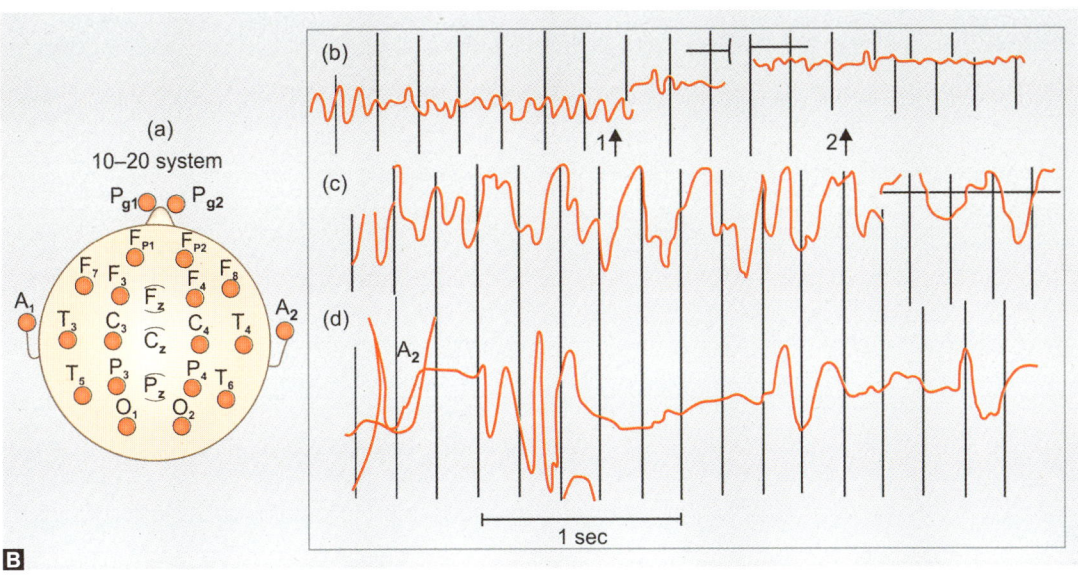

Figs. 3.14.1A and B: (A) 10–20 system for the placement of electrodes on the scalp; (B) Electroencephalogram: (a) The international "10–20" (ten-twenty) system of electrode placement, (b) Normal record showing alpha rhythm, (c) Delta rhythm; low frequency high amplitude waves in a patient of focal epilepsy, (d) Grand mal epilepsy, spike wave pattern, (1) Effect of opening the eyes (alpha block), (2) Effect of closing the eyes once again when the alpha rhythm is restored.

INTERPRETATION OF ELECTROENCEPHALOGRAM

The interpretation of EEG depends on the frequency, amplitude and distribution of the wave activity in various leads. Each record is then graded according to different systems.

CLINICAL APPLICATIONS OF ELECTROENCEPHALOGRAM

EEG has not only contributed a great deal to our understanding of the functioning of the brain, but is also an important tool in the study of patients of epilepsy, brain tumors, head injuries, brain attacks, etc. The EEG has its limitations in that a normal record may be obtained in spite of strong clinical evidence of organic disease. Also, an abnormal record may not always indicate an organic disease. Still, EEG is useful in the following disorders:

1. **Epilepsy:** In epilepsy, an excessive discharge from some part of the cerebrum is commonly associated with abnormalities of consciousness.
    - In **grand mal epilepsy,** there are generalized tonic-clonic convulsions of the muscles followed by unconsciousness. The EEG shows high-voltage, high-frequency synchronous waves during tonic stage and slower and larger waves during clonic stage.
    - In **petit mal epilepsy**, there are brief (lasting a few seconds) episodes of loss of contact with surroundings and the patient has a vacant look. The EEG shows a "spike and dome" pattern.
    - In **psychomotor** or **temporal lobe epilepsy**, there are behavioral changes (they indicate involvement of the limbic system). The EEG may show low-frequency rectangular waves.
2. **Brain tumors and abscess:** Abnormal EEG recorded from a region overlying a tumor or abscess can help in the localization of these lesions.
3. **Head injuries and vascular lesions:** Serial EEG recordings can help in following the course of head injuries, e.g. an expanding hematoma.
4. Encephalitis, meningitis and congenital defects of brain.
5. **Electroencephalogram organic and functional disorders:** Electroencephalogram may prove useful in differentiating between organic and functional disorders, i.e. nonorganic psychiatric disorders. However, its role in functional disorders is doubtful.

QUESTIONS

Q.1. How is EEG recorded? Describe the key features of the different EEG waves.
Q.2. What is alpha block?
Q.3. What do you mean by "desynchronization"?
Q.4. What is the physioclinical significance of EEG?

Section 3: Human Experiments

STUDY NOTES

Teacher's Signature

CHAPTER 3.15

Electroneurodiagnostic Tests

INTRODUCTION

Electroneurodiagnostic technique includes stimulating, recording, displaying, measuring and interpreting action potentials (APs) and other electrical changes occurring in:
1. **Peripheral nerves:** nerve conduction studies (NCSs)
2. **Muscles:** electromyography (EMG)
3. **Central nervous system (CNS):** evoked potentials.

APPARATUS

1. **Cathode ray oscilloscope:** It is a type of electronic test instrument, that graphically displays varying signal voltages, usually as a two-dimensional plot of one or more signals as a function of time. The display can be photographed or recorded directly on an ink-writing oscillograph.
2. **Amplifiers:** A variable degree of amplification is required in most applications because:
   - Biological signals are very small because of intrinsic impedance (resistance) of the recording electrodes.
   - Also the impedance of the electrode—skin contact point tends to reduce the amplitude of potential changes.
   - Amplification also minimizes distortion of waveforms and improves noise rejection. The sensitivity of the amplifier can be adjusted as required.

> **NOTE**
> **Impedance** is defined as the resistance offered to the current flow. The resistance offered by the intervening tissue to the current flow is measured in kilo ohms or mega ohms. **Voltage** represents the difference of potential between two points. It is measured in millivolts (mV) or microvolts (μV). **Current** is measured in milliamperes. **Time** is measured in milliseconds (ms or msec) and microseconds (μsec).

3. **Filter:** It is a device that removes unwanted frequencies (**high or low**) from a signal and allows only desired frequencies to pass through.
4. **Averager:** This extracts small signals that are buried or hidden in large noise. For example, evoked potentials buried in electroencephalography (EEG) noise, sensory nerve APs hidden in EMG noise.
5. **Stimulators:** Stimulators are required in most applications in neurophysiology. They are of two general types:
   a. *Electronic/electrical stimulators:* They can provide variable constant current or constant voltage, single pulse or repeated stimuli.
   b. *Magnetic stimulators:* These are employed for noninvasive stimulation of motor cerebral cortex, spinal cord and peripheral nerves. Low-intensity stimulation causes current flow mainly in superficial soft tissues. With stronger stimuli, more current enters tissues at the cathode which may be painful in some persons.

> **NOTE**
> **Stimulus artifact:** When a stimulus is applied, there is a brief, irregular deflection of the baseline, this is called a stimulus artifact and is due to leakage of current from the stimulating to the recording electrodes. It is employed for measuring the latent period (latency).

6. **Electrodes:** Electrodes are made of metal—platinum, silver, gold, stainless steel, chromium, nickel, etc. Silver and gold electrodes have the advantage of stable electrode polarizing potentials that give noise-free recordings.
   a. **Recording electrodes (REs):** In clinical practice, the following two types of electrodes are used:
      i. **Surface electrodes:** They are in the shape of discs, cups or rings and are used for recording activity from body surface. They are "attached" (applied) in place with electrode paste or jelly that is gently rubbed on the skin to reduce the resistance at electrode-skin contact point. In general, these electrodes are preferred as there is least chance of infection.
      ii. **Concentric needle electrode:** The concentric (or coaxial) needle electrode (usually 24 gauge) is a bipolar electrode, one pole of which is formed by the shaft and the other by a teflon-coated wire threaded through the shaft. The electrode records activity at its tip, the recording area being 150–500 μm^2, thus sampling a restricted area in a muscle. The monopolar needle electrode is solid steel, 22–24 gauge needle and coated with varnish or Teflon except at its tip. The reference electrode is placed on the skin. These electrodes have higher impedance.

> **NOTE**
> The action potential is measured between **active** and **reference** electrodes while the **ground** electrode serves as a "zero" voltage reference point.

   b. **Stimulating electrodes (SEs):** Stimuli of various duration and intensity can be applied through these electrodes. They are in the shape of cups, discs or rings.

PRECAUTIONS

1. The main supply must be checked to confirm adequate voltage.
2. Proper earthing of the equipment must be ensured.
3. The subject should also be properly grounded.
4. The procedure should be explained to the subject.
5. Loose wire and cable connections as well as the electrode placement may cause distorted APs.
6. A very important precaution is to ensure that the subject is not using a cardiac pacemaker, a cochlear implant or has a history of epilepsy.

A. NERVE CONDUCTION STUDY

PRINCIPLE

When a current is passed through two electrodes placed on the skin, some of it penetrates deep into the tissues. If it is strong enough and in the neighborhood of a nerve, then it will stimulate enough fibers to produce a recordable muscle response. Nerve conduction velocity determination requires stimulation of a nerve at two places along its length. **The velocity in m/sec can be calculated from the difference in the latent periods of the two responses and the length of the nerve segment between the two points stimulated.**

Nerve conduction studies are carried out in both motor and sensory nerves. The nerves commonly tested are:
1. **In the upper limbs:** Median, ulnar, radial and brachial plexus.
2. **In lower limbs:** Sciatic, femoral, common peroneal, tibial and sural nerves.

PHYSIOCLINICAL SIGNIFICANCE

1. Nerve conduction tests are useful in nerve injuries during accidents, fractures of bones, dislocations of joints, local pressure on nerves by tumors or by ligaments, arthritis, neuropathies in diabetes mellitus, demyelination (multiple sclerosis), vitamin B deficiency, leprosy and so on.
2. Testing of conduction velocities in both motor and sensory nerves provides early and accurate diagnosis. There may be an increase in the latency or even complete block of nerve impulses.

NERVE FIBER TYPES AND FUNCTION

Table 3.15.1 shows a classification of nerve fibers, their type, location and function, diameter and conduction velocity (**Erlanger and Gasser's classification**).

Table 3.15.1: Nerve fiber type and function.

Fiber type		Location/Function	Diameter (μm)	Conduction velocity (m/sec)
A	α	Somatic motor, proprioceptor	12–20	70–120
	β	Touch, pressure and motor	5–12	30–70
	γ	Motor to muscle spindle	3–6	15–30
	δ	Pain, touch and cold	2–5	12–30
B		Preganglionic autonomic	1–3	3–15
C	Dorsal root	Pain, temperature and some mechanoreception reflex responses	0.4–1.3	0.5–2
	Sympathetic	Postganglionic sympathetic	0.3–1.3	0.7–2.3

A and B fibers are myelinated, while C fibers are nonmyelinated.

MOTOR NERVE CONDUCTION

The procedure to determine median nerve conduction velocity has been described here.

Median nerve (C-6, 7, 8; T-1): It is a mixed nerve and arises from the brachial plexus. Its motor branches supply most of the flexor-pronator muscles of the forearm. It enters the hand through the carpal tunnel to supply the thenar muscles. It is sensory to the lateral palm and lateral two- and half fingers and their distal ends. It has no innervation in the upper arm.

Apparatus

1. Cathode ray oscilloscope (CRO)
2. Preamplifier
3. Electronic stimulator
4. Stimulating and recording electrodes
5. Electrode jelly
6. Spirit swabs.

Procedure

1. Ask the subject to sit on a chair and explain the procedure to him.
2. Clean the skin over the thenar muscle pad and the areas over the median nerve at the elbow and the wrist. Rub electrode jelly over these areas (Fig. 3.15.1).
3. Apply the cup recording (active) electrode (A) over the motor point of abductor pollicis brevis and the reference electrode (R) about 3 cm away from it.

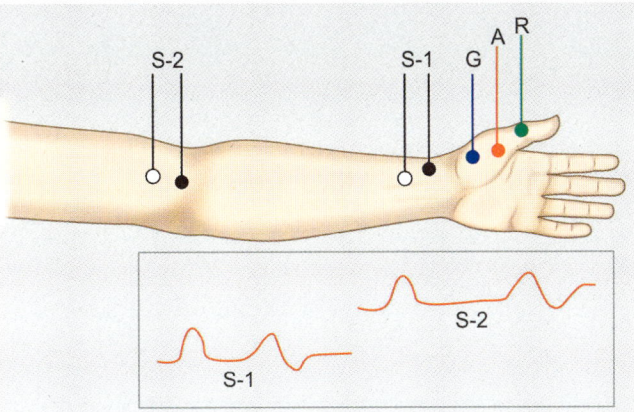

Fig. 3.15.1: Measurement of motor nerve conduction velocity in median nerve.
[S-1: stimulation at wrist; S-2: stimulation at elbow; A: recording (active) electrode; R: reference electrode; and G: ground electrode]

4. Place the ground electrode (G) between recording and stimulating electrodes (S-1).
5. Connect the recording electrodes to the CRO through the preamplifier.
6. Apply the stimulating electrodes on the wrist 3 cm above the distal wrist skin crease (S-1) and apply a supramaximal stimulus. Note the response of the thenar muscles.
7. Now shift the electrodes to the elbow and apply a stimulus (S-2). Note that at both the sites of stimulation (S-1 and S-2), the cathode is the stimulating electrode and it is placed distal to the anode.
8. The motor nerve conduction velocity is calculated by measuring the distance between two points of stimulation in mm, which is divided by the latency difference in ms.
   Normal value: The normal velocity of motor fibers of median nerve in humans is 55–65 m/sec.

Observations and Results

In both cases, there is a stimulus artifact at the beginning of the sweep, followed by a latent period and a biphasic AP with initial negativity, this is called **a biphasic muscle potential or compound muscle action potential (CMAP).**

Compound muscle action potential: It includes the onset latency, duration and the amplitude of the biphasic AP, as shown in Figure 3.15.2.

1. **Onset latency:** It is the time from the stimulus artifact to the start of the first negative deflection. It is a measure of speed of conduction in fastest nerve fibers and includes neuromuscular transmission time, spread of AP over the muscle fibers and the process of excitation-contraction coupling.

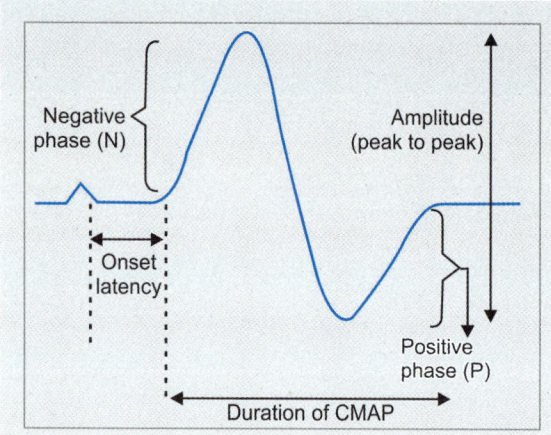

Fig. 3.15.2: Compound muscle action potential (CMAP).
[N: negative phase; P: positive phase; 1. Onset latency, 2. Amplitude (peak to peak) and 3. Duration of CMAP]

2. **Amplitude of compound muscle action potential:** It is measured from baseline to the negative peak (base to peak) or between negative to positive peaks (**peak to peak**).
3. **Duration of compound muscle action potential:** It is measured from onset to the negative or positive peaks or the final return of the waveform to the baseline.

Physioclinical Significance

The median nerve while entering the hand passes through a tunnel formed between the carpal bones and the flexor retinaculum—a band of connective tissue. The tunnel gets constricted or thickened due to fracture of the wrist or thickening of the retinaculum. The resulting compression can cause pain, paresthesias (sensations of pins and needles), wasting and paralysis of thenar muscles and trophic changes in fingertips. This relatively common condition, called **"carpal tunnel syndrome"** is treated by cutting through the retinaculum to relieve the pressure. Testing the conduction velocity in median nerve provides early diagnosis (the latent period at the wrist may increase from the normal values of 3–5 ms to 8–10 ms or even more).

> **NOTE**
> Working for long periods at the keyboard of a computer may also cause of carpal tunnel syndrome.

SENSORY NERVE CONDUCTION

The procedure to determine ulnar nerve conduction velocity has been described here.

Ulnar nerve: The ulnar nerve, like the median nerve, is also a mixed nerve. It arises from C-7 to T-1 segments of the spinal cord, passes behind the medial epicondyle of humerus and then down the ulnar side of the forearm. It gives **motor** branches to muscles in the forearm and in the hand to the hypothenar and other muscles. Its **sensory** branches supply the skin of the medial half of the hand and of the little and ring fingers.

> **NOTE**
> In the body, sensory nerve fibers conduct nerve impulses (APs) only in one direction, i.e. from the sensory receptors toward the CNS (**orthodromic conduction**). But when they are stimulated artificially, say, through the skin, they can conduct APs in the opposite direction as well, i.e. toward the sensory receptors (**antidromic conduction**).

Apparatus

1. Cathode ray oscilloscope with storage facility
2. Electronic stimulator
3. Stimulating silver ring electrodes
4. Recording silver cup electrodes
5. Electrolyte paste
6. Spirit swabs.

Procedure (Orthodromic Conduction)

1. Clean the areas of the little finger where electrodes are to be applied and rub electrode jelly over these points.
2. **Stimulating electrodes:** Place silver ring electrodes, one on the middle phalanx (active electrode) and the other on the terminal phalanx.
3. **Recording electrodes:** Apply two silver cup recording electrodes about 2–3 cm apart, proximal to wrist skin crease. Apply the ground electrode between the SE and the RE on the palm. Connect all these to the CRO through the preamplifier.
4. Adjust the settings: Filter = low cut: 5–10 Hz; high cut: 2–3 kHz; gain = 1–5 mV/div; sweep speed = 1–2 ms/div or as desired.
5. Apply a supramaximal stimulus and note the response. Record a time tracing and note the distance between the SE and the RE.
6. For antidromic conduction, simply reverse the connections of SE and RE.
7. The sensory conduction velocity is calculated by dividing the distance between the stimulating and the recording site by the latency.
   Normal value: The normal velocity of sensory fibers of ulnar nerve in humans is 50–65 m/sec.

Observations and Results

Figure 3.15.3 shows a sensory nerve action potential (SNAP). It has a stimulus artifact, onset latency, amplitude and duration.

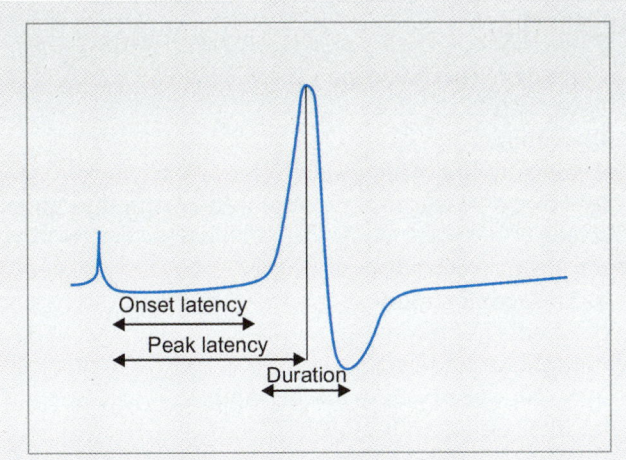

Fig. 3.15.3: Latency, amplitude and duration of sensory nerve action potential.

> **NOTE**
> The orthodromic and antidromic conduction velocities provide similar information in clinical practice. The duration of SNAP gives information about the number of slow-conducting fibers, while amplitude reveals the density of nerve fibers. Both are affected in nerve injuries, neuropathies, vitamin efficiencies, leprosy, etc.

> **NOTE**
> Sensory nerve conduction velocity can also be determined in median nerve by placing stimulating ring electrodes on the index finger and recording electrodes at the base of the thumb. This will record orthodromic conduction velocity. Antidromic velocity can be recorded by reversing the locations of the electrodes.

QUESTIONS

Q.1. Name the equipment employed in electroneurodiagnostic techniques.
Q.2. What is the basis of working of a cathode ray oscilloscope?
Q.3. What are the electrodes employed for in these studies?
Q.4. What is a waveform and what are its components?

B. ELECTROMYOGRAPHY

INTRODUCTION

Electromyography is a recording of the electrical activity occurring in a muscle during voluntary contraction. It is the sum of APs of many muscle fibers. This change of potential sets up a current field that can be recorded either with needle electrodes or by surface electrodes. EMG is useful in the detection of lower motor neuron diseases and disorders of neuromuscular transmission from certain muscle disorders such as muscular dystrophy.

In a contracting muscle, the muscle fibers do not contract individually but as part of a motor unit consisting of a variable number of innervated muscle fibers. Thus, the motor unit is the functional unit of muscle activity. A resting muscle is electrically silent, i.e. it does not show any electrical potential. When it contracts, however, such changes can be recorded.

> **NOTE**
> **Motor unit:** A motor unit consists of one anterior gray column motor neuron of the spinal cord (or the equivalent motor cranial neuron in the brainstem), its axon and all its branches as it enters a muscle and all the muscle fibers innervated by these branches. The number of muscle fibers in a motor unit varies from a few (external ocular muscles) to many hundreds (muscles of the back, thighs, etc.). *While a normal muscle fiber shows a RMP at rest and an Action Potential when stimulated for contraction, a denervated muscle fiber shows unstable potential and spontaneous twitching.*

MOTOR UNIT POTENTIAL

The motor unit potential (MUP) is the potential change produced by the excitation of muscle fibers of a motor unit. Since these fibers discharge synchronously (at the same time) near the needle electrode, the MUP has higher amplitude and a longer duration than the AP produced by a single muscle fiber.

Characteristics of Motor Unit Potential

A MUP is characterized by its firing frequency, duration, amplitude, phases and rate of rise.

1. **Frequency:** With mild contraction, the MUP shows a frequency of 5–15 Hz. With stronger contractions, there is recruitment of additional motor units (and so of MUPs) that depends on the **size principle**—the smaller motor units being recruited first, then larger and larger units are brought into action.
2. **Duration:** The duration of a MUP is measured from the initial take-off of the potential to the point of return to the baseline (Fig. 3.15.4). It varies from 5 ms to 10 ms, being shorter in children and longer in adults. The duration of MUP is a measure of conduction velocity, length of muscle fibers, membrane excitability and synchronization of response of muscle fibers.

a. *Short-duration MUPs* are found in myopathies, myasthenia gravis and early stage of reinnervation after nerve injuries.
b. *Long-duration MUPs* are seen in lower motor neuron lesions and myopathies.
3. **Amplitude:** It is measured from peak to peak and the normal value is 0.5–2.0 mV. It depends on the size, density and type of muscle fibers, synchrony of firing, nearness of needle to muscle fibers, age of the subject and temperature of the muscle.
4. **Phases:** The MUP recorded by needle electrodes shows a triphasic potential, i.e. positive-negative-positive sequence, as shown in Figure 3.15.4. A phase is the part of a MUP between the departure and return of the potential to the baseline. A MUP with more than four phases is called polyphasic. Some potentials show directional changes without reaching baseline—these are called *turns*. Polyphasic potentials and turns are more commonly seen in myopathies when regeneration is occurring.
5. **Rise time:** The rise time of a MUP is the duration from the initial positive to the next negative peak. The usual rise time is up to 500 ms and indicates the distance of the needle from the muscle fibers. A greater rise time indicates increased resistance of the intervening tissues.

Factors Affecting Motor Unit Potential

1. **Technical factors:** These include: Type of needle electrode and its location (superficial, deep or near endplate of muscle fiber; the amplitude is smaller when it is superficial), preamplifier and amplifier and method of recording, etc.
2. **Physiological factors:** These are: Age—the amplitude and duration increases while firing rate decreases as age advances. Sex and the temperature of muscle also affect MUPs.

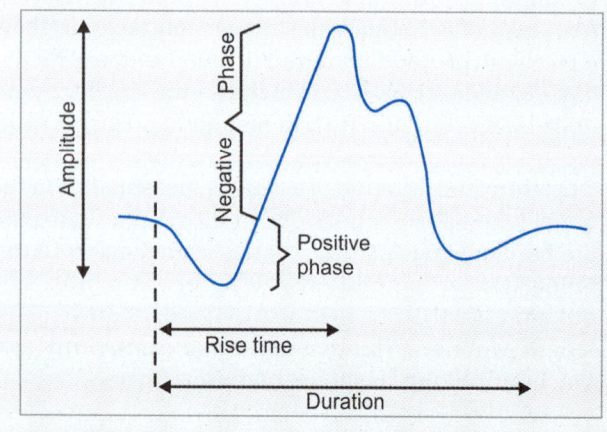

Fig. 3.15.4: Normal motor unit potential (MUP) recorded by needle electromyography (EMG).

APPARATUS

1. Cathode ray oscilloscope:
2. Polygraph
3. Preamplifier
4. Audio amplifier with speaker
5. Electrode paste, 70% alcohol and cotton and gauze swabs.
6. Recording electrodes:
   a. Surface electrodes
   b. Needle electrode.
7. Equipment settings:
   a. Sweep speed = 5–10 ms/division
   b. Filter setting = 20–10,000 Hz
   c. Amplitude = 50 mV/division for spontaneous activity and 200 mV for MUPs.

PROCEDURE FOR SURFACE ELECTROMYOGRAPHY

1. With the subject lying supine on a couch and the arm extended, clean the skin over the biceps with alcohol. Tell him/her to relax and that the procedure will be painless.
2. Using electrode paste, fix a set of three electrodes over a small area of the skin, one for grounding and the other two for recording (one active, one reference). Connect the electrodes through the preamplifier to the CRO, the recorder and the audio amplifier. Observe if there is any electrical activity.
3. Ask the subject to flex the arm and then pronate and supinate the forearm, first gently, then with greater force. Note the potentials.

PROCEDURE FOR NEEDLE ELECTROMYOGRAPHY

1. Clean the skin with alcohol and let it dry and fix the ground electrode on the skin. Tell the subject that an injection needle will be inserted into the muscle.
2. Insert the concentric needle gently into the muscle and advance it by steps to several depths.
3. Make the following observations at each depth: Activity evoked by insertion, activity produced by moving the needle, activity of relaxed (resting) muscle with the needle undisturbed and activity during weak and then during stronger and stronger voluntary contractions.

OBSERVATIONS AND RESULTS

Note the following activities and draw diagrams:
1. **Insertion activity:** There is a brief burst of electrical activity of 0.5–1.0 ms due to mechanical damage by the needle, appearing as positive or negative bursts of high-frequency spikes.
2. **Spontaneous activity:** There is no spontaneous electrical activity except that when the needle electrode is near

the endplate region when miniature endplate potentials (MEPPs) may be recorded. They are monophasic negative waves of up to 100 mV and of 1-2 ms durations.
3. **Voluntary contractions:** With weak contractions, MUPs of 5-15 Hz are recorded. With stronger contractions, potentials of 0.3-2 mV and 5-15 ms are recorded. With still stronger contractions, the potentials run into each other and the resulting confused tracing is called interference pattern.
4. **Audio signals:** As audio signals, the MUPs produce knocking or thumping sounds on the loudspeaker.

QUESTIONS

Q.1. Define the term EMG. What is its relevance in clinical physiology and medical diagnosis?

Q.2. Why are resting muscles electrically silent?
The resting muscle fibers only show a steady RMP across their cell membranes, negativity on the inside and positivity on the outside. So, when the recording electrode lies near them, no potential difference is recorded and they are electrically silent. They show APs only when they are reactivated by signals arriving along their motor nerves. This electrical activity is then followed by the mechanical activity of contraction.

Q.3. How is force of contraction graded?
The varying force of reflex or voluntary contraction of skeletal muscles depends on:
1. Number of motor units activated.
2. Frequency of nerve impulses.
3. Synchronization of nerve impulses.
4. Initial length of muscle fibers.

Q.4. How can recruitment of motor units be demonstrated experimentally without needle electrodes?
This can be done by placing recording electrodes on the skin over thenar region and then asking the subject to move the thumb slowly at first and then with greater force. MUPs of different amplitude and shape will be recorded.

C. EVOKED POTENTIALS

INTRODUCTION

Electrical potentials can be produced (evoked) in the cerebral cortex by the stimulation of sensory receptors or sensory nerves. But since these cortical potential changes are small and buried in the background of spontaneous electrical activity (EEG), their details can only be studied and evaluated by repeated stimulation and averaging the responses obtained after each stimulation by a computer.

The commonly tested evoked potentials are:
1. **Brainstem auditory evoked potentials (BAEPs)**
2. **Visual evoked potentials (VEPs)**
3. **Somatosensory evoked potentials (SEPs)**
4. **Motor evoked potentials (MEPs)**.

BRAINSTEM AUDITORY EVOKED POTENTIALS

The BAEPs represent an objective test for hearing. They are a series of potentials generated by sequential activation of different parts of the auditory pathway. These APs cannot only be recorded from along this pathway but also from the body surface, especially from the scalp.

Apparatus

1. Cathode ray oscilloscope
2. Preamplifier
3. Electroencephalography electrodes
4. Electrode paste
5. Alcohol or ether swabs
6. Headphones.

Procedure

1. The test is carried out preferably in a soundproof room. Ask the subject to sit in a chair, with his back to the apparatus and relax.
2. Clean the skin where electrodes are to be applied. Place the recording (active) electrodes on both earlobes or on the mastoid processes. Place the reference electrode at the vertex (C_z position) and the ground electrode on top of the forehead.
3. Connect the REs to the amplifier. Use amplification of 200,000-500,000; set low filter at 100 Hz and high filter at 3,000 Hz.
4. Apply brief click stimuli of 70 dB intensity above the subjects threshold, at a rate of 10/sec and of 0.1 ms duration (the stimuli are usually square wave pulses; the pulse wave can move the diaphragm of the earphone either toward or away from the ear, i.e. condensation or rarefaction stimuli).
5. The sound clicks stimulate not only the ipsilateral ear but also travel to the opposite ear by bone and air conduction to stimulate that ear at an intensity of 40-50 dB lower than the ipsilateral ear.

6. Observe the effect of intensity of stimulation on the BAEPs.

Observations and Results

The auditory nerve and BAEPs are "volume conducted" to the surface recording electrodes. At the vertex and earlobes, they form vertex positive and vertex negative potentials. A sequence of five or more distinct waveforms (vertex positive peaks) labeled I–V (Fig. 3.15.5) is recorded within 10 ms of the application of stimulation. If the recording is continued, a few more positive and negative waves are recorded. The origin of the waveforms is:

- **Wave I:** From the peripheral part of auditory nerve.
- **Wave II:** From cochlear nuclei.
- **Wave III:** From superior olivary nucleus.
- **Wave IV:** From lateral lemniscus.
- **Wave V:** From inferior colliculi.
- **Wave VI:** From medial geniculate body.
- **Wave VII:** From auditory radiation.

Measurement of brainstem auditory evoked potential waveforms: The features noted are—absolute latency, amplitude, interpeak latencies, inter-ear-interpeak differences and amplitude ratio of V/I.

Factors affecting brainstem auditory evoked potentials: These include—age, sex, height, temperature, drugs (alcohol and barbiturates prolong the latency of wave V) and hearing loss.

Physioclinical Significance

1. The auditory responses provide an objective assessment in infants and young children suspected of being deaf.
2. The BAEPs aid in assessing the degree of hearing loss.

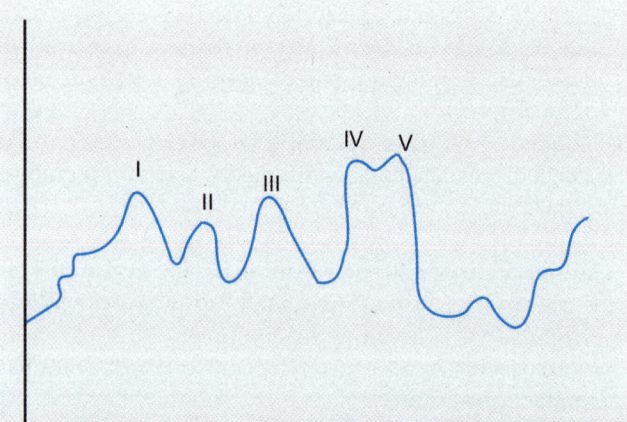

Fig. 3.15.5: Brainstem auditory evoked potentials in normal individual. Interpeak latencies are measured from the top of one peak to the other. Refer to text for the origin of different waveforms.

3. The latencies of waveforms provide information in patients of vestibular nerve and brainstem tumors, demyelination and in distinction of various kinds of coma and drug-induced and traumatic disease processes.

VISUAL EVOKED POTENTIALS

The VEPs are the potential changes recorded from the scalp in response to visual stimuli. They represent the resultant responses of cortical and subcortical structures to photostimulation. Normal VEPs indicate the intactness of the entire visual pathway. They can detect abnormality, if any, but cannot exactly locate the site of lesion. The VEPs primarily represent the activity originating in the central 3–6° of visual field that is relayed to the visual cortex (area 17) (impulses from peripheral retina project to the visual cortex buried in the calcarine fissure).

Procedure

1. Photic stimulation by black and white checkered board or vertical grating at rates of 1, 3, 6, 10 and 20 flashes per second is employed.
2. One eye is tested at a time and standard disc EEG recording electrodes at O_z, F_{pz} and C_z are employed.
3. A series of waveforms of opposite polarity, i.e. N (negative) and P (positive) are recorded and their latency, duration and amplitude determined and evaluated.

SOMATOSENSORY EVOKED POTENTIALS

In humans, event-related, "far-field SEPs" are simultaneously recorded from several electrodes placed over the popliteal fossa, lumbar and thoracic vertebrae (spinal evoked potentials) and over the parietal region of the opposite side. The SEPs are generated mainly by the large diameter (12–20 μm) fibers in response to repeated stimuli applied to them anywhere along their course in peripheral nerves or in ascending tracts in CNS [large fibers carry mainly proprioceptive impulses, while small diameter fibers (0.5 mm) carry pain and temperature].

Though SEPs can be obtained by stimulation of any large peripheral nerve; in clinical practice they are generally recorded from **median nerve** (median SEPs) and the **posterior tibial nerve** (tibial SEPs). The method can prove useful in the evaluation of spinal defects such as multiple sclerosis, spinal injuries, etc.

MOTOR EVOKED POTENTIALS (MEPs)

Sensory evoked potentials (auditory, visual and somatosensory) are recorded from the scalp or from sensory pathways after sensory stimulation. The MEPs, on the other hand, are recorded from target muscles as EMG following stimulation of motor cortex or spinal cord. The stimuli used may be electrical or magnetic. Since electrical transcranial stimuli can be painful, magnetic stimuli are applied over the vertex and cervical and lumbar regions. The target muscles include deltoid, biceps, thenar muscles, tibialis anterior and abductor hallucis brevis.

HOFFMANN'S REFLEX (H-REFLEX)

Introduction

Tendon jerks or deep reflexes (tested clinically) are reflex contractions of skeletal muscles in response to stimulation of their stretch receptors located in their muscle spindles. The stimulus is the sudden stretch of their muscle spindles that sends impulses via Ia (Aα) afferents to the spinal cord where they stimulate the anterior horn cells (AHC) that supply the muscle. The H-reflex is the electrical equivalent of a tendon jerk. It confirms the integrity of the reflex pathway.

Apparatus

1. Cathode ray oscilloscope
2. Electronic stimulator
3. Stimulating and recording electrodes
4. Swabs moist with alcohol or ether.

Procedure

1. Apply the stimulating electrodes on the skin over the tibial nerve behind the knee and recording electrodes on the skin overlying soleus muscle in the calf region.
2. Apply a minimum strength of stimulus. Since the threshold of stimulation of Ia sensory fibers is much lower as compared to motor fiber, the H-wave (H-reflex) will be recorded, as shown in Figure 3.15.6. It has a long latency because the Ia signals are conducted orthodromically (arrow 1) to monosynaptically stimulate AHC that innervate soleus.
3. Increase the strength of stimulus to stimulate both sensory and motor fibers. Note that two responses are recorded from the muscle. The first waveform is the *"M-wave"* resulting from direct stimulation of motor fibers (arrow 2), while the second response is the *"H-wave"* due to H-reflex resulting from excitation of Ia sensory fibers.

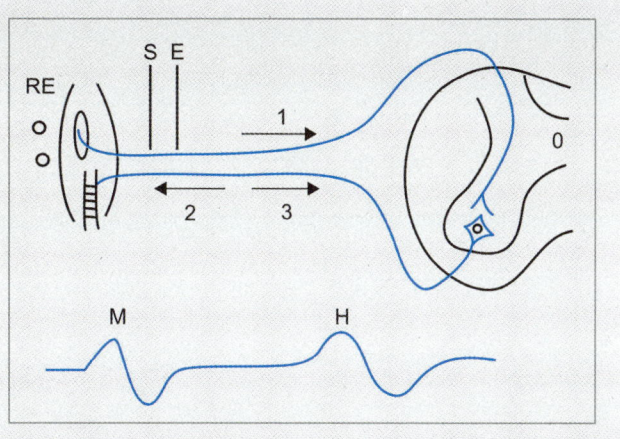

Fig. 3.15.6: Recording of H-reflex.
[SE: stimulating electrodes on skin over tibial nerve; RE: recording electrodes on skin over the muscle; M: M-wave due to direct (orthodromic) stimulation of muscle; and H-wave: due to H-reflex]

4. Increase the strength of stimulus still further and note that the H-wave gradually decreases and then disappears, leaving only the M-wave. The APs in motor nerves, in addition to normal orthodromic conduction toward the muscle, are also conducted antidromically (arrow 3) to cause depolarization of AHC so that when Ia signals arrive they find the motor neurons refractory—thus canceling their reflex response.

> **NOTE**
> Two clinical signs are associated with Hoffmann's name:
> 1. **Hoffmann's sign:** Flicking the distal phalanx of the index finger causes clawing movement of fingers and thumb. This response in the upper limb is equivalent to the Babinski response in the sole of the foot in upper motor neuron (UMN) lesions.
> 2. **Hoffmann's sign of tetany:** Electrical or mechanical stimulation of a sensory nerve produces muscle spasm (the ulnar nerve is usually selected for this test in parathyroid tetany).

QUESTIONS

Q.1. Describe the different waveforms in the recording of BAEP. What is the physiological basis of BAEP?
Q.2. Name the factors affecting BAEP. What is the clinical significance of BAEP?
Q.3. Describe the different waveforms of VEP. What is the physioclinical significance of VEP?

Section 3: Human Experiments

STUDY NOTES

Date ....

CHAPTER 3.16

Study of Human Fatigue by Mosso's Ergograph and Handgrip Dynamometer

AIM

To study the phenomenon of human fatigue and to calculate the work done using Mosso's ergograph.

INTRODUCTION

Fatigue is defined as a temporary and reversible loss of the physiological property of contraction of skeletal muscles. This is a subjective feeling of tiredness so the onset of fatigue can be somewhat delayed by motivation. However, with rest fatigue is completely reversible.

FACTORS THAT AFFECT ONSET OF FATIGUE

The degree, duration and type of work done are the important factors that in general affect the onset of fatigue.
1. The weight to be lifted.
2. Frequency of contractions.
3. Motivation.
4. Blood supply to contracting muscles.
5. Training.
6. Obesity.
7. Environmental factors such as temperature, humidity and pollution affect the onset of fatigue.

> **NOTE**
> **Effect of isometric exercise:** The effect of isometric exercise can be demonstrated by using handgrip dynamometer. The subject can be asked to sustain the force at 30% of the maximum voluntary contraction (MVC) for 1 minute. BP and HR can be recorded immediately following it.

Human fatigue can be studied by using:
1. **Mosso's ergograph**
2. **Handgrip dynamometer.**

APPARATUS

1. Mosso's ergograph
2. Metronome
3. Sphygmomanometer
4. Weights
5. Kymograph.

Mosso's Ergograph

Mosso's ergography is done to record the voluntary **isotonic contractions** of a skeletal muscle. **Erg** is the unit of work and **ergograph** is the apparatus used for recording voluntary contractions of skeletal muscle in humans. The Mosso's ergograph is employed not only to assess the performance of hand and forearm muscles but also to study the phenomenon of fatigue and the factors that affect fatigue.

Parts of Mosso's Ergograph

1. It consists of a flat wooden board with two pairs of clamps (curved plates) to fix the forearm of the subject (Figs. 3.16.1A and 3.16.2).
2. There is a pair of metal tubes (finger holders) into which index and ring fingers are inserted.
3. A sliding plate with a chart holder is fitted which can move to and fro and it carries a lever system to record muscle exertions.

Section 3: Human Experiments

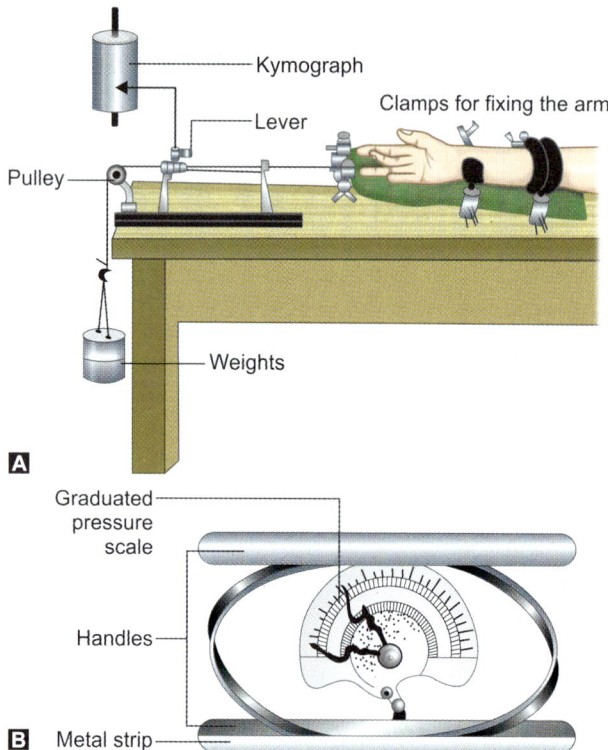

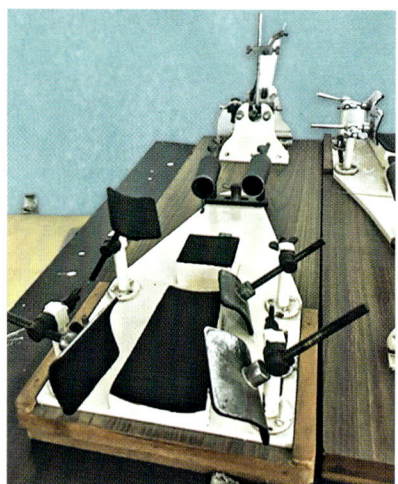

Figs. 3.16.1A and B: (A) Mosso's ergograph; (B) Dynamometer.

Fig. 3.16.2: Mosso's ergograph.

4. A pencil can be fitted vertically over the chart paper and adjusted so as to write on the chart paper when the chart holder moves.
5. One end of the sliding plate is connected through a sling to the middle finger of the hand. The other end of the sliding plate is attached to thick cord which passes over a pulley. The lower end of the thick cord has a hook for suspending the weights.

> **NOTE**
> If the ergograph is not equipped with chart holder the cord is made to move a lever, the movements of which are recorded on a kymograph.

6. When the middle finger is flexed, the load is lifted up and the distance, through which the load is lifted, is marked by the writing lever on the chart paper.

Metronome: It is timing device which functions as a "variable interrupter" to deliver the sounds at a preselected frequency of up to 200/minute. In older models, there is a thin metal rod bearing a scale with a sliding clip which can set the desired frequency to provide beats at which the sound can be delivered. Nowadays, electronic metronomes with digital display are used (Fig. 3.16.3).

Procedure

1. Explain the procedure to the subject and seat the subject beside the table.
2. Fix the forearm in supination on the ergograph and insert the index and ring fingers in the finger holders.
3. Slip the loop at the end of the cord on to the middle finger of the subject positioning it at the distal interphalangeal joint.
4. Apply weights of 1–2 kg on the hook.
5. Ask the subject to flex the middle finger and check that the system works freely.
6. Set the beat of the metronome at 30/minute, i.e. one beat every 2 seconds.
7. Ask the subject to pull the cord by flexing the middle finger maximally and rhythmically, following each beat of the metronome.
8. Continue the procedure until the muscle is fatigued and the weight can no longer be lifted.
9. ***Effect of venous occlusion:*** After a rest for 15 minutes, apply the blood pressure (BP) cuff on the upper arm and **raise the pressure to 40 mm Hg to stop venous return**. Repeat the whole procedure. Fatigue sets in

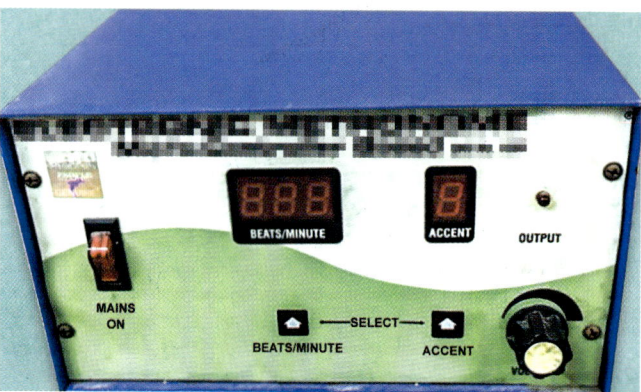

Fig. 3.16.3: Metronome.

earlier because of accumulation of waste products in the exercising muscles.

10. **Effect of arterial occlusion:** After another period of rest, **raise the BP to about 160–170 mm Hg to stop arterial blood flow [the pressure increased should be above the systolic blood pressure (SBP)]**. Tell the subject to repeat the procedure. Fatigue sets in much earlier now because there is not only an accumulation of waste products but also a deficiency of oxygen and other nutrients.

Calculation of work done: Calculate the work done in each case as shown in Figure 3.16.4:

Work done (W) = F × D
F: Weight lifted (in kg)
D: Total distance moved (in metres)
D = No. of contractions × average height contraction (A), where

$$A = \frac{\text{Area of triangle } [\frac{1}{2} \times \text{base (b)} \times \text{height (h)}] + \text{Area of rectangle } [\text{length (a)} \times \text{breadth (h)}]}{\text{Total length of base (a + b)}}$$

Express the result of work done in Joules.

Handgrip Spring Dynamometer

The handgrip dynamometer (Figs. 3.16.1B and 3.16.5) uses a spring to measure maximum **isometric contractions** of the hand and forearm muscles. The device has a handle and a graduated pressure scale. The results need to be read manually from the scale. The dial hand (needle) displays the maximum force and needs to be reset to zero after each test.

Procedure

1. Show the use of the instrument to the subject before testing. Ask the subject to stand, with arms at the sides and elbows slightly bent.
2. Ask him/her to hold it in the dominant hand to get a full grip of it.

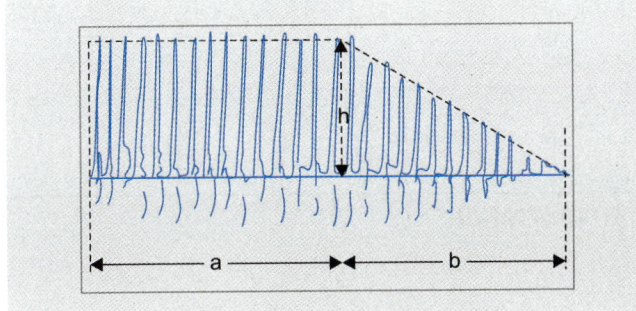

Fig. 3.16.4: Calculation work done.

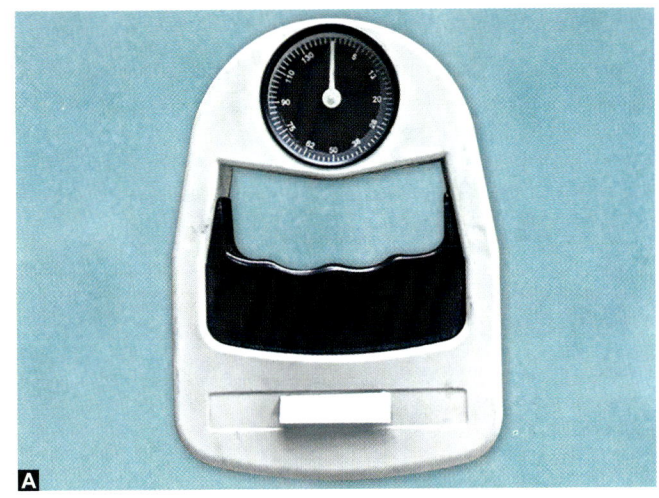

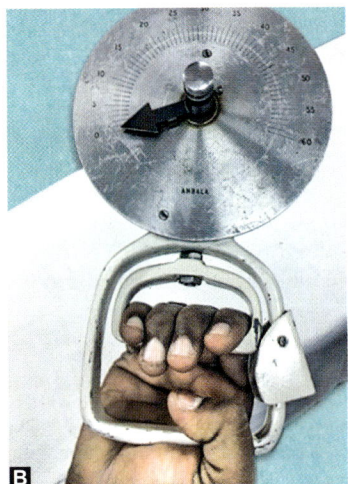

Figs. 3.16.5A and B: Handgrip dynamometer.

3. Then ask him/her to close the eyes and to squeeze only once. Note the tension developed.
4. Tell him/her to make two more trials with a pause of about a minute between them to avoid fatigue. Take the mean of these readings; this is called **Tmax (maximal isometric tension)**.
5. Determine the **endurance time** for 60–80% of Tmax. This is the time of the onset of fatigue after starting the exercise on the dynamometer.
6. After a rest of 2–3 minutes, measure the endurance time for 60–80% of Tmax first after occlusion of veins and then after occlusion of arteries with a BP cuff on the upper arm.

Results

The Tmax depends on many factors such as sex, age, muscle strength, hand dominance, time of the day, nutrition, fatigue and pain. There is a slight difference in values between the two hands.

Section 3: Human Experiments

Physioclinical Significance

Venous occlusion decreases the work done due to accumulation of metabolites in the muscle. Arterial occlusion further decreases the work done and brings in an early onset of fatigue as it prevents the supply of nutrients to the muscle. The performance of a person can be increased by encouragement and motivation.

Objective Structured Practical Examination–I

Aim: Calculate the work done using Mosso's ergograph.
Procedural steps: See text above.
Checklist:
1. Instruct the subject to give his/her effort.
2. Insert the index and the ring finger into fixed tube holder in Mosso's ergograph.
3. Set the metronome to oscillate (at a fixed frequency).
4. Connect the sling to the middle finger at distal interphalangeal joint (IPJ).
5. Ask the subject to lift the load by maximal contraction of the flexors of the middle finger.
6. Ask the subject to continue to lift the load till onset of fatigue.
7. Repeat the entire procedure with arterial and venous occlusions.

Objective Structured Practical Examination–II

Aim: To measure your own endurance time for 60–80% of your Tmax by using the provided handgrip dynamometer.
Procedural steps: See text above.
Checklist:
1. Check the instrument and hold it in the dominant hand to get a feel of it. (Y/N)
2. Close the eyes and then squeeze the handle with her maximum effort. Take a reading. (Y/N)
3. Wait for about a minute and then take the second reading of maximum tension. (Y/N)
4. Take the mean of the two readings (Tmax). (Y/N)
5. Measure the endurance time for 60–80% of the Tmax. (Y/N)

QUESTIONS

Q.1. Define the term fatigue. What are the factors that affect the onset of fatigue?

Q.2. How does motivation improve muscular performance?
Encouragement improves performance for a short time. This shows that cerebral cortex is involved in fatigue in humans. In sports physiology, motivation plays an important role in enhancing performance.

Q.3. What is the site of fatigue in humans?
The first site of fatigue in humans is central nervous system (CNS). This is proved by the fact that encouraging the person enhances the performance and delays the onset of fatigue. The next site of fatigue is the muscle followed by the neuromuscular junction.

Q.4. How will you demonstrate the site of fatigue in an intact muscle?
After the flexors of the fingers are fatigued, they will still contract on peripheral nerve stimulation. This will show that fatigue is a "central" phenomenon involving synapses.

Q.5. How does fatigue in this experiment compare with fatigue in frog's nerve-muscle preparation?
In frog's preparation, there is no blood supply. Hence, fatigue sets in early. Also, the seat of fatigue is neuromuscular junction. In the present experiment, the seat of fatigue appears to be a central phenomenon.

Q.6. Name a clinical condition where venous or arterial occlusion can impair muscular performance.
In thrombosis of leg veins due to thrombophlebitis, the venous return is decreased so that fatigue sets in early. Arterial occlusion occurs in Buerger's disease (said to be due to chronic smoking); there is pain while walking. The narrowed vessels cannot keep pace with increased demands of muscles for oxygen. In coronary artery disease, the ischemic muscle pain has a similar mechanism.

Q.7. How will the results be affected if the rate of work done is increased by setting metronome faster? Give reasons.
Onset of fatigue is earlier if the rate of work done is increased. This is because of increased accumulation of metabolites and increased degree of hypoxia.

Q.8. How is the work done affected following venous and arterial occlusions? Give reasons.

Q.9. What is the difference in the mode of muscular contraction in Mosso's ergography and handgrip dynamometry?

OBSERVATION AND RESULT

1. Mosso's Ergograph

Sl. No.	Weight	Metronome frequency	Circulation	Onset of fatigue	
				Duration	Work done
1.	2 kg	30/min	Intact		
2.	2 kg	30/min	Venous occlusion		
3.	2 kg	30/min	Arterial occlusion		

2. Handgrip dynamometer

Sl. No.	Circulation	Endurance time for 60–80% Tmax
1.	Intact	
2.	Venous occlusion	
3.	Arterial occlusion	

INTERPRETATION

....
....
....
....
....

STUDY NOTES

CHAPTER 3.17

Autonomic Function Tests

INTRODUCTION

1. The term ***autonomic nervous system*** (ANS) was suggested by Langley over 100 years ago for that part of the nervous system that controls visceral activities, i.e. cardiac muscle, smooth muscle and glands. Most visceral activities are not under our control (hence called autonomic) and cannot be easily altered or suppressed.
2. The ANS is divided into the sympathetic nervous system (SNS) and parasympathetic nervous system (PSNS).
3. Both SNS and PSNS have preganglionic and postganglionic neurons.
4. In SNS, the preganglionic neurons are myelinated and cholinergic. The postganglionic neurons are unmyelinated and adrenergic except these innovating the sweat glands and some skeletal muscles and blood vessels (sympathetic vasodilator system) are cholinergic.
5. Sympathetic preganglionic neurons synapse with postganglionic neurons in the paravertebral sympathetic chain of ganglia. The parasympathetic preganglionic neurons synapse with the postganglionic neurons, near or in the viscera.
6. **Divisions of autonomic nervous system:** Depending on the anatomical location of connector or preganglionic neurons, the ANS is divided into **craniosacral (parasympathetic)** and **thoracolumbar (sympathetic)** components (Fig. 3.17.1).
7. The PSNS conserves and stores energy and is **anabolic** while the SNS is **catabolic** and prepares the body for emergency situations.
8. The effects of PSS are localized and short-lived, the effects of SS are prolonged and widespread.

CLASSIFICATIONS OF AUTONOMIC FUNCTION TESTS

In general, changes in blood pressure (BP) are monitored for assessing the sympathetic function, while heart rate (HR) changes are monitored for assessing parasympathetic function.

Tests for Sympathetic Functions

QT-QS2 Ratio

This test is an index of sympathetic excitation of the heart.

Procedure

1. Ask the subject to lie down supine on the couch and relax. Attach ECG leads and place the contact microphone on the carotid artery to record heart sounds [phonocardiogram (PCG)].
2. Record lead II of ECG and PCG simultaneously at a paper speed of 50 mm/sec.
3. Measure QT interval from the beginning of QRS complex to the end of T wave. Measure QS2 from the beginning of QRS to the first major vibration of aortic component of second heart sound in PCG. Determine the QT/QS2 ratio.

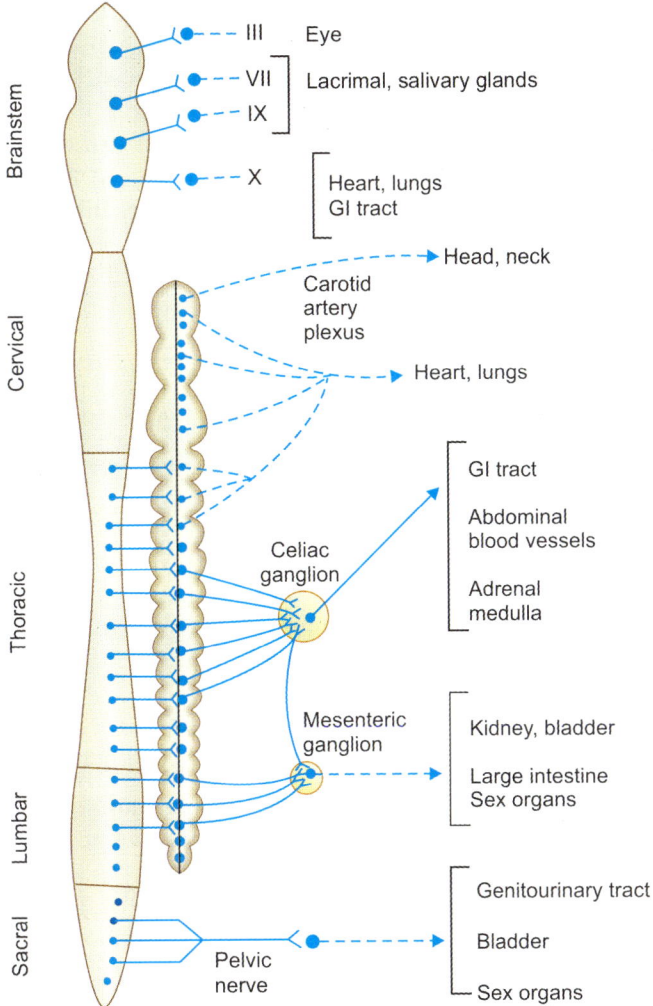

Fig. 3.17.1: Diagram to show the efferent pathways of the autonomic nervous system. The preganglionic neurons are shown as solid lines, postganglionic neurons as dashed lines.
(GI: gastrointestinal)

> **COMMENTS**
> QS2 is the total electromechanical systolic interval. A high value indicates greater sympathetic tone, while a low value represents low sympathetic tone.

Sympathetic Skin Response (SSR)

Rationale
The sweat glands distributed over the entire body are innervated by sympathetic postganglionic cholinergic fibers (except in palms and soles which are innervated by noradrenergic sympathetic fibers). The stratum corneum of the skin, which is punctured by the ducts of sweat glands, offers maximum resistance to the passage of current through the skin. However, when the sweat glands are activated, the ducts get filled with sweat (which is an electrolyte), so that an electric current can easily pass through the skin due to a fall in skin resistance.

Change in skin potential in response to stimuli causing sympathetic activation is called **sympathetic skin response**. It is also called **galvanic skin response** (GSR).

Procedure
An EMG machine and a CRO are generally adequate to record the response to application of current. However, a polygraph may be used.
1. Set the preamplifier to GSR and EMG machine: Frequency response = 0.1–1,000 Hz, gain = 0.5 mV/div and set the sweep speed to record 5 seconds after the stimulus.
2. After cleaning the skin and applying small amounts of paste, place the active electrode (disk type) on the palm (or sole of foot), reference electrode on the dorsum of the hand (or foot), with the ground electrode between the two.
3. Apply a constant current of 5 µA and note the response and calculate its latency and amplitude. Estimate the skin resistance in millivolts from the recording pen deflection (the deflection resulting from 1 mV to the amplifier is equal to a resistance change to 10 kΩ).
4. Give a stimulus in the form of startling sound (say, a sudden handclap near the head of the subject) and record the response, i.e. the SSR potentials, their latency and amplitude (the stimulus will activate the SS).

> **NOTE**
> The SSR may be mono, di or triphasic and the potentials may be 1.1–1.5 mV in amplitude and about 1.5 seconds in latency in the hands and 0.7–0.9 mV and 2.0–2.5 seconds in the feet. Abnormal SSR is usually seen in progressive autonomic dysfunction.

Cold Pressure Response

Rationale
Physical or mental stress causes stimulation of SS. Plunging a hand in cold water act as a pain stimulus and causes rise in BP.
1. Explain the test to the subject and seat him/her in a chair: Record the baseline BP.
2. Ask the subject to immerse one hand in cold water at 4–5°C for 2 minutes. Record the BP from the other arm at 30 seconds intervals.
3. Note the maximum increase in systolic and diastolic pressures (DPs) and compare with the pretest readings. The systolic pressure (SP) may increase by 20 mm Hg, while the DP rises by 10 mm Hg.

Results
Reduced sympathetic activity is indicated by a smaller rise of BP. In some normal persons, there may be no significant rise in BP.

Handgrip Test (Isometric Exercise)

Sustained handgrip causes a rise in HR and BP. An ECG machine, a sphygmomanometer and a handgrip spring dynamometer will be required for this test.

1. Apply the BP cuff on the nonexercising arm and lead II of ECG for recording HR. Record the resting BP and HR at 30 seconds intervals for 4 minutes. Then ask the subject to hold the dynamometer in the dominant hand and take a full grip on it.
2. Ask the subject to exert maximum force and note the maximum tension developed. Repeat three times at intervals of 2 minutes. Take the highest reading and note it as *maximum isometric tension (Tmax)*.
3. Now ask the subject to maintain a tension of 30% of Tmax for 5 minutes. During this procedure, record the BP and ECG at 30 seconds intervals.
4. Note the diastolic blood pressure (DBP) at the point just before the release of handgrip.
5. Note the mean resting value of DBP readings during the last 3 minutes before starting the exercise.

Results

The rise in DBP in normal subjects is more than 15 mm Hg but less than 10 mm Hg in sympathetic insufficiency.

Tests for Parasympathetic Functions

Standing Test (30:15 RR Ratio)

Rationale

Upon sudden standing from supine, there is pooling of blood in the lower parts of the body. This is followed by a sequence of events: fall of venous return → decrease in cardiac output and BP → decreased baroreceptor activity → increase in sympathetic tone and decrease in parasympathetic activity. This causes reflex increase in HR and peripheral vasoconstriction, after which the HR falls.

Thus, HR rises immediately on standing and continues to rise for the next 15–20 seconds, after which it slows down to a maximum degree as a result of variations in vagal tone.

Procedure

1. Ask the subject to lie supine on the couch and relax for 15 minutes. Apply ECG leads and the BP cuff (or the wrist BP monitor).
2. Record ECG (lead II) for noting HR and BP. Then ask the subject to stand (without support, i.e. not leaning against the wall) and remain motionless for 3 minutes, recording the ECG continuously. Record BP at the end of 1st and 3rd minutes after standing. Mark the point of standing on the ECG paper.
3. Calculate the HR from R-R interval at 15th beat (fastest HR; shortest R-R interval) and at 30th beat (slowest HR; longest R-R interval) after standing.
4. Determine the 30:15 ratio, which is considered a **cardiac vagal effect**. Normal value is more than 1.04. An R-R ratio of less than 1.0 indicates autonomic insufficiency.
5. In normal persons, the fall in systolic blood pressure (SBP) on standing should not be more than 10 mm Hg.
    a. In orthostatic hypotension, the SBP and DBP fall more than 20 mm Hg and 10 mm Hg respectively.
    b. In vasovagal syncope, hypotension is accompanied by paradoxical bradycardia because cardiac vagal supply is overactive.

> **NOTE**
> Similar responses can be better studied by passively tilting the subject on a tilt table from supine position to an inclination of 80° (head up) for a period of 3–4 minutes.

Standing to Lying Ratio (S/L Ratio)

Rationale

When a normal person lies down from a standing position, there is at first a rise in HR which is followed by a slowing of the heart. This rise and fall of HR is due to changes in vagal tone.

Procedure

1. Explain the procedure to the subject. Connect ECG leads for recording lead II. Ask the subject to stand quietly for 2 minutes and then to lie down supine without any support.
2. Record ECG for 20 beats before and for 60 beats after lying down. Note the point of change of position on the ECG paper.
3. Repeat three times at intervals of 5 minutes.
4. **Calculation of S/L ratio:** Take the average R-R interval during five beats before lying down and shortest R-R interval during 10 beats after lying down. The maximum ratio of the three trials is reported. Any abnormally low ratio indicates parasympathetic insufficiency.

Valsalva Ratio

Valsalva maneuver (effort) is forced expiration against a closed glottis. This straining, associated with changes in HR and BP, is a simple test for baroreceptor activity (Fig. 3.17.2).

Procedure

1. Seat the subject on a stool and explain the procedure. Connect ECG leads and BP cuff on him/her and close the nostrils with a nose clip.
2. Disconnect the cuff from another BP apparatus and ask the subject to take a deep breath, blow into the manometer and maintain the pressure of 40 mm Hg for 15 seconds (recall the 40 mm Hg test for lung functions).

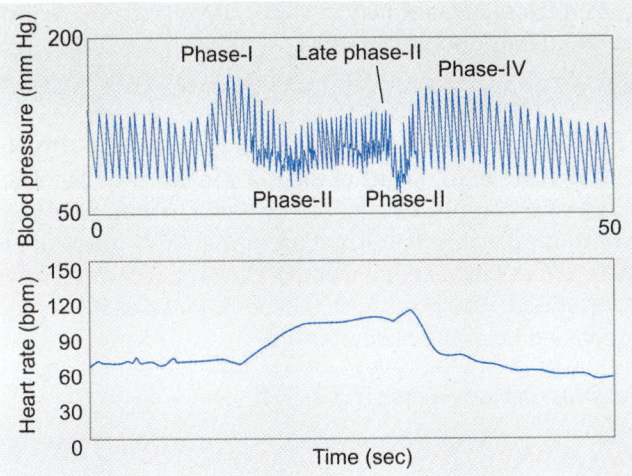

Fig. 3.17.2: Heart rate and blood pressure during Valsalva maneuver. (bpm: beats per minute)

3. Record ECG (lead II) for 1 minute before the straining, for 15 seconds during straining and for 45 seconds after the release of strain. It may also be calculated as the ratio of longest R-R interval after the strain to the shortest R-R during the strain.

Observations

The Valsalva maneuver has four phases:
1. **Phase I:** It is onset of strain. In this phase, there occurs transient decrease in BP. Mechanical compression of the great vessels and increased intrathoracic pressure contributes to this rise. There is not much change in HR.
2. **Phase II:** During straining, there is decrease in venous return, fall in cardiac output and BP and inhibition of baroreceptors, followed by tachycardia and vasoconstriction. The HR increases throughout straining due to vagal inhibition initially and sympathetic activation later.
3. **Phase III:** At the release of strain, there is a transient fall of BP without significant change in HR.
4. **Phase IV:** After further release of strain, the BP slowly rises with decrease of HR. These, in turn, stimulate baroreceptors causing bradycardia and drop in BP to normal levels.

The maximum Valsalva ratio of three trials is taken as the index of autonomic activity. A ratio of greater than
- 1.45 is normal, 1.20–1.45 is borderline and less than
- 1.20 indicates autonomic disturbance.

Clinical Significance

Failure of HR to increase during straining suggests sympathetic insufficiency, while failure of HR to slow down after the effort suggests a parasympathetic insufficiency.

Tachycardia Ratio

This ratio is related to Valsalva ratio and is defined as the ratio of shortest R-R interval during Valsalva effort to the longest R-R interval before the effort. It is believed to be a better index of vagal activity.

Deep Breathing Test

The HR increases during inspiration (due to decreased cardiac vagal activity) and decreases during expiration (due to increased vagal activity). This is a normal phenomenon and is called *sinus arrhythmia*.

Procedure

There are two methods to show the effect of breathing on HR. In one method, a single deep breath is taken and its effect noted. In the other method, the subject breathes deeply for 1 minute.
1. Explain the procedure to the subject and ask him to lie down supine and relax, with the head raised to 30°.
2. Attach the ECG leads for recording lead II. Then ask the subject to breathe deeply and slowly at a rate of 6 breaths/min, with 5 seconds for inspiration and 5 seconds for expiration. Record ECG before and during deep breathing.
3. Determine the maximum and minimum HR with each respiratory cycle and note the average HR in inspiration and in expiration.
4. Calculate the expiration to inspiration ratio (E:I ratio). This is the mean of maximum R-R intervals during expiration (slow HR) to the mean of minimum R-R intervals during deep inspiration (fast HR).
6. In normal persons, the fall in HR should be more than 15 beats/min. In vagal insufficiency, the HR slows less than 10 beats/min.

Other Tests

The smooth muscle of the iris and ciliary body are supplied by both SNS and PSNS nerve fibers. Sympathetic activity causes pupillary dilation while parasympathetic activity causes pupillary constriction, accommodation, lacrimation and salivation.

Test for Pupillary Function

Sympathetic activity causes pupillary dilatation while parasympathetic activity causes pupillary constriction, accommodation, lacrimation and salivation. Local application of pharmacologic agonists is helpful in establishing pupillary denervation—resulting in denervation hypersensitivity.

Denervation Hypersensitivity

This is the phenomenon in which an effector tissue (muscle, in this case) becomes hypersensitive to a neurotransmitter 2–3 weeks after denervation of that tissue.

1. Put a drop or two of 0.125% pilocarpine drops in the eye of the subject. Normally, this causes minimal pupillary constriction. In parasympathetic denervation, there is a strong constriction of the pupil.
2. In a similar way, 2–3 drops of 0.1% solution of epinephrine put three times in the eye at 1 minute intervals causes minimal dilatation of the pupil. But in sympathetic denervation, there is strong pupillary dilatation (checked at 15, 30 and 45 minutes).

Test for Lacrimation (Schirmer's Test)

Take a strip of filter paper, 25 mm long and 5 mm wide and place its one end between the lower eyelid and sclera, allowing its other end to hang down over the cheek.

Measure the length of its wetting after 5 minutes. In normal persons, the filter paper wets by about 15 mm while less than 10 mm suggests parasympathetic insufficiency.

APPARATUS

1. Electrocardiogram (ECG) machine
2. Blood pressure apparatus
3. Multichannel polygraph
4. Cathode ray oscilloscope (CRO)
5. Electrodes
6. Electronic stimulator
7. Electromyography (EMG) machine and preamplifier.

HEART RATE VARIABILITY

Heart rate variability is defined as the cardiac beat-beat variation and represents the variation in cardiac cycle length during respiratory cycles at rest.

Heart rate variability (HRV) is a highly sensitive noninvasive indicator of autonomic functions. It is mainly important for assessment of sympathovagal balance. This is mainly used for prediction of cardiovascular dysfunction. The methodology is based upon the calculation of successive R-R intervals. These can then be plotted as frequency histogram (**time domain**) or undergo power spectral analysis to yield information in the **frequency domain**. The physiological phenomenon of variation in the time interval between heart beats is known as **HRV**. It describes oscillation in consecutive cardiac cycles.

Heart Rate Variability Analysis

The variations in HR can be evaluated by the following two HRV indices:

1. Time domain analysis
2. Frequency domain analysis.

Time Domain Analysis (Fig. 3.17.3)

This is one of the simplest methods to access the HRV. In this, the HR at any point of time or the intervals between successive complexes are determined. A continuous ECG record is taken and a normal to normal (N-N interval, i.e. all intervals between adjacent QRS complexes) interval is determined. The term N-N is used in place of R-R as the processed beats are normal beats.

Frequency Domain Analysis (Fig. 3.17.4)

The HRV is comprised of various frequencies. Frequency domain analyzes this by viewing different frequency components of the waveform. The main frequency components that represent autonomic activity are:
- **High frequency (HF): 0.15–0.4 Hz**
- **Low frequency (LF): 0.04–0.15 Hz**
- **Very low frequency (VLF): 0.0–0.04 Hz.**

The LF and HF components are relative indices of cardiac sympathetic and vagal activity, respectively.

High frequency component is because of vagal tone during respiratory cycle.

Low frequency component results from self-oscillation in the sympathetic component of the baroreceptor reflex loop as a result of negative feedback.

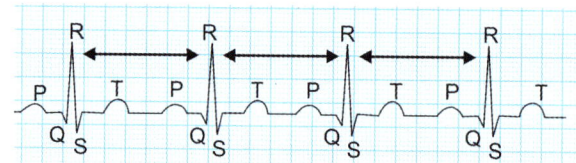

Fig. 3.17.3: Time domain analysis of heart rate variability (HRV) using R-R interval.

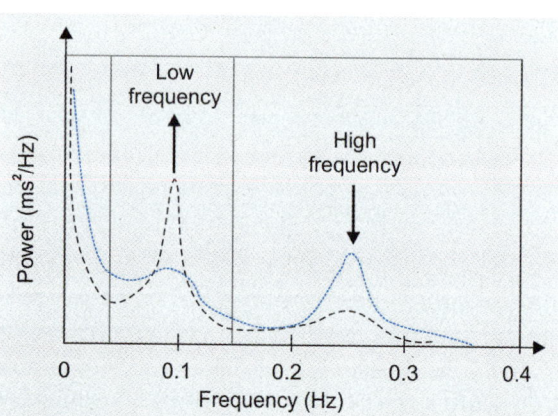

Fig. 3.17.4: Frequency domain indices of heart rate variability (HRV) analysis.

All other HR changes such as associated with thermoregulation and humoral mechanisms are accounted by VLF components.

Heart Rate Variability Recording

Two types of HRV recordings are done:
1. Short-term (5 minutes) recording
2. Long-term (day-night) HRV recording.

For research and clinical investigations, short-term HRV recording is preferred, although long-term HRV recording is more reliable.

After 5 minutes of supine rest, lead II ECG recording is obtained from the subject at a rate of 1,000 samples/sec using computer software (data acquisition system). This data is further processed with the help of another software to get HRV analysis.

Physiological Significance

1. Heart rate variability analysis assesses the efficiency of vagal control precisely. During inspiration, vagal tone is inhibited thereby leading to increase in HR. The HR shows fluctuations with a frequency similar to the respiratory cycle. The vagal tone is inhibited during inspiration because of the irradiation of impulses from the respiratory to the cardiovascular center.
2. It also provides information about sympathovagal balance.
3. Heart rate variability alterations have also been seen during yoga and traditional exercise.
4. Heart rate variability is used as a prognostic tool after myocardial infarction and cardiac transplantation.
5. Decreased HRV is seen in many cardiovascular diseases.
6. There is a good correlation between decreased HRV and risk for sudden cardiac death in patients of heart disease.

QUESTIONS

Q.1. What are the divisions of autonomic nervous system?
Q.2. Describe the functions of parasympathetic and sympathetic divisions of the ANS.
Q.3. Name the various conventional autonomic function tests.
Q.4. Discuss the physiological basis of clinical tests in assessing autonomic dysfunction.
Q.5. Which is the most sensitive autonomic function tests?
Q.6. Give the common causes of autonomic dysfunction.

In progressive autonomic dysfunction both preganglionic and postganglionic neurons undergo degeneration. This leads to **orthostatic or postural hypotension** (inability to maintain BP in the erect posture), constipation, sexual dysfunction, incontinence of urine, disturbances of sweating, etc.

Common causes of autonomic neuropathy are diabetic neuropathy, alcoholic neuropathy and uremic neuropathy.

Q.7. What is HRV? What is its physioclinical significance?
Q.8. What do the time domain and frequency domain indices of HRV represent?

STUDY NOTES

UNIT 5: REPRODUCTIVE SYSTEM

Date ....

CHAPTER 3.18

Semen Analysis

AIM

To perform semen analysis of the given sample.

INTRODUCTION

Semen (spermatic fluid) is studied for sterility, i.e. the inability of a male to impregnate a normal female. It is a routine test to determine if the sterility is due to a defect in the semen. Study of semen is also done to confirm the completeness of vasectomy, a procedure commonly adopted for control birth.

CHARACTERISTICS OF NORMAL SEMEN

A sample of semen collected after 2–3 days of sexual abstinence has the following features:

1. **Volume:** Normal volume is 2.5–5 mL. It decreases in functional disorders or inflammation of the male genital tract.
2. **Physical characteristics:** White, opalescent, mucoid and sticky.
3. **pH:** About 7.2–7.7. The alkaline pH brings the vaginal pH of 3.5–4.5 to about 6–6.5, the pH at which sperms show maximum motility.
4. **Morphology:** Normal sperms are actively motile. They are one of the smallest cells (5-6 mm), in contrast to an ovum, which is the largest cell of the body (about 120 μm). They have a head, neck, body and tail.
   Abnormalities in shape include: Bifid or absent heads, bifurcated tails, etc. If present in more than 70% of sperms, it indicates some pathology.
5. **Motility:** More than 80% sperms show a good forward motility due to "flail-like" movements of their tails. More than 70% of sperms in a specimen should show active motility within 3 hours of collection of specimen. Less than 40% motile sperms indicate sterility.
6. **Count:** Normal count is 60–120 million/mL, with an average of 100 million/mL. Counts between 20 million/mL and 40 million/mL indicate borderline infertility. Counts below 20 million/mL indicate sterility.
7. **Clotting and liquefaction:** Normal semen clots within 5 minutes of ejaculation. There is no thrombin or prothrombin (The clotting is due to the conversion of fibrinogen into fibrin). However, the exact mechanism is not known. It undergoes secondary liquefaction due to the presence and activation of plasmin and other proteolytic enzymes, such as prostate-specific antigen (PSA), pepsinogen, hyaluronidase and amylase.
8. **Fructose:** Normal semen contains fructose. It is used by sperms for production of adenosine triphosphate (ATP) via Krebs cycle.

Other components include: Calcium, citric acid, clotting proteins different from those of blood clotting, hyaluronidase, acid phosphatase and prostaglandins.

PRINCIPLE OF SPERM COUNTING

Semen is collected from the subject, diluted 20 times in a white blood cell (WBC) pipette and the sperms are counted in a Neubauer's chamber.

APPARATUS

1. **Microscope:**
   - Improved Neubauer's chamber
   - White blood cell pipette
   - Coverslips
   - Slides
   - Plasticine.
2. **Diluting fluid:** About 5% sodium bicarbonate in 1% phenol solution.

PROCEDURE

1. Collect a fresh sample of semen (after 2 days of abstinence) in a petri dish or a small beaker.
2. Wait for 25–30 minutes for secondary liquefaction. Observe if the liquefaction is uniform. Measure its volume.
3. **Assessing sperm motility:** Place a drop of semen on a coverslip and invert it on the rim of a small circle of plasticine previously made on a slide. Examine under low and high power and watch the motility of sperms. Try to assess the percentage of motile to nonmotile sperms. Also note their morphology.
4. **Counting the sperms:** Gently shake the sample to assure uniformity.
   - Draw semen to 0.5 mark in the WBC pipette, then draw the diluting fluid to the mark 11. Mix the contents of the bulb for 2–3 minutes.
   - Discard the first few drops, then charge the counting chamber and count the sperms under high power in the four WBC squares, as was done for total leukocyte count (TLC) (Refer Chapter 1.6).
5. **Calculation:**
   Number of sperms in 64 squares (volume = $4/10$ mm^3) = N
   Then, number of sperms in 1 mm^3 of undiluted semen
   = N × 10/4 × 20
   To get sperm count in 1 mL = N × 50 × 1,000
   Normal count = 60 – 120 million/mL
   Report: Morphology ....
   Count = ... million/mL.

QUESTIONS

Q.1. What is semen? Where are sperms formed?
Semen is a mixture of spermatozoa and a liquid consisting of the secretions of seminiferous tubules, seminal vesicles, prostate and bulbourethral glands. The liquid part provides nourishment and a transport system.

About 60 million sperms are manufactured daily in about 1,000 seminiferous tubules in each testis, each tubule being 50–60 cm long. Leydig cells of testis secrete testosterone, the male sex hormone that promotes spermatogenesis, in addition to primary and secondary "male" sex characteristics.

Q.2. What are the indications for sperm analysis?
Semen is examined for three main purposes:
1. To determine whether a male is fertile or not.
2. In the investigation of genetic disorders like cryptorchidism and Klinefelter syndrome.
3. To diagnose inflammatory or neoplastic diseases of the genital tract.
4. To confirm the completeness of vasectomy.

Q.3. What is the composition of semen? Name some features of the sperms.

Q.4. Why is abstinence advised for 2 days before collecting a sample of semen?
Since the volume and sperm count of semen decrease rapidly with frequent ejaculations, it might give a misleading low-count result if this precaution is not taken.

Q.5. What is the significance of clotting and liquefaction of semen?
These two features of semen—(1) clotting and (2) secondary liquefaction—appear to play a biological role. The initial coagulation helps to retain semen in the vagina, while the subsequent liquefaction aids the sperms to swim up the female genital tract.

Q.6. When is a male considered infertile?
The male infertility (or sterility) is the inability of a person to fertilize a secondary oocyte. It may be due to a low sperm count (<20 million/mL) or a high percentage of nonmotile or abnormal sperms.

Infertility should not be confused with impotence (erectile dysfunction), i.e. inability to perform the sexual act.

Q.7. For how long can sperms remain capable of fertilization in the female genital tract?
The maximum duration of fertilization capacity of normal sperms varies between 24 hours and 48 hours.

Q.8. Define the terms oligospermia, azoospermia and necrospermia.
Oligospermia refers to a count less than 20 million/mL, azoospermia means total absence of sperms and necrospermia refers to dead (nonliving) sperms in the semen.

Q.9. For how long sperms may appear in the semen after bilateral vasectomy?
For the first 2 months after vasectomy, viable sperms may be released from their storage in ampullae of seminal vesicles.

STUDY NOTES

Date ....

CHAPTER 3.19

Pregnancy Diagnostic Tests

INTRODUCTION

The laboratory tests of pregnancy are based on detection human chorionic gonadotropin (hCG) in the urine of the pregnant female. The hCG appears in the urine within 2 weeks after conception. The hCG concentration of about 25 mIU/mL in the urine is considered positive for pregnancy.

The tests can be classified into:
1. Biological tests
2. Immunological tests
3. Other tests

Biological Tests

These tests are no longer routinely used as they are time consuming and expensive.
1. Aschheim-Zondek test
2. Kuppermann test
3. Hogben test
4. Friedman test
5. Galli-Mainini test.

Immunological tests

The immunological tests are the most commonly used in laboratory.
1. Gravindex test
2. Radioimmunoassay (RIA)
3. Enzyme-linked immunosorbent assay (ELISA).

IMMUNOLOGICAL TESTS

Gravindex Test

Principle

Injection of hCG into a rabbit produces antibodies to hCG. The antiserum can then be used to detect the presence of hCG in the urine or the serum of the pregnant women by complement fixation, precipitation tests or by hemagglutination tests.

Procedure

Urine containing hCG is added to the hCG antisera, causing the hCG to combine with its antibody. This neutralizes the antibody, so when hCG coated tanned red cells or latex particles are added no agglutination occurs. This is called as a **positive test**.

If the hCG antisera to urine which does not contain hCG, the antibodies will not be neutralized. Thus, the antibody will remain available to agglutinate with the hCG coated tanned red cells or latex particles. In this case, agglutination will occur and this is called as a **negative test** for pregnancy.

> **NOTE**
> **False negative tests** occur if the urine hCG is low or if the test is taken very early in pregnancy. **False positive tests** can be seen in cases of hydatidiform mole, disorders affecting the pituitary gland especially in perimenopausal women and at menopause.

Radioimmunoassay (RIA)

RIA is a more sensitive method and it can detect the presence of hCG in the serum as early as 7–10 days following fertilization.

Principle

A known amount of labeled antigen and antigen in the specimen are mixed and reacted competitively with the constant amount of antibody. When the immune reaction reaches its equilibrium the mixture is washed for removing unreacted conjugates. The antigen and the immune complex are then separated. A graph is then plotted between the concentration of unlabeled antigen and the ratio of bound to total labeled antigen (Flowchart 3.19.1).

A mixture of radioactive antigen and antibody is prepared. The standard reference curve for RIA is shown in Fig. 3.19.1.

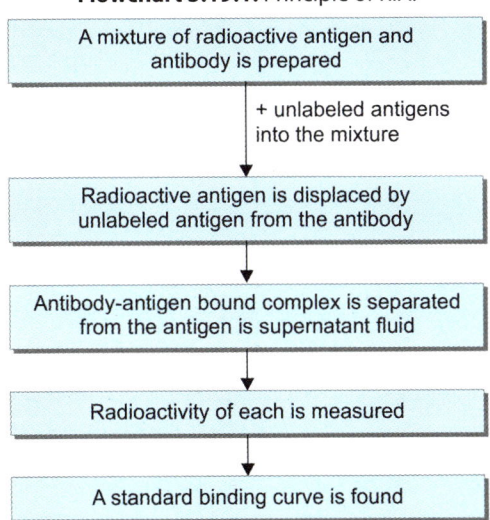

Flowchart 3.19.1: Principle of RIA.

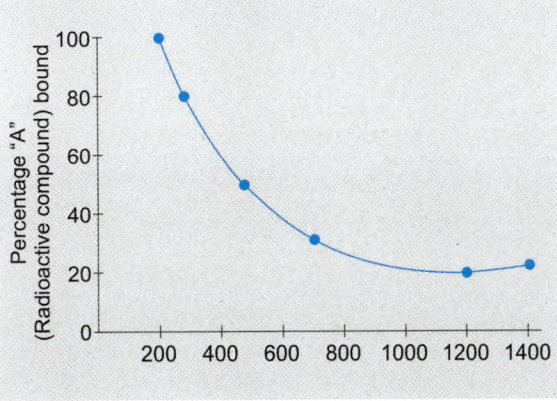

Fig. 3.19.1: Standard reference curve for RIA.

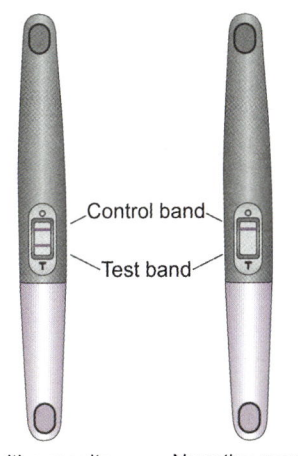

Fig. 3.19.2: ELISA for pregnancy diagnostic test.

Enzyme-Linked Immunosorbent Assay (ELISA)

This is widely used for the detection of various antibodies and antigens. It is as sensitive as RIA and requires very small quantities of reagents.

Principle

The principle of ELISA is nearly the same as that of RIA. Here instead of a radioactive substance an enzyme is used.

Procedure

A mixture of purified hCG linked to an enzyme and the test sample (urine) are added to the test system. If no hCG is present in the test sample, then only the linked enzyme binds to the solid surface. If more hCG is present in the urine sample it will cause a reaction and show up on the test plate as a colored line or a positive (+) mark. This is called as a **Positive test** for pregnancy (Fig. 3.19.2).

> **NOTE**
> A monoclonal antibody assay is used in ELISA to detect hCG in urine.

OTHER TESTS

Radiological investigations: This is the most reliable of all the pregnancy diagnostic tests.
1. *Transvaginal ultrasound:* The gestational sac can be detected by ultrasonography as early as 5th week of pregnancy.
2. *Abdominal ultrasound.*

This test is useful in determination of:
1. Gestational age
2. Any congenital fetal abnormalities

3. Multiple pregnancy
4. Position of placenta.

PHYSIOCLINICAL SIGNIFICANCE

1. Helps in early diagnosis of pregnancy.
2. Positive pregnancy test is seen in cases of hydatidiform mole or vesicular mole (benign tumor of placenta).
3. High levels of hCG are seen in choriocarcinoma (malignant tumor of placenta).

QUESTIONS

Q.1. Name the different pregnancy diagnostic tests.
Q.2. Why are immunological tests preferred over biological tests?
Q.3. Give the physiological basis of the immunological pregnancy diagnostic tests.
Q.4. Name the most reliable tests for pregnancy diagnosis.
Q.5. Give the physioclinical significance of pregnancy diagnostic tests.

STUDY NOTES

Teacher's Signature

CHAPTER 3.20

Birth Control Methods

INTRODUCTION

Birth control is the procedure employed to restrict the number of children by various methods that control fertility and prevent pregnancy. **Contraceptives** are temporary or permanent measures employed to prevent pregnancy in spite of sexual intercourse.

Birth control methods are employed not only for limiting the number of children but also for the spacing of pregnancies because repeated pregnancies pose danger not only to the health of the mother, but also to that of the offspring.

METHODS BASED ON PHYSIOLOGICAL PRINCIPLES

1. **Rhythm method ("safe period"—periodic abstinence):** Normally, only one viable ovum is released per menstrual cycle and it remains viable for about 24 hours, while the sperms, after entering the uterus survive for about 48 hours. Thus, there is a minimum period of 3 days during which intercourse must be avoided to prevent pregnancy.

    For this method to be effective, the time of ovulation must be known. In most women who have regular periods, ovulation usually occurs **14 days before the onset of the next menstruation** (not the 14th day from the 1st day of a cycle). For example, if the cycle starts on the 1st day of a month and lasts 30 days, the time of ovulation would be the 16th of that month. Pregnancy is unlikely to occur if coitus is avoided 4 days before and 4 days after the expected day of ovulation.

    > **NOTE**
    > The rhythm method, though physiological, is the most unreliable method because pregnancy has been reported to occur from coitus on every day of the cycle.

2. **Withdrawal method:** Withdrawal of penis just before ejaculation (orgasm or climax) though practiced is not reliable, the failure rate of this method (coitus interruptus) being about 20%.

BARRIER METHODS (CONDOM AND DIAPHRAGM)

Since it is very cheap and effective, the condom (a rubber sheath worn over the penis during coitus), is the most widely used method by the males. An added advantage is the protection it gives to the male against sexually transmitted diseases (STDs) like acquired immunodeficiency syndrome (AIDS), hepatitis, syphilis and gonorrhea.

A similar barrier, the rubber diaphragm, is fitted over the cervix by the female.

In addition to these mechanical barriers, a spermicidal jelly is used by many couples at the same time.

USE OF SPERMICIDAL AGENTS

Use of creams, jellies, foams, suppositories, etc. in the female before coitus and vaginal douches after intercourse may be combined with barriers.

INTERRUPTION OF THE NORMAL PATHS OF SPERMS OR OVUM (SURGICAL STERILIZATION)

Interrupting the normal paths of sperm or ovum by vasectomy in males and tubectomy in females, appear to be the ideal methods suitable for our poor and illiterate population. However, restoration of the patency of these tubes, if required later on, has few chances of success.

INTRAUTERINE DEVICES

Intrauterine devices (IUDs) or intrauterine contraceptive devices (IUCDs) are foreign bodies (plastic or metal) that are placed in the uterus and left there. "Copper T" and "loop D" (stainless steel) are the common devices used. They possibly make the endometrium unsuitable for implantation of fertilized egg by causing "aseptic inflammation" and/or by increasing uterine motility. IUDs have long-term use (6–10 years), can be removed when desired and are as effective as tubectomy (the copper in **copper T** may also be spermicidal).

ORAL CONTRACEPTIVES (HORMONAL METHODS)

It has been known for long that various doses of synthetic estrogens and progesterone given during the first half of menstrual cycle inhibit release of follicle stimulating hormone (FSH) and luteinizing hormone (LH) by negative feedback. This, in turn, reduces the levels of the normal ovarian estrogens and progesterone, the midcycle LH surge does not occur and ovulation is not triggered. Even if ovulation does occur, changes in cervical mucus and in the endometrium prove hostile for sperms and implantation.

The pills are started early in the cycle, continued beyond the expected day of ovulation and then stopped to allow menstruation to occur. The contraceptive "pills" are 100% effective and are used by millions worldwide. The hormonal methods include:
- **Classical pill:** It contains orally active progesterone-like substance—gestagen and a small dose of estrogen. In addition to inhibiting ovulation, these pills also render the cervical mucus hostile to sperm penetration. They may also induce endometrial changes which prevent implantation of the fertilized egg.
- **Sequential pill:** It has a high dose of estrogen for 15 days followed by estrogen plus gestagen for 5 days. This pill inhibits ovulation by suppressing both LH and FSH.
- **Luteal supplementation pill:** These pills contain low doses of gestagen throughout the entire cycle. It controls fertility without inhibiting ovulation. The hormone may be acting on the cervical mucus or on the endometrium or perhaps by reducing the motility of the fallopian tubes.
- **"Morning-after pill" [emergency contraception (EC)]:** These pills have high doses of estrogens and progestin. They inhibit FSH and LH and stop the secretion of ovarian estrogens and progesterone. The sudden fall of these hormones causes shedding of uterine endometrium, thus blocking implantation.

  When two pills are taken within 72 hours of unprotected coitus and another two tablets after another 12 hours, chances of pregnancy are greatly reduced.

Other Hormonal Methods

- Subcutaneous implantation of hormone-containing capsules (they slowly release the drug into the circulation and are effective for about 5 years).
- Intramuscular injection of progestin (e.g. Depo-Provera) every 3 months.
- Once-a-month intramuscular injection of estrogen and progesterone, skin patches containing these hormones, once a week for 3 weeks of the cycle.

QUESTIONS

Q.1. How can the time of ovulation be determined?

The anterior pituitary hormone FSH is responsible for the early maturation of the ovarian follicle, while LH is responsible for its final maturation. A burst of LH secretion at the midcycle causes the release of the ovum and the initial formation of corpus luteum. It is important to know the time of ovulation for the rhythm method to be effective in preventing pregnancy. The following methods are employed to determine the time of ovulation:

1. **Change in the basal body temperature:** A fairly reliable and convenient indicator of the time of ovulation is a rise in the basal body temperature at the time of ovulation. Using a thermometer with wide graduations and before getting out of bed in the morning, the oral temperature is recorded every day and charted on a temperature chart. The temperature continues to fall during the first half of the cycle and then it starts to rise from the time of ovulation till the onset of the next cycle, the difference being 0.5–1.0°C. The cause of temperature rise is probably the increase in progesterone secretion, since this hormone is thermogenic.
2. **Examination of cervical secretions:** It shows thick, cellular mucus that does not form a fern pattern.

Q.2. What is meant by MTP? How is it carried out?

The procedure of deliberately evacuating the uterus before 28 weeks of pregnancy is called "induction of abortion".

Under certain conditions such as cases of rape, threatened abortion, fetal abnormalities, etc. pregnancy may be legally terminated (aborted)—a procedure called "medical termination of pregnancy (MTP)". Some of the methods employed are:

1. **Dilatation and curettage (D and C; up to 12 weeks):** The cervix is dilated with graduated metal dilators and a curette is used to evacuate the uterine contents.
2. **Vacuum aspiration:** The cervix is dilated and the uterus is evacuated with an electrical suction pump. The method is suitable up to 12 weeks of pregnancy.
3. **Menstrual syringe:** A plastic syringe and cannula, called menstrual regulator (MR) syringe, is used to aspirate the uterine contents, up to 6 weeks of pregnancy.
4. **Intra-amniotic hypertonic saline solution (13–20 weeks):** About 200 mL of 20% saline or 80 g of urea in 200 mL of water, are injected into the amniotic cavity to cause abortion.
5. **Extra-amniotic ethacridine lactate (13–20 weeks):** About 10 mL/week of pregnancy of this dye solution is introduced via a catheter placed in the cervix.
6. **Prostaglandins (13–20 weeks):** Prostaglandin PGE, PGF2 or their analogs are instilled intra-amniotically to cause strong uterine contractions which cause expulsion of fetus.
7. **Pitocin (oxytocin):** Pitocin drip, 10–20 units in 500 mL of 5% dextrose solution is used for inducing or augmenting abortion.

Q.3. How can safe period be determined when the menstrual periods are irregular?

If the periods are irregular, the safe period can be calculated as indicated by the following examples:

Woman A: Menstrual cycles regular, duration of a cycle is 29 days.

Menstrual cycle: 29 days.

Ovulation: 15th day of the cycle (14 days before the onset of the next cycle).

Safe period: Extends up to 11th day and continues from 19th day onward to the end of the cycle.

Woman B: Menstrual cycles *irregular*, duration of cycles varies between 26 days and 33 days (to calculate the safe period in women with irregular menstrual cycles during the preovulatory phase, 18 is subtracted from the shortest recorded cycle. During the luteal phase, 11 is subtracted from the longest recorded cycle).

Safe period: 26 – 18 = 8 and 33 – 11 = 22

Therefore, in this woman, the safe period extends up to the 8th day of any cycle and continues from day 22 onward till the end of the cycle (the first day of the menstrual cycle is the day when the menstrual bleeding starts).

STUDY NOTES

Section 4

Clinical Examination

CHAPTERS

- 4.1 History Taking and General Physical Examination
- 4.2 Clinical Examination of the Respiratory System
- 4.3 Clinical Examination of the Cardiovascular System
- 4.4 Clinical Examination of the Abdomen
- 4.5 Clinical Examination of the Nervous System
    - A: Examination of Higher Functions
    - B: Examination of the Cranial Nerves
    - C: Examination of the Motor System
    - D: Reflexes
    - E: Examination of the Sensory System

Date ....

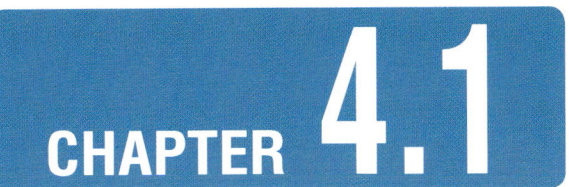

History Taking and General Physical Examination

While making a diagnosis the first step is observation of the patient which includes **history taking, general physical examination** and other investigations. The second step is interpretation of the obtained knowledge. An exhaustive general examination is an important part of clinical examination of the patient. It should be performed before proceeding to the **systemic examination.**

CLINICAL EXAMINATION

There are two basic steps in clinical examination of a patient/subject:
1. **History taking:** History taking is perhaps the most important and skilled part of clinical examination. The patient is asked for a description of what has happened. The history taking includes:
   a. Age and address
   b. Marital status
   c. Social and occupational history
   d. History of previous illness
   e. Family history
   f. Presenting complaints
   g. History of present illness
   h. Treatment history
2. **Physical examination:** It is an orderly examination for evaluation of the patient's body and its functions. It includes the noninvasive methods, along with measurement of vital signs. It has two components:
   a. General physical examination
   b. Systemic physical examination.

Prerequisites for a Satisfactory Physical Examination

1. Establish a good rapport (sympathy) with the patient. He/she will be relaxed and reassured.
2. The room should be comfortable, with adequate natural daylight as artificial light may mask the changes in skin color.
3. If the patient is a female, the husband, female relative or a female nurse must be present.
4. The patient should be asked to expose the area which is to be examined.
5. The doctor, if right handed, must always stand on the right side of the patient.

General Physical Examination (GPE)

GPE necessitates a general examination of the patient from head to toe in order to have vital information. This should include:
1. General appearance
2. Whether the patient is conscious/unconscious
3. Orientation in time and space
4. Whether the patient is depressed/sad, cheerful
5. Whether the patient is dyspneic or not
6. Gait
7. General examination of hair, eyes, face, mouth, pharynx, neck and limbs.
8. Position of the trachea and apex beat.
9. Whether there is pallor, icterus, cyanosis, clubbing, lymphadenopathy and edema

10. Whether the jugular venous pressure (JVP) is raised or not
11. Taking vitals (temperature, pulse rate, blood pressure and respiratory rate).

General appearance: Does the patient look healthy, unwell or ill? Apparent age, weight and height, body build, body mass index (BMI) and nutrition status.

$$BMI = \frac{Weight\ (kg)}{[Height\ (m^2)]}$$

Note if breathing is comfortable.

Posture in bed: In congestive heart failure there is orthopnea (i.e. the patient is more comfortable sitting rather than lying down).

Gait: Some diseases are obvious by the gait, e.g. drunken *(zigzag)* gait of cerebellar ataxia and the rigid gait of Parkinsonism.

Facies and speech: Note the expression, symmetry and color of the face. Does he/she speak or is silent? Is the speech hysterical?

Skin: Look for the color, texture, eruptions, petechiae and scars. There is pallor in anemia (color of oral mucosa and creases of palm give a better idea of paleness); yellowish in jaundice and hypercarotenemia; and bluish in cyanosis (due to presence of at least 5.0 g of reduced Hb in the skin capillaries).

Neck: Look for enlarged lymph glands; thyroid; pulsations of vessels, venous distension; position of trachea.

Chest: Shape; deformities, curvature of spine at the back. Note rate of breathing (Normal = 12–16 breaths/min).

Note the odor of breath: breath may be sweet and sickly in diabetes and ketosis; ammoniacal in uremia; halitosis (bad breath) in poor dental and oral hygiene.

Abdomen: Note the contour, skin, scars and pulsations.

Hands: Look for tremors, skin, nails, clubbing of fingers and trophic changes.

Limbs: Look for scars, wounds, deformities, edema and prominent leg veins.

Vitals:
- Pulse rate: Count for complete one minute. Note if there is tachycardia or bradycardia (Normal range = 60–90 beats/min).
- Temperature: Keep the thermometer under the tongue for 2 minutes (Normal range = 97.2–98.8°F). Oral cavity temperature approximates the core body temperature (In children, the axillary or groin temperature is less by about 1.0°F).
    - Core temperature refers to the measurement of temperature of body cavities.
    - Hyperpyrexia is said to occur when the core temperature exceeds 107°F.
    - Hypothermia is said to occur when the core temperature goes down below 95°F.
- Respiratory rate: The respiration is counted for full 1 minute by observing the subjects abdominal movements (Normal range = 12–16 respirations/min)
- Blood pressure: Record the blood pressure after a short period of rest.

The average systolic blood pressure (SBP) in a healthy adult is 100–140 mm Hg, the average diastolic blood pressure (DBP) is 60–90 mm Hg. In elderly both the values, i.e. SBP and DBP reach or even exceed the higher figure. In children both SBP and DBP approximate to be lower figure. The difference between SBP and DBP is called pulse pressure. Normal pulse pressure is 30–60 mm Hg.

"PICKLE"—Pallor, Icterus, Cyanosis, Clubbing, Lymphadenopathy and Edema

1. **Pallor:** It is the paleness of skin which is usually detected by retracting the lower eyelids and examining the lower palpebral conjunctiva (Fig. 4.1.1). It is seen in conditions where the blood flow to the capillaries is diminished or when the hemoglobin content in the blood is decreased. The degree of pallor is expressed as:
    - Pallor 0: No anemia
    - Pallor +: Mild anemia
    - Pallor ++: Moderate anemia
    - Pallor +++: Severe anemia.

2. **Jaundice/icterus:** It is the yellowish discoloration of sclera, skin and mucous membrane of the body due to presence of excess bilirubin in the blood (Fig. 4.1.2). While examining for icterus/jaundice the preferred site is sclera which is rich in collagen fibers. They have high affinity for bilirubin leading to yellow discoloration of sclera in jaundice. Normal serum bilirubin concentration—0.2 to 0.8 mg/100 mL of blood. When serum bilirubin levels exceed 2 mg% jaundice is said to appear clinically.

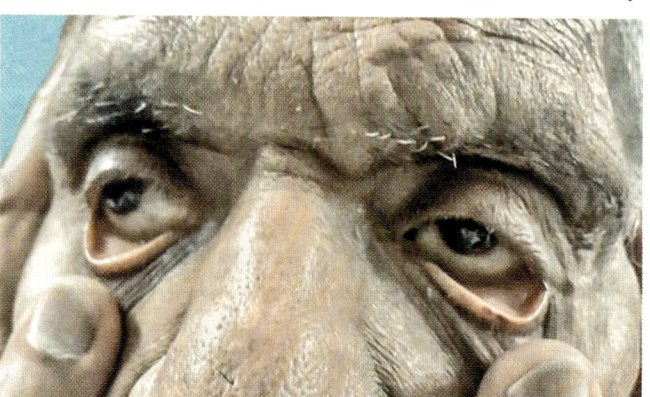

Fig. 4.1.1: Looking for pallor.

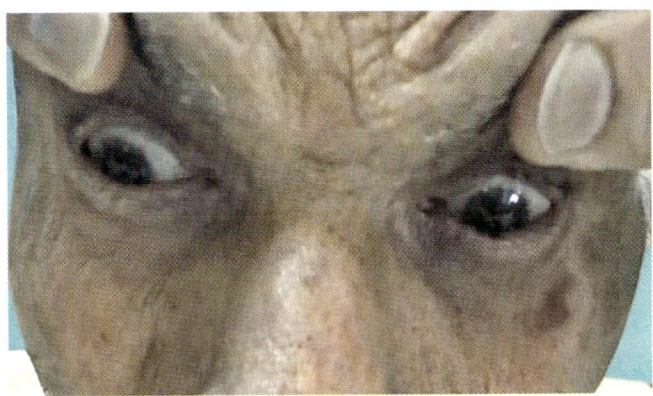

Fig. 4.1.2: Looking for icterus.

3. **Cyanosis:** It is the bluish discoloration of the skin and mucous membranes that occurs when the absolute concentration of deoxygenated/reduced hemoglobin is more than 5 g%. It is of two types:
   a. *Central cyanosis:* It is seen at the lips and tongue. Anemic or hypovolemic patients rarely have central cyanosis because severe hypoxia is required to produce the necessary concentration of deoxygenated hemoglobin. Patients with polycythemia can become cyanosed at normal arterial oxygen saturation.
   b. *Peripheral cyanosis:* It is seen in the hands, feet or ears, usually when they are cold. It is also found with central cyanosis, but is most often seen with poor peripheral circulation due to shock, heart failure, peripheral vascular disease, Raynaud's phenomenon and venous obstruction, e.g. deep vein thrombosis.
4. **Clubbing:** It is the bulbous enlargement of the soft parts of the terminal phalanges, the tissues at the base of the nail are thickened and the angle between the base of the nail and the adjacent skin of the finger is lost (Fig. 4.1.3).

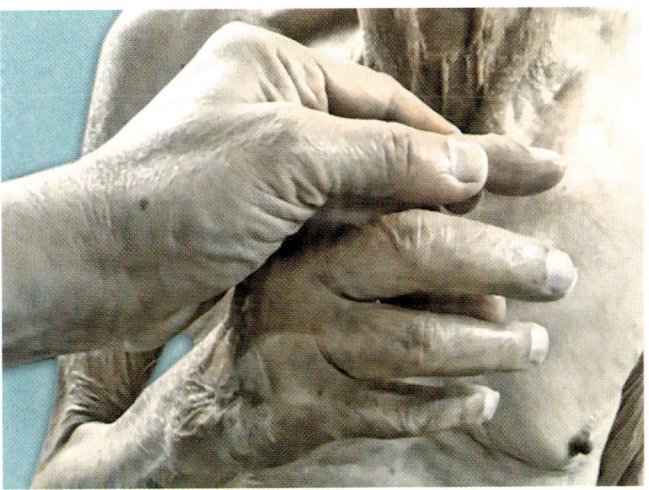

Fig. 4.1.3: Looking for clubbing.

Thus, the nail becomes convex both transversely and longitudinally. Clubbing can be detected by any of the following signs:
   a. *Fluctuation test:* Holding the base of the nail from both sides and gently press the tip of the nail to elicit fluctuation which increases in clubbing.
   b. *Curving of the nails:* The nail becomes convex both transversely and longitudinally due to the hypertrophy of the nail bed tissue.
   c. *Schamroth's sign:* The two fingers are held together with their nails facing each other a space is seen at the nail fold, which is lost in clubbing.
   d. *Base angle:* Normally the angle between the base of nail and the adjacent portion of the dorsum of the terminal phalanx is an obtuse angle of about 160°. However, in clubbing this angle gets obliterated and increases.

Causes of clubbing:
   a. Cyanotic heart disease and infective endocarditis
   b. Bronchiectasis, bronchial carcinoma
   c. Inflammatory bowel disease.

Degree of clubbing:
   a. **1st degree:** Increased fluctuation of the nail bed.
   b. **2nd degree:** Curving of nail bed along with increased fluctuation of nail bed.
   c. **3rd degree:** Increased fluctuation, increased curving and obliteration of base angle of nail.
   d. **4th degree:** All of the above plus subperiosteal thickening of the wrist and ankle bones along with the presence of definite transverse ridge at the root of the nails.

5. **Lymphadenopathy:** Lymph nodes may be palpable in normal people, especially in the submandibular, axilla and groin. Areas on both the sides should be examined. Lymph nodes in the neck are examined by standing behind the subject keeping the head slightly flexed. The different groups of lymph nodes are examined. Distinguish between normal and pathological lymph nodes.

   Pathological lymphadenopathy may be local or generalized and is of diagnostic and prognostic significance in the staging of lymphoproliferative diseases and other malignancies. The lymph nodes are palpated to check for their size, shape, consistency, mobility and tenderness.

   The most common cause of lymphadenopathy in India is tuberculosis. Other causes include: Connective tissue disorder (e.g. systemic lupus erythematosus and sarcoidosis), endocrine disorders (e.g. Addison's disease) and drug induced (e.g. phenytoin, carbamazepine).

Examine lymph nodes under the following headings:
- **Size:** Normal lymph nodes in adults are seldom <0.5 cm in diameter.
- **Consistency:** Normal lymph nodes feel soft. In Hodgkin's disease they are characteristically "rubbery", in tuberculosis they may be "matted" and in metastatic cancer they feel hard.
- **Tenderness:** Acute viral or bacterial infection, including infectious mononucleosis, dental sepsis and tonsillitis, cause tender, variably enlarged lymph nodes.
- **Fixation:** Lymph nodes fixed to deep structures or skin suggests malignancy.

6. **Edema:** It is the swelling of skin and subcutaneous tissues due to accumulation of free fluid in excess in the interstitial tissue spaces. It is diagnosed by usually pressing the skin against the bone in the dependent parts of the body. It can be of two types:
   a. *Pitting edema:* Congestive heart failure, cirrhosis of liver, nephrotic syndrome (facial edema).
   b. *Non-pitting edema:* Filariasis.

Systemic Physical Examination

Observation is a very essential faculty in medical practice that has to be cultivated rigorously, is the hallmark of inspection.

1. **Inspection:** It should be carried out in good light, the part of the body should be fully exposed and looked at from different angles. Note, if there are any changes in the body that deviate from the normal.
2. **Palpation:** It is carried out by placing the right hand flat on the body part, with the forearm and wrist in the same horizontal plane. Apply a gentle pressure with the fingers, moving them at the metacarpophalangeal joints.

> **NOTE**
> Never "poke" the patient's body with your fingers. The ulnar border of your hand may also be used for palpation.

3. **Percussion:** It means giving a sharp tap or impact on the surface of the body, usually with the fingers. Its purpose is to set up vibrations in the underlying tissues and listening to the echo.

   Rules of percussion:
   - The middle finger (**pleximeter finger**) of the left hand is placed firmly in contact with the skin keeping the other fingers well separated apart.
   - The back of its middle phalanx is struck with the tip of the striking middle finger (**percussing finger**) of the right hand, two or three times in a perpendicular direction.
   - The striking finger must also be lifted immediately after the stroke to avoid damping of the resulting vibrations.
   - The movement of the hand should be at the wrist joint and not at the elbow or shoulder joint.

> **NOTE**
> Percussion is always carried out from resonant toward the dull area.

The following things are noted on percussion:
a. Character of the sound produced
b. The characteristic feeling imparted to the pleximeter finger.

4. **Auscultation:** It refers to listening to the sounds in order to assess the functioning of certain organs. A stethoscope is used to amplify the sounds. For example, listening to heart sounds and breath sounds.

COMMONLY USED TERMS IN CLINICAL EXAMINATION

1. **Symptoms:** These are subjective disturbances in the body function resulting from disease, which a patient experiences and which cause him to feel he is not well. These subjective changes that are not visible to an observer are called symptoms.
2. **Physical signs:** These are objective marks of diseases that a trained person can see and measure using his senses, generally unaided, though the aid of a stethoscope is usually allowed under this definition (e.g. fever, high BP and paralysis).
3. **Syndrome:** Constellation of symptoms which occur together and characterize a particular abnormality or condition.
4. **Disorder:** The term refers to any abnormality of structure or function.
5. **Disease:** It is a more specific term for an illness characterized by specific recognizable set of symptoms and signs. Thus, it is any specific change from the state of health. A disease may be a local one, affecting a part or limited region of the body. Or it may be a systemic disease affecting either the entire body or several parts of it.
6. **Diagnosis** (Dia = through; gnosis = knowing). It is the science and skill of distinguishing one disorder or disease from another. The patient's history of illness and physical examination (and sometimes various tests) and their correct interpretation builds up a picture of the patient's illness. Sometimes the diagnosis is only "provisional", which is usually confirmed after laboratory and/or special investigations.
7. **Prognosis:** After considering all aspects of a patient's illness, the doctor may be able to give an opinion about

the possible future course of the disease, i.e. the degree of cure possible (or otherwise). This comment on the future course of the disease is called prognosis.

8. **Vital signs:** This term refers to the four signs which can be seen, measured and recorded in a living person. They include: **Pulse, blood pressure, respiratory rate** and **body temperature**. The former three are controlled by the "vital centers" located in the medulla, while the body temperature is controlled by the hypothalamus. The vital signs must always be checked during general physical examination.

QUESTIONS

- Q.1. What is the importance of GPE? What are the prerequisites before proceeding for GPE?
- Q.2. How do you detect jaundice clinically?
- Q.3. What are the causes of yellowish discoloration of skin and mucous membrane?
- Q.4. Define cyanosis. What are the different types of cyanosis? Discuss its physiological basis.
- Q.5. Why natural light is preferred over artificial light for doing a clinical examination?
- Q.6. What is clubbing? How is it detected?
- Q.7. What are the causes of clubbing?
- Q.8. What are vital signs?
- Q.9. Define edema. What are the different types of edema?
- Q.10. What is lymphadenopathy?

OBSERVATION AND RESULT

Perform the general physical examination of the given subject and note down the observations in a tabular form.

INTERPRETATION

STUDY NOTES

CHAPTER 4.2

Clinical Examination of the Respiratory System

IMPORTANT SIGNS AND SYMPTOMS OF RESPIRATORY DISEASE

1. **Dyspnea:** Breathlessness which is out of proportion to the level of physical exertion and is unpleasant is known as **dyspnea**. Dyspnea may be present at rest also.
2. **Cough:** It may be dry or productive.
3. **Expectoration (sputum):** Look for the amount, color, whether watery or frothy; whether contains pus or blood.
4. **Hemoptysis:** It means coughing out of blood in the sputum. It usually indicates some serious pathology like pulmonary tuberculosis or lung carcinoma.
5. **Wheezing:** The patient must be asked if any additional sounds come from the lungs during breathing.
6. **Pain:** Apart from pain from the muscles and skeleton of the chest, pain due to lung disease comes usually from the pleura.
7. **Other signs:** Like cyanosis, clubbing and lymphadenopathy.

NOTE
Always take family history, occupational history and the smoking history.

Important landmarks: Vertical lines dawn on the front and back of the thorax constitute some of the important landmarks. These are: Midsternal line; midclavicular lines; anterior axillary, midaxillary and posterior axillary lines; midspinal and midscapular lines (Figs. 4.2.1A and B).

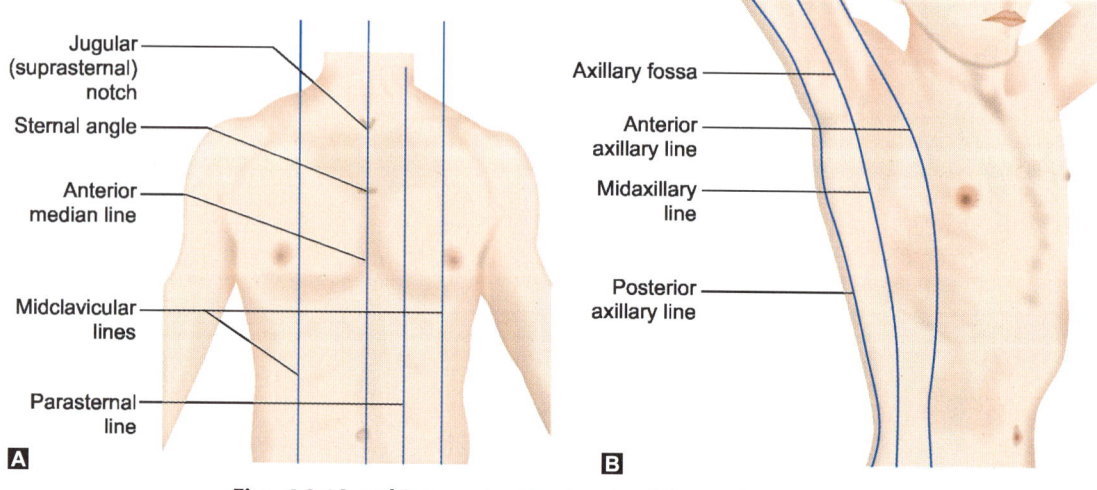

Figs. 4.2.1A and B: Important landmarks of the respiratory system.

Examination of the Respiratory System

This is to be done as under the following headings:
- **General physical examination:** Any systemic examination is preceded by general physical examination.
- **Systemic examination:** This is to be done under the following headings:
    - Inspection
    - Palpation
    - Percussion
    - Auscultation
- The subject is examined in good light, stripped to the waist and preferably in sitting position. The chest should be inspected from all sides.

Inspection

Shape of the Chest (Figs. 4.2.2A to F)

1. **Normal chest:** Elliptical in cross-section and bilaterally symmetrical.
   Normal ratio of transverse to anteroposterior diameter (Hutchinson's index) = 7:5
2. **Abnormal forms of chest:**
   a. *Pigeon-shaped chest or pectus carinatum* (elliptical chest with prominent sternum seen in children with rickets).
   b. *Barrel-shaped chest:* Anteroposterior diameter more than the transverse diameter. The sternum is arched and the lungs are overinflated as seen in emphysema.
   c. *Funnel-shaped chest or pectus excavatum:* It is characterized by a depression in the lower half of the sternum. This is also known as sunken chest.
   Kyphosis (forward bending of the vertebral column) and **scoliosis** (lateral bending of the vertebral column) also lead to the asymmetry of the chest.

Respiratory Movements

1. **Rate:** The rate should be counted surreptitiously, while keeping the fingers on the radial pulse, because a nervous patient may breathe rapidly and irregularly. The normal rate of respiration is 12–16 breaths/min, one inspiration and one expiration making up one cycle. It is faster in children and in old age. The rate bears a definite ratio to pulse rate of about 1:4, which is usually constant in the same person.

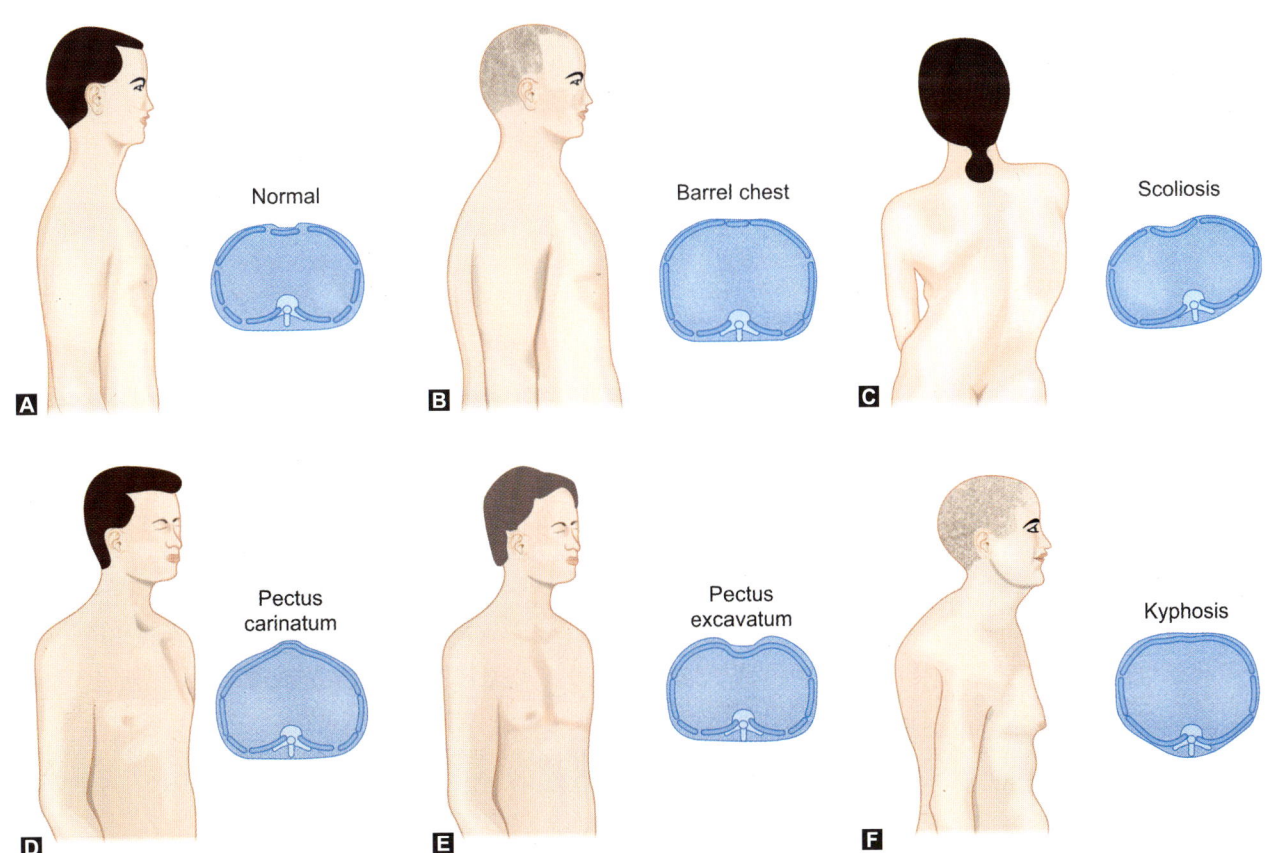

Figs. 4.2A to F: Shapes of chest.

2. **Depth**: The rate and depth usually increase or decrease together. They are regulated by the respiratory center via reflexes arising in the thorax and the great vessels. Look whether the respiration is shallow or deep. In bronchial asthma, the respiration is shallow and it is deep when there is brain damage or uremia.
3. **Rhythm**: Normal respiration is regular. Irregular breathing may be seen during brain damage, after voluntary hyperventilation or in left ventricular failure. It may also occur in obstructive airway disease.
4. **Type (manner) of breathing**: The respiration can be predominantly thoracic or abdominal. In women the respiration is **thoracoabdominal** while in males it is **abdominothoracic**.
5. **Expansion of chest:** Both sides move equally, symmetrically and simultaneously. Asymmetric expansion of the lungs may be seen when the underlying lung is diseased. Fibrosis, consolidation, collapse or pleural effusion can all decrease chest expansion on the affected side though other physical signs will also be present.

Position of Trachea and Apex Beat

Inspection may not show the position of trachea, though cardiac pulsation may be visible; the lowermost and outermost point on which would be the apex beat. It will be **confirmed by palpation**.

Palpation

1. **Position of trachea:**
   - Put the tip of the index and the ring finger of the right hand on the sternal head of the clavicle and then gently move the middle finger upward from the suprasternal notch to feel the tracheal rings.
   - The trachea can also be palpated by placing the index finger in the suprasternal notch and try to judge the space between it and the insertion of sternomastoid muscle on either side of it.
   - Normally, trachea is in the midline or slightly to right side. However, in diseases, it may be pulled to the affected side (fibrosis, lung collapse) or pushed away from the affected side (pneumothorax, pleural effusion).
2. **Position of apex beat:** Displacement of trachea and apex beat indicates shifting of the mediastinum.
3. **Presence of lymph nodes:** Note the presence or absence of lymph nodes in the axilla and supraclavicular regions, because these may be the only evidence of carcinoma of the lungs.
4. **Expansion of chest:**
   - The expansion of the chest when measured with a tape placed around the chest just below the level of the nipples is 4–8 cm after a deep breath.
   - Chest expansion can also be tested by placing the fingertips of either hand at the patients sides in such a way that the tips of the two thumbs meet in the midline. The patient is then asked to inspire deeply. The increase in distance between the thumbs indicates the extent of chest expansion (Fig. 4.2.3).
5. **Vocal fremitus:** The detection of vibrations transmitted to the hands from the larynx through bronchi, lungs and chest wall during the act of phonation is called vocal fremitus (Fig. 4.2.4).
   - The ulnar border of the hand is placed on the intercostal spaces while the patient is asked to say "ninety nine" or "ek do teen".
   - The vibrations felt by the hand are compared on identical points, from above downward, on the front, axillary region and on the back of the chest.
   - Vocal fremitus may be **diminished** if the voice is feeble or when a bronchus is blocked by a new growth

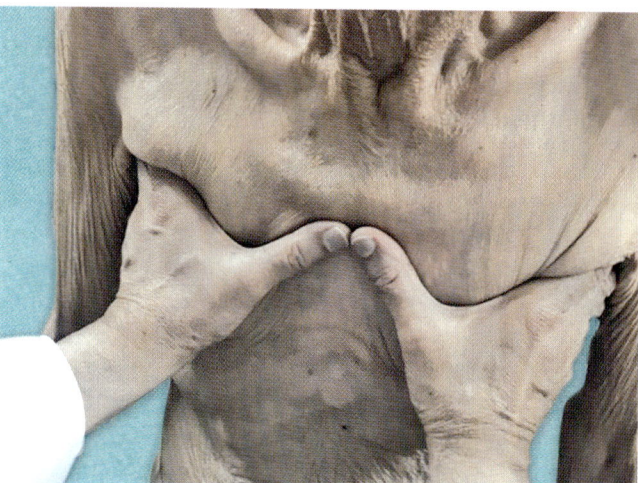

Fig.4.2.3: Chest expansion.

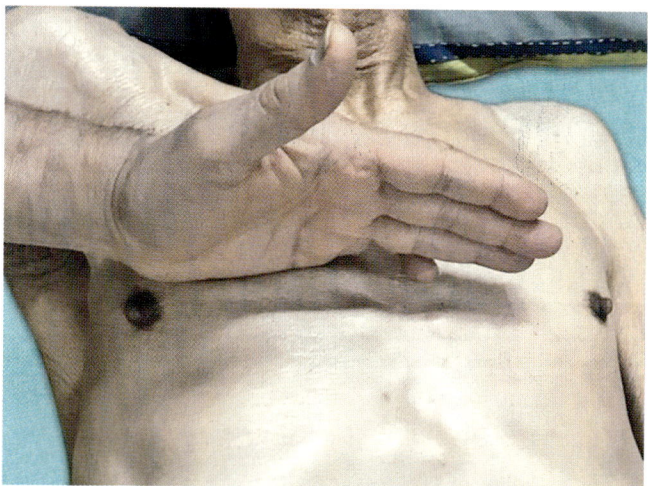

Fig. 4.2.4: Eliciting vocal fremitus.

which interferes with the passage of vibrations or when the vibrations are dampened by fluid or air in the pleural cavity.
- It is **increased** when the vibrations are better conducted, as through solid lung (consolidation due to pneumonia).
6. **Tenderness:** Palpate all the regions of the chest wall to elicit tenderness if any. It may be seen in injury or inflammatory conditions of the chest wall.

Percussion

Percussion is the procedure employed for setting up artificial vibrations in a tissue by means of a sharp tap, usually delivered with the fingers (Fig. 4.2.5).

- **Rules of percussion:** Discussed under General Physical Examination (GPE) (*Refer* Chapter 4.1).
- The striking finger **(percussing finger)** should lie, almost over and parallel to the pleximeter finger, should be relaxed and should not be lifted more than 2 or 3 inches. It must also be lifted clear immediately after the blow to avoid damping of the resulting vibrations.

Percussion is done for determining:
a. The condition of the underlying tissues—lungs, pleura.
b. The borders of the lungs.

The following two things are to be noted during percussion:

1. **The character of the sound produced.** It differs in quality and quantity over different tissues.
   - When the air in cavity of sufficient size and appropriate shape is set into vibration the sound which is produced is known as resonant sound. Air-containing organs, such as lungs, thus produce a resonant sound.

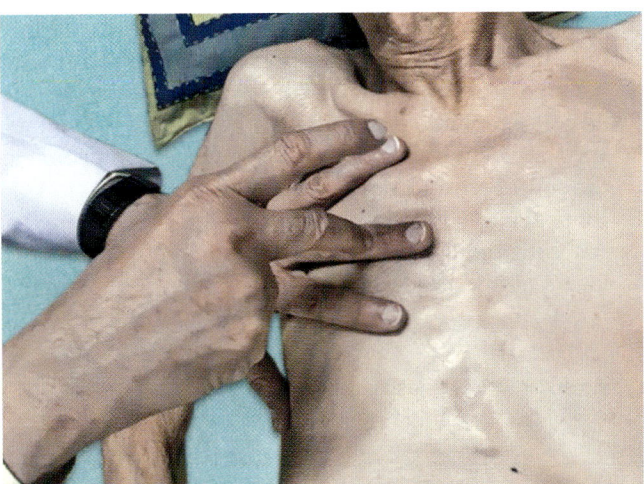

Fig. 4.2.5: Percussion.

- An increase in resonance (**hyperresonance**) though difficult to detect may be produced when there is air in the peural cavity, i.e. pneumothorax.
- The opposite of resonance, i.e. lack of note, called **dullness**, is found over solid viscera like heart and liver or when the lung becomes solidified as in pneumonia, growth or fibrosis.
- An extreme form of dullness is called **stony dullness**, in which a feeling of resistance is felt by the tapping finger along with a dull note; such dullness is found by percussing over the thigh and is encountered in pleural effusion.
- The percussion note changes to **tympani** when air fills the pleural cavity or when air is contained unloculated in a large lung cyst or in stomach.

2. **The characteristic feeling imparted to the pleximeter finger.** The student should practice percussing over different parts of his/her body and over various objects like wooden and steel furniture and so on.

The following precautions are to be taken while doing percussion:

1. When the boundaries of organs are to be defined, percussion is done from resonance to dullness and from more resonant to less resonant areas.
2. The direction of percussion should be at right angles to the edge of the organ.

Apical percussion: It is carried out in the supraclavicular fossae to determine the upper borders of the lungs which lie 3–4 cm above the clavicles.

Basal percussion: The lower limits of lung resonance are determined by percussing the chest from above downward, with the pleximeter finger parallel to the diaphragm. With light percussion and in quiet respiration, the lower border of the right lung lies in the midclavicular line at the 6th rib, in the midaxillary line at the 8th rib and in the scapular line at the 10th rib. Posteriorly, on both sides and anteriorly on the right side, the percussion note changes from resonant to dull, while anteriorly on the left side, the percussion note changes from resonant to tympanic.

Auscultation

Auscultation of Lungs and Trachea

Auscultate the chest with the diaphragm and not the bell of the stethoscope. This is because the chest sounds are relatively high-pitched and the diaphragm is more sensitive than the bell.

- Auscultation is done all over the lungs—front, axillary regions and back—and sounds at corresponding points on the two sides are compared.
- Since breath sounds during quiet breathing are insufficient for study, the patient is asked to breathe

deeply through an open mouth. The following points are noted:
a. *The type or character of breath sounds*—whether vesicular or bronchial.
b. *Intensity of breath sounds*—whether diminished or absent.
c. *Added or adventitious sounds*—crepitations, rhonchi, pleural rub, etc.
d. *Character of vocal resonance.*

Type or character of breath sounds
Figure 4.2.6 shows the types or character of breath sounds.

Differences between vesicular and bronchial breath sounds are discussed in Table 4.2.1.

Intensity of breath sounds
The intensity or loudness of breath sounds may be normal, reduced or increased.
1. **Reduced breath sounds**: Localized airway narrowing, extensive lung damage, e.g. emphysema, pleural thickening, pleural fluid.
2. **Increased breath sounds**: It may be heard in very thin persons.

Vocal resonance
Vocal resonance refers to the sounds heard over the chest during the act of phonation. The vibrations set up by the vocal cords are transmitted along the airways and through the lung tissues to the chest wall.

The subject is asked to repeat "ninety nine" or "ek do teen" in a normal, clear and uniform voice; and the sounds heard are compared on the identical regions on the two sides.
- The normal intensity of vocal resonance gives the impression of being produced near the chest piece of the stethoscope.
- When the intensity is increased and the sounds appear to come from near the earpiece of the stethoscope, they are called **bronchophony**.
- It is heard over consolidation of lung tissue as in pneumonia, in tuberculosis or over lung apex when the upper lobe is collapsed and trachea is pulled to that side.
- When the words are clear and appear to be spoken (whispered) right into the ears and the words can be clearly identified, the condition is called **whispering pectoriloquy**.

Table 4.2.1: Differences between vesicular and bronchial breath sounds

	Vesicular breath sounds	Bronchial breath sounds
Origin	Larger airways: When there is normal air filled healthy lung present between the airways and the chest wall	Larger airways: When there is no air containing lung tissue between the airways and the chest wall, e.g. consolidation, fibrosis, lung collapse
Location	Heard over the healthy lung especially in the axillary and infrascapular regions	• Normally over the trachea • Also in areas where the bronchus is patent but alveoli are not filled with air
Character	• Low-pitched and rustling • No distinct pause between end of inspiration and beginning of expiration	• High-pitched, louder and harsh • There is a gap between the end of inspiration and beginning of expiration
Relative duration	Expiration is less than inspiration	Both inspiration and expiration are equal

- Vocal resonance may be decreased or even abolished when there is fluid in the pleural cavity, pneumothorax or emphysema.

Adventitious or "added" sounds
The sounds which do not form an essential part of the usual breath sounds are called adventitious (extra) or "added" sounds. They are generally of three types:
1. **Rhonchi:** These are **"dry sounds"** and are produced by the passage of air though narrowed or partially blocked respiratory passages.
2. **Crepitations (or "moist sounds"):** They are discontinuous "bubbling" or "crackling" sounds produced by the passage of air through fluid in the small airways and/or alveoli. Crepitations may be "fine" or "coarse" (If you rub your hair between your thumb and a finger near your ear, the sound produced resembles fine crepitations).
3. **Pleural rub (or "friction sound"):** It is a "creaking" or "rubbing" sound produced by friction between the two layers of inflamed and roughened pleura. It is mainly

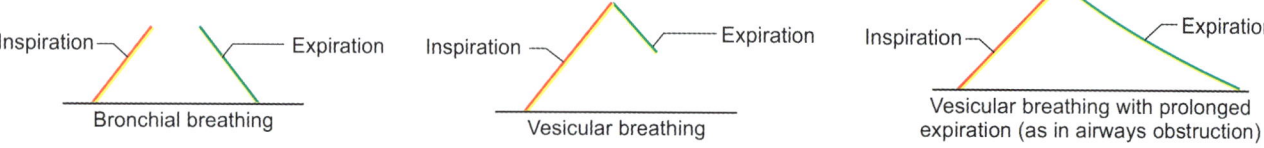

Fig. 4.2.6: Two main types of breath sounds.

produced during that part of respiration when the rough surfaces rub against each other, i.e. during deep inspiration. The pleural rub disappears when there is accumulation of fluid in the pleural cavity.

QUESTIONS

Q.1. What are the different abnormalities of the shape of the chest?
Q.2. What are the different types of breath sounds? How do you differentiate between them?
Q.3. Why is the diaphragm of the stethoscope preferred while listening to the breath sounds?
Q.4. What is vocal fremitus?
Q.5. What do you mean by vocal resonance? Name few conditions in which it is increased or decreased?
Q.6. What are adventitious or "added" sounds?

OBSERVATION AND RESULT

Examine the respiratory system under the following headings:

Inspection

Palpation

Section 4: Clinical Examination

Percussion

Auscultation

INTERPRETATION

STUDY NOTES

Date ....

CHAPTER 4.3

Clinical Examination of the Cardiovascular System

IMPORTANT SIGNS AND SYMPTOMS OF CARDIOVASCULAR DISEASE

1. **Chest pain:** Chest pain may be due to myocardial ischemia (most common symptomatic manifestation of myocardial ischemia is angina), myocardial infarction, pericarditis and aortic aneurism. Other causes of chest discomfort are esophageal spasm, pneumothorax and musculoskeletal pain.
2. **Dyspnea:** It is an abnormal awareness of breathing occurring at rest or on low level of exertion. It may be of cardiac or respiratory origin. It is a major symptom of left heart failure. In **orthopnea,** the patient is more comfortable in sitting than in lying down position.
3. **Palpitation:** Awareness of ones own heart beat is common during exercise or heightened emotions. Under other circumstances, unpleasant awareness of heart beat may indicate abnormal rhythm.
4. **Syncope and dizziness:** The cause could be drug related, arrhythmias or left ventricular outflow obstruction.
5. **Edema:** Pitting edema is the chief feature of congestive heart failure.
6. **Tachycardia** and/or other arrhythmias, headache, fatigue, postural hypotension, cyanosis are the other symptoms.

Anatomical Landmarks

Precordium: It is refers to the anterior aspect of the chest wall overlying the heart.

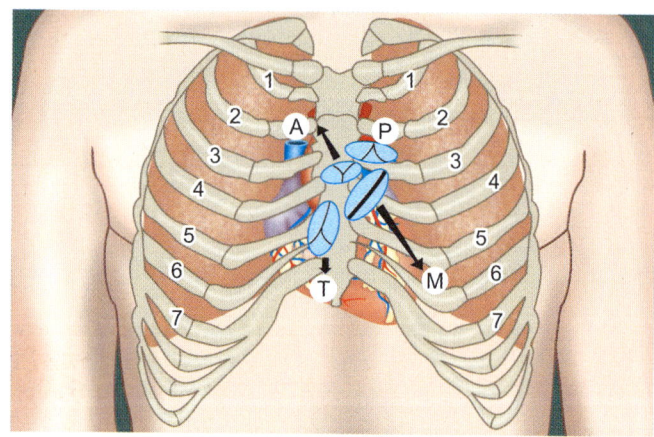

Fig. 4.3.1: Diagram showing the auscultatory areas. P—pulmonary area, A—aortic area, T—tricuspid area and M—mitral area.

The positions of the valves and the different borders of the heart are delineated on the precordium (Fig. 4.3.1) for the clinical examination of cardiovascular system (CVS).

EXAMINATION OF THE CARDIOVASCULAR SYSTEM

1. General physical examination.
2. Systemic examination:
   a. *Examination of the arterial pulse*
   b. *Examination of venous pulse*
   c. *Examination of the precordium.*

Examination of the Venous Pulse

Both arterial and venous pulsations may be seen in the neck, especially in thin persons.

Jugular venous pulse (JVP) differs from carotid arterial pulse in the following aspects (Table 4.3.1).

Jugular venous pulse characteristics can also be remembered by the mnemonic **POLICE**, i.e.:
Palpation—not palpable
Occlusion—easily occluded
Location—between the heads of sternocleidomastoid muscle
Inspiration—height of JVP drops with inspiration
Contour—biphasic waveform
Erection/Position—height decreases on sitting.

The venous pressure can usually be estimated by watching the degree of distension of peripheral veins, especially the neck veins. For example, **in normal, resting, sitting individuals, the neck veins are not distended**. However, when the right atrial pressure rises, as in congestive heart failure, the veins become distended. The pressure in the right internal jugular vein is studied to assess the jugular venous pressure.

Jugular Venous Pressure (Figs. 4.3.2A and B)

- The presence of venous valves prevent external jugular vein being a pure conductor of the central venous pressure changes. **It is not routinely examined because it is prone to kinking and partial obstruction as it travels across the deep fascia of the neck.**
- The **internal jugular vein** (the larger of the two veins) passes down the neck, from near the ear lobe and behind the angle of the jaw, lateral to internal and common carotid arteries and medial to clavicular head of sternomastoid muscle to empty into the subclavian vein.
- **The internal jugular vein is almost in line with right atrium and therefore acts as a better manometer.**
- Right internal jugular vein reflects all right atrial pressure changes, thus providing important information about this pressure, which represents the **"central venous pressure"**.

Table 4.3.1: Differences between carotid arterial pulse and jugular venous pulse.

Carotid arterial pulse	Jugular venous pulse
Palpable	Not palpable
Independent of respiration	Height of pulsation varies with respiration
Cannot be easily occluded	Can be easily occluded
Independent of abdominal pressure	Height increases with abdominal pressure
Independent of position of patient	Varies with position of patient
Rapid outward movement	Rapid inward movement
1 peak per heart beat	2 peaks per heart beat

Procedure for examination of JVP

1. The subject is made to lie on his back, with the upper part of the body supported at an angle of 45° to the horizontal (Figs. 4.3.2A and B), so as to relax the neck muscles especially the sternocleidomastoid. Turn the neck slightly to the left.
2. The neck veins are then inspected carefully in good light by looking across the neck from the side of the patient.
3. When reclining at an angle of 45° the top of the pulsation is normally just at the level of clavicle.
4. If the pulsations are not seen normally manual pressure can be applied over the right upper abdomen for 5–10 seconds **(hepatojugular reflux)**. This increases the venous return and thereby increasing the right atrial pressure.
5. Focus on the right internal jugular vein and look for pulsations in the right side of the neck.
6. Identify the highest point of venous pulsation. Extend a long rectangular card/ruler horizontally from this point and a centimeter ruler vertically from the sternal angle (make an exact right angle)

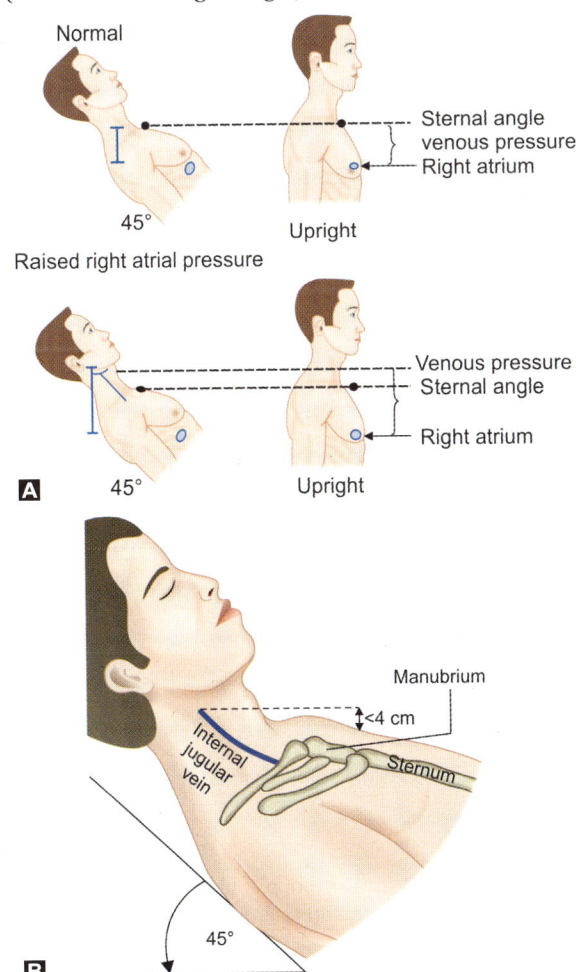

Figs. 4.3.2A and B: Jugular venous pressure.

7. Measure the vertical height (in centimeters) above the sternal angle where the horizontal card meets the ruler.
8. Add to this distance 4 cm (the distance from the sternal angle to the center of the right atrium).

Normal JVP: 6 to 8 cm above the right atrium.
Abnormal/elevated JVP is >9 cm above the right atrium (>4 cm above the sternal angle).

Jugular Venous Waveform (Fig. 4.3.3)

The normal waveform consists of:
1. **Three positive waves**—
   - **"a" wave:** "a" wave is due to atrial systole. It occurs just before the first heart sound. Prominent "a" wave is seen in conditions when there is restriction of blood flow from the right atrium to the right ventricle. Cannon waves or giant "a" waves are produced when the right atrium contracts against closed tricuspid valve, e.g. in complete heart block. The "a" wave disappears in atrial fibrillation.
   - **"c" wave:** The "c" wave is due to the bulging of the tricuspid valve (atrioventricular or AV valve) toward the atrium at the beginning of isovolumetric (isometric) phase of ventricular systole.
   - **"v" wave:** The "v" wave is caused by atrial filling during ventricular systole when the tricuspid valve is closed. A prominent "v" wave is characteristics of tricuspid regurgitation.
2. **Two negative waves or descents**—
   - **"X" descent:** The "a" wave is followed by the "X" descent which is interrupted by the "c" wave.
   - **"Y" descent:** The decline in atrial pressure as the tricuspid valve opens to allow ventricular filling produces the "Y" descent.

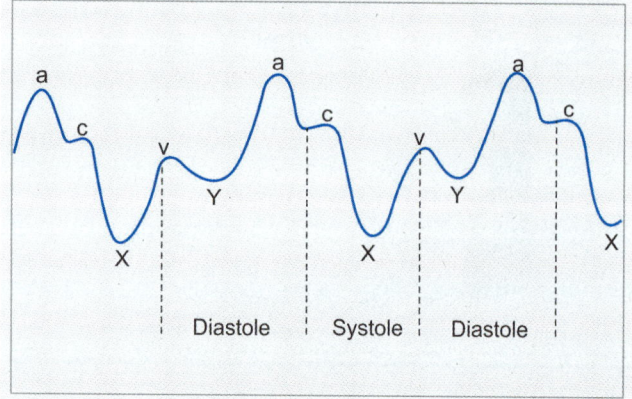

Fig. 4.3.3: The normal jugular venous pulse tracing showing three positive waves—(1) a, (2) c and (3) v and two negative waves or descents—(1) X and (2) Y.

Examination of the Precordium

Examination of the precordium is done under the following headings:
- Inspection
- Palpation
- Percussion (Not very important in examination of cardiovascular system. This is used to define the cardiac borders)
- Auscultation.

Inspection

Precordium is the area of the chest wall lying in front of the heart. The subject should be examined in the recumbent and sitting position and in good light. The following observations are made:
1. **Shape of the chest:** Note for any **deformity**, such as **kyphosis** (forward bending of spine), **scoliosis** (sideward bending of spine) or **bulging** of the precordium (enlargement of heart).
2. **Apex beat:** It is the lowest and the outermost point of definite cardiac pulsation. It is usually visible and palpable and is located 8–10 cm from the midsternal line or 1 cm internal to the midclavicular line in the left 5th intercostal space.

The apex beat may not be visible in some normal persons because:
- It may be located behind a rib.
- The chest wall may be thick due to fat or muscle.
- The emphysematous lung may cover part of the heart.
- The breast may be pendulous.

Inspection for other visible pulsations:
- Arterial pulsations in the neck may be visible in hyperdynamic circulation, as in anxiety, hyperthyroidism, aortic regurgitation and hypertension.
- Pulsations to the right or left of the upper sternum may be due to aortic aneurysm.
- Enlargement of the right ventricle or enlarged left atrium due to severe mitral regurgitation may cause pulsations in the left upper parasternal region.
- Pulsations in the epigastrium are most commonly due to pulsations of abdominal aorta increased by emotional excitement in thin individuals or enlargement of the right ventricle or due to hepatic pulsations from tricuspid regurgitation.
- Pulsations in the superficial arteries of thorax may be visible in coarctation of aorta.

Palpation

1. **Position of the trachea**
2. **Apex beat (Fig. 4.3.4):**

- For locating the position of the apex beat by palpation, the flat of the hand is placed over the heart to feel for the apical impulse.
- Once the cardiac pulsation is felt, the ulnar border of the hand and then the tip of the index finger is used to locate and confirm the point of apex beat already defined by inspection (Fig. 4.3.4). The apex beat should then be marked by a marker pen.
  a. **Position of apex beat:** The apex beat is located 8–10 cm from the midsternal line, in the left 5th intercostal space. To locate the 5th space:
     - The sternal angle (angle of Lewis)—the junction between manubrium sterni and body of sternum is first located.
     - The second costal cartilage articulates with sternum at this level.
     - The 2nd intercostal space lies below the 2nd rib.
     - The 5th intercostal space can now easily be counted downward and located.
     - If the apex beat is not palpable, the patient is then turned over to the left side or sits up and bends forward. However, despite all efforts the apex beat may still not be palpable for the reasons already mentioned above.

> **NOTE**
> One should always make it a habit, especially if the apex beat is not palpable in its usual place, to palpate the chest on both sides, with hands placed on either side, so as not to miss the **dextrocardia**.

  b. **Character of apex beat:** In normal persons, the apex beat gently raises the palpating finger. The strength of this thrust increases after exercise, in nervousness, in hyperthyroidism or in left ventricular hypertrophy.

Significance of Palpating the Apex Beat
- Enlargement of the heart due to hypertrophy or dilatation may shift the apex beat.
- Pulling or pushing of the mediastinum due to lung disease may shift the position of the apex beat.
- Diffuse, sustained and more forceful thrust indicates left ventricular hypertrophy or hyperkinetic circulation.
- A "tapping" or "slapping" apex beat may be seen in mitral stenosis.
- If the apex beat is not palpable the causes may be: obesity, apex lying under a rib, dextrocardia, shift of the mediastinum to the right, pneumothorax, pericardial effusion, left-sided pleural effusion.

3. **Thrills:** A palpable murmur is called a thrill. Murmur are due to the turbulence in the blood flow at or near a valve or an abnormal communication within the heart. The thrill feels like placing ones hand on a purring cat.
4. **Parasternal heave:** This is indicative of right ventricular hypertrophy. This can be elicited by placing the ulnar border of hand just left to the sternum and feel for the pulsations (Fig. 4.3.5).

Percussion

It is of little significance and carried out sometimes to demarcate the extent of cardiac dullness in conditions like pericardial effusion. Nowadays, it has been replaced by the chest X-ray and echocardiography.

Auscultation

Auscultate the different cardiac areas (mitral, tricuspid, aortic and pulmonary areas) using stethoscope and identify the different heart sounds (Fig. 4.3.6).
- It is good practice to palpate the carotid artery while listening to the heart sounds because the carotid pulse coincides with the first heart sound.
- As a routine, the four cardiac areas, **named according to the valves from which sounds arise (***See* **Fig. 4.3.1)**,

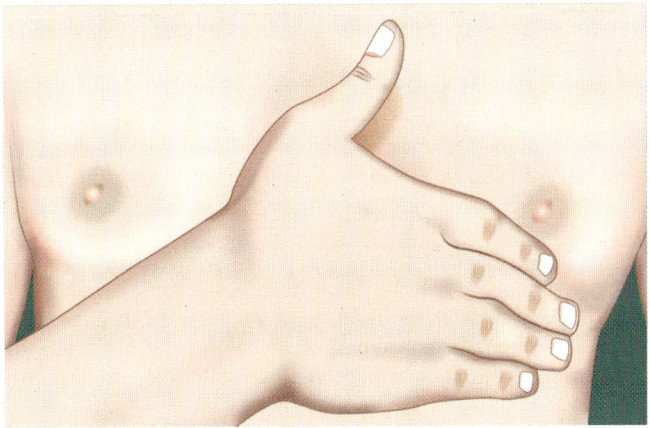

Fig. 4.3.4: Apex beat.

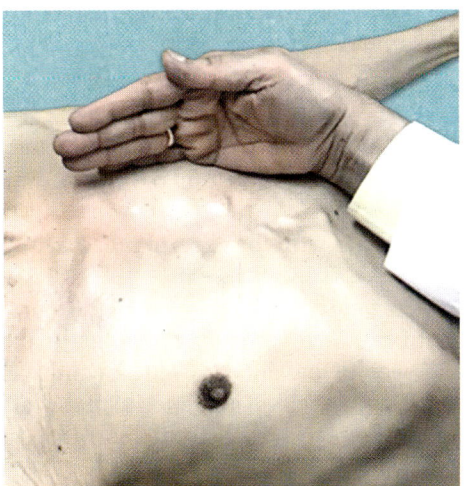

Fig. 4.3.5: Parasternal heave.

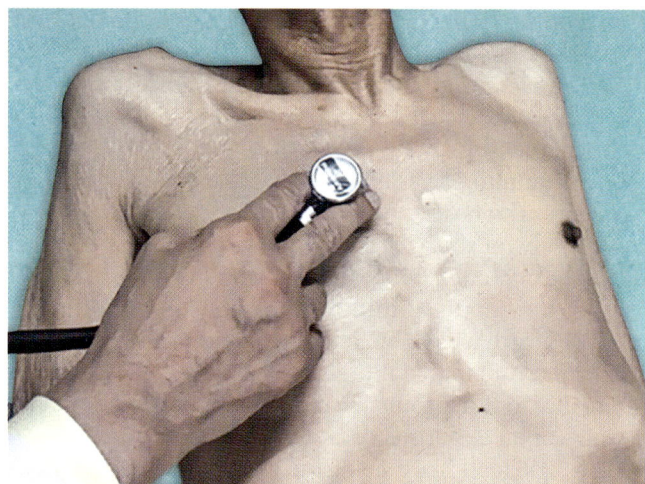

Fig. 4.3.6: Auscultation.

are auscultated first. This is followed by auscultation in between these areas. The different areas are:

- **Mitral area:** The mitral area corresponds to the apex beat, i.e. 5th intercostal space about 8–10 cm from the midsternal line.
- **Tricuspid area:** This area lies just to the left of the lower end of the sternum.
- **Aortic area:** It lies to the right of the sternum in the 2nd intercostal space.
- **Pulmonary area:** It lies to the left of the sternum in the 2nd intercostal space.

> **NOTE**
> The corresponding valves of the heart do not lie under these areas; only the sounds produced by these valves are heard best over these areas.

Over all these areas of auscultation, both the first and the second heart sounds are heard clearly, though the first sound is heard better in mitral and tricuspid areas while the second sound is heard better in aortic and pulmonary areas.

Heart Sounds

1. The heart sounds are **always** timed with the simultaneous palpation of carotid artery pulsation. The **1st heart sound coincides with the carotid pulse.** The 2nd heart sound follows a little later.
2. The **1st heart sound**, which is due to the simultaneous closure of the atrioventricular valves, is prolonged (0.1–0.17 sec), of low pitch (20–40 Hz) and booming in character. Phonetically, it is likened to the syllable "LUB". It is synchronous with the carotid artery pulsation and coincides with the "R" wave of the ECG and is best heard over the mitral area.
3. The **2nd heart sound**, which is due to the closure of aortic and pulmonary valves, is shorter, abrupt and clear and of high pitch. Phonetically, it resembles the spoken sound "DUB". It may precede, coincide or follow the T wave of the ECG and is best heard over aortic and pulmonary areas.
4. The time interval between the 1st and the 2nd heart sounds is shorter than the time interval between the 2nd sound and the next 1st sound. The sequence is thus: LUB-DUB pause, LUB-DUB pause and so on as shown in Figure 4.3.7.
5. **3rd and 4th sounds:** These sounds occur during early and late diastole. They can best be heard with the **bell of the stethoscope**, with the patient leaning slightly forward.
6. The **3rd sound** is normally heard in children and in adults with hyperdynamic circulation. It is associated with rapid distension of the ventricles in early diastole.
7. The **4th sound**; whenever present is pathological. It is usually heard if atrial systole is particularly forceful.

> **NOTE**
> The opening of the heart valves does not produce any sounds; only their closure produces sounds; e.g. clapping of the hands produces a sound while opening the palms does not.

Deviations of Heart Sounds from the Normal

1. **Intensity of the sounds:** The 1st heart sound may be accentuated in exercise, hypertension, anemia and beriberi (hyperkinetic circulation). It may be diminished in shock, myocardial infarction and pericardial effusion. 2nd heart sound may be increased in systemic and pulmonary hypertension and diminished in aortic and pulmonary stenosis.
2. **Splitting of heart sounds:** Splitting of the 1st heart sound is difficult to detect by auscultation because the two components are very close together. Splitting of the second heart sound is easier to appreciate because of a wide gap between the aortic and pulmonary

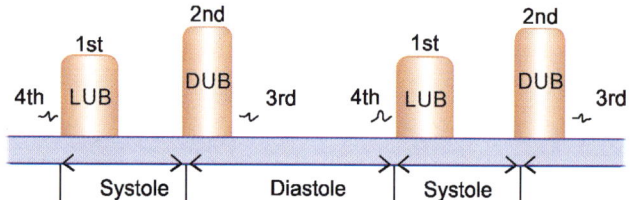

Fig. 4.3.7: Diagrammatic representation of heart sounds. LUB and DUB—phonetic representation of 1st and 2nd heart sounds respectively. The diagrammatic representation of 3rd and 4th heart sounds is to indicate that they have a lower frequency than the 1st and 2nd sound.

components. It is most easily heard in children and splitting becomes more prominent during inspiration.

3. **Triple rhythm** (gallop rhythm when the heart rate is above 100 beats/min): Splitting of heart sounds must be differentiated from triple rhythm, which is produced by the addition of 3rd or 4th heart sounds to the normal 1st and 2nd sounds and which may be imitated by "LUB-DUB-DUB" (Though phonocardiography shows that a 3rd and a 4th (atrial) sounds are generally present, they are difficult to hear with a stethoscope. When either of these is prominent and audible, they produce a triple rhythm, as in left ventricular failure).

4. **Adventitious or extra added sounds:** These sounds may occur along with or replace the heart sounds.
   - **Murmurs**, which are longer than heart sounds and may be systolic or diastolic and these can have a "blowing" or "swishing" quality. When a murmur is palpable, it is called a **"thrill"**.
   - Their time of occurrence, region of maximum intensity, direction of propagation and their character should be noted.
   - They are caused by turbulent flow and eddy currents within the heart or great vessels.
   - Valvular defects (change in size, deformities) are the usual causes of murmurs.
   - **Pericardial friction** or **rub** gives an impression of two pieces of dry leather being rubbed together. It occurs in pericarditis.
   - **Opening snap** is commonly heard in mitral stenosis.
   - **Ejection clicks** are produced due to stenosis of the aortic or pulmonary valve.
   - **Mid-systolic clicks** are heard in mitral valve prolapsed.

Objective Structured Clinical Examination–I

Aim: To locate the apex beat of the subject provided.
Procedural steps: See text above.
Checklist:
1. Stand on the right side of the subject and expose the chest completely and inspect the precordium to see if there is any cardiac pulsation. (Y/N)
2. Place the flat of the hand over the precordium, its base on the base of the heart and fingers toward the apex. (Y/N)
3. Use the ulnar border of her hand to locate the apex beat. (Y/N)
4. Use the tip of the forefinger to confirm the apex beat and mark it. (Y/N)
5. Count the intercostal spaces and report the exact position of apex beat. (Y/N)

Objective Structured Clinical Examination–II

Aim: To auscultate the mitral area for the heart sounds.
Procedural steps: See text above.
Checklist:
1. Stand on the subject's right side and completely expose the chest. (Y/N)
2. Check for the correct functioning of the stethoscope. (Y/N)
3. Locate the apex beat and mark its position. (Y/N)
4. Apply the stethoscope to the ears and place its diaphragm on the mitral area. (Y/N)
5. Listen to the heart sounds and check these with carotid artery pulse. (Y/N)

QUESTIONS

Q.1. How would you proceed to examine the cardiovascular system?
Q.2. Examine the neck veins of the subject provided for jugular venous pressure.
Q.3. Inspect the precordium in the subject provided and give your findings.
Q.4. Palpate the chest of the subject provided for apex beat. What is its significance?
Q.5. Auscultate the heart sounds over the mitral, tricuspid, aortic and pulmonary areas.

OBSERVATION AND RESULT

Examine the cardiovascular system under the following headings:

Inspection

....
....
....
....
....
....
....
....
....
....

Palpation

Percussion

Auscultation

INTERPRETATION

STUDY NOTES

CHAPTER 4.4

Clinical Examination of the Abdomen

IMPORTANT SIGNS AND SYMPTOMS OF GASTROINTESTINAL TRACT DISEASE

- **Dysphagia**—difficulty in swallowing
- **Hematemesis**—vomiting of blood
- **Dyspepsia**—indigestion
- **Loss of appetite**
- **Burning sensation behind sternum or in epigastrium**
- **Flatulence**
- **Distension** and **tenderness of abdomen**
- **Nausea** and **vomiting**
- **Diarrhea, constipation, rectal bleeding, melena** ("black" stools)
- **Jaundice, loss of weight** and **fever.**

> **NOTE**
> Oral cavity should always be checked for the health of the teeth and gums, tongue, tonsils and oropharynx.

Examination of the Gastrointestinal Tract

1. **General physical examination.**
2. **Systemic examination:** This is to be done under the following headings:
   - Inspection
   - Palpation
   - Percussion
   - Auscultation.

Prerequisite for GIT Examination

- The subject should be lying flat on his back, arms by the sides, on a firm bed.
- The subject should be relaxed, with hips and knees flexed and head turned to one side.
- The subject is asked to take deep breaths through the mouth.
- The subject is examined from the right side.
- Before palpating the abdomen, the patient is asked about any pain or tenderness (pain on pressure) and such areas are the last to be palpated.
- Palpation is generally started in the left iliac fossa and worked anticlockwise to end in the suprapubic region.

EXAMINATION OF ABDOMEN

It is customary to divide the abdomen into nine regions by two horizontal (B and C) and two lateral vertical lines (A and A'). Each vertical line is taken from midclavicle to midinguinal point. The upper horizontal line passes across the abdomen at the lowest points on the costal margin (10th costal arch). The lower horizontal line joins the tubercles of iliac crests.

Abdominal regions: The regions marked by these lines are shown in Figure 4.4.1.

In the upper abdomen: (1) right hypochondrium; (2) epigastrium; (3) left hypochondrium.

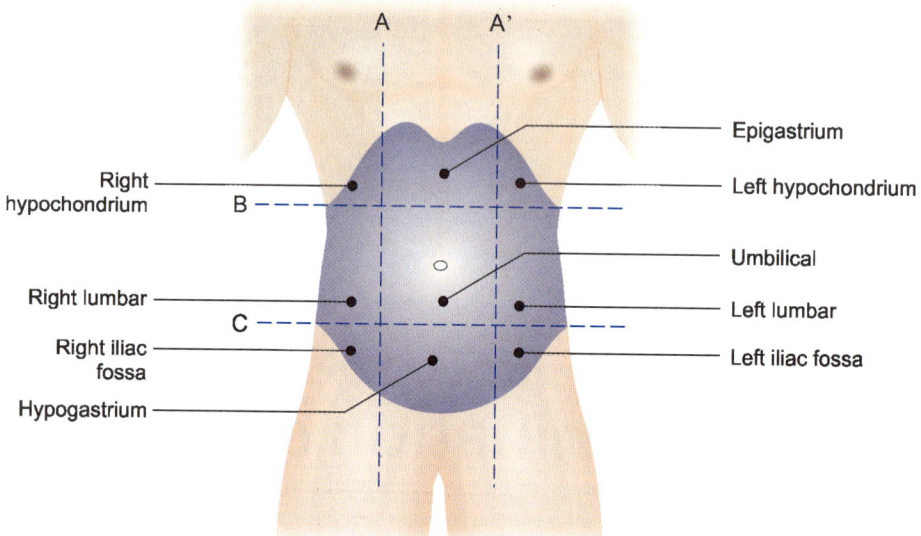

Fig. 4.4.1: Abdominal regions

In the middle abdomen: (4) right lumbar; (5) umbilical; (6) left lumbar.

In the lower abdomen: (7) right iliac fossa; (8) hypogastrium; (9) left iliac fossa.

INSPECTION

On inspection of the abdomen the following are observed:
1. **State of the skin:** Whether stretched; presence of scars (previous operations) and striae (due to gross stretching); and pigmentation.
2. **Contour or shape:** There are three main types of abdominal contours:
   a. **Flat abdomen:** The rib margins and the abdominal wall are at about the same level.
   b. **Globular or round abdomen:** A generalized and symmetrical fullness (i.e. a forward convexity) may be due to fat (obesity), fluid (ascites), flatus (gas), fetus (pregnancy) or feces (chronic constipation). There may be sagging of the abdominal wall due to loss of muscle tone.
   c. **Scaphoid (sunken) abdomen:** It is seen in extreme starvation, wasting diseases, carcinoma, especially of esophagus and stomach and sometimes in very thin individuals.
3. **Abdominal asymmetry:** The normal abdomen is symmetrical. Asymmetric localized distention or bulging may be due to gross enlargement of liver, spleen or ovary or due to tumors.
4. **State of umbilicus:** Normally the umbilicus is slightly retracted and inverted or level with the skin surface. It may be everted or ballooned out in umbilical hernia, raised intraabdominal pressure or it may be transversely stretched in ascites (fluid in the peritoneal cavity).
5. **Movements of the abdominal walls with respiration:**
   - The abdomen moves freely with respiration, rising gently during inspiration and falling during expiration (In females, the respiratory movements are mainly thoracic).
   - The abdominal movements may be restricted in generalized peritonitis, inflammation of diaphragm or injury to the abdominal muscles and in tense ascites.
6. **Visible pulsations:** Epigastric pulsations of abdominal aorta are frequently visible in nervous, thin individuals. Pulsations from a pulsating liver or from right ventricle may also be seen in the epigastrium.
7. **Visible peristalsis:** Peristalsis may be visible as movement of a slow wave on the abdomen in persons with thin abdominal wall, in malnourished children and cachexia. Visible peristalsis may be an indication of pyloric and small and large intestinal obstruction.
8. **Hernial sites:** The hernial sites in the groin should be checked for any swelling on straining or coughing.
9. **Presence of prominent veins:** Presence of prominent veins on the abdomen and chest wall is seen in obstruction of vena cava. Presence of prominent veins

around the umbilicus (caput medusa) is seen in portal hypertension.

PALPATION

Protocol for Palpation

- The right hand is placed flat on the abdomen, with the wrist and the forearm in the same horizontal plane.
- The relaxed hand is "molded" to the abdomen, not held rigidly, with the fingers almost straight with slight flexion at the metacarpophalangeal joints (Fingers are never "poked" in the abdomen).
- On palpation, the normal abdomen is soft and there is no tenderness.

Palpation for Liver (Fig. 4.4.2)

1. The palpation for the liver starts in the right iliac fossa and then gradually worked up to the right costal margin.
2. As the patient inspires deeply, the fingers are pressed firmly inward and upward.
3. If the liver is palpable, it meets the radial aspect of the index finger as a sharp regular border.
4. It is sometimes palpable in children and adults, but generally, it is palpable only when it is enlarged.
5. If palpable, the character of its surface is noted—whether soft and smooth, very firm or hard and irregular.
6. The liver is enlarged (**hepatomegaly**) in congestive heart failure, amebic hepatitis, liver abscess, viral hepatitis, malignancy, leukemias and so on.

Palpation of Spleen (Fig. 4.4.3)

1. The flat of the right hand is placed on the right iliac fossa and the left hand is placed over the left lowermost rib cage posterolaterally.

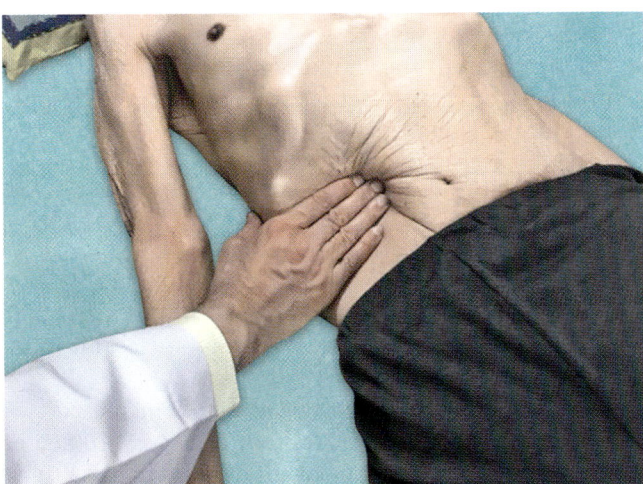

Fig. 4.4.2: Palpation of liver.

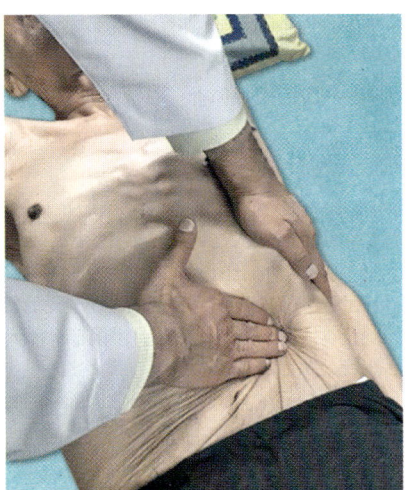

Fig. 4.4.3: Palpation for spleen.

2. The left hand presses medially and downward while the right hand presses deeply toward the left costal margin to feel for the spleen (when the spleen enlarges, it does so toward the right iliac fossa).
3. The normal spleen is not palpable until it increases two or three times its normal size.
4. Enlarged spleen (**splenomegaly**) is seen in malaria, kala-azar, typhoid, portal hypertension and portal cirrhosis, acute leukemias, chronic myeloid leukemia and some anemias.

Palpation of the Kidneys

Since both kidneys are located behind the peritoneum, the examiner employs both hands for their palpation.

Palpation of Left Kidney

1. The right hand is placed anteriorly in the left lumbar region while the left hand is placed posteriorly under the costal margin.
2. As the subject takes a deep breath, the left hand presses forward and the right hand presses backward, upward and inward; and an attempt is made to feel for the kidney between the pulps of the fingers of the two hands.
3. The left kidney is not usually palpable unless enlarged or low in position.

Palpation of Right Kidney

1. The right hand is placed anteriorly in the right lumbar region with the left hand placed posteriorly in the right loin.
2. As the subject takes a deep breath, the left hand presses forward and the right hand pushes inward and upward; and an attempt is made to feel for the kidney between the fingers of the two hands.

3. The lower pole of the right kidney is commonly palpable in thin subjects as a smooth, rounded swelling which descends on inspiration.

PERCUSSION

- Using light percussion, all the nine regions of the abdomen are percussed systematically.
- A resonant (tympanitic) note is heard all over the abdomen except over the liver where the note is dull.
- The percussion note varies depending on the amount of gas in the intestines.
- Ascites, tumors, enlarged liver or spleen, enlarged glands, etc. give a dull note.

Clinical Significance of Percussion

The principal value of abdominal percussion is to distinguish between distension due to gas, ascites, cystic or solid tumors. The collection of free fluid in the peritoneal cavity is called **ascites.** Over 1,500 mL of fluid must accumulate before it can be detected by physical examination. Ascites has to be differentiated from two other common causes of diffuse enlargement of the abdomen, namely, a massive ovarian cyst and obstruction of distal small bowel, large bowel or both.

In the case of *intestinal obstruction,* the percussion note is tympanitic all over. In the case of a large ovarian cyst, the percussion note is resonant in the flanks and dullness with convexity upward, over the pelvis.

Test for the Presence of Free Fluid in the Peritoneum (Ascites)

Shifting Dullness

- The fluid gravitates to the dependent parts, it flows into the flanks and the intestines float in the umbilical region when the patient lies on his back.
- The abdomen is percussed first with the patient lying on his back, when both flanks show dullness, while the umbilical region shows a tympanitic note.
- The subject is then rolled on to his left side; a resonant note is now obtained from the right flank while the left flank sounds a dull note due to shifting of fluid to the left flank and the intestines floating up to the right flank.
- A similar procedure is repeated with the patient rolled on to his right side, when the left flank will now give a resonant note.
- The shift of the fluid and the accompanying dullness is called "shifting dullness", i.e. dullness due to shifting of fluid with a change in the position of the subject.

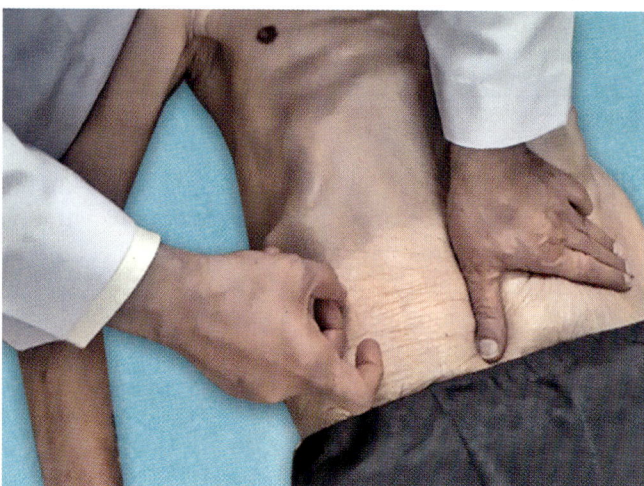

Fig. 4.4.4: Test for detection of fluid thrill.

Fluid Thrill (Fig. 4.4.4)

- The patient lies supine.
- One hand is placed over the lumbar region of one side and a sharp tap or flick is given over the opposite lumbar region.
- A wave or fluid thrill is felt by the detecting hand.
- A similar sensation may be felt if the abdominal wall is very fat. To avoid this, the subject is asked to place the ulnar edge of his hand firmly along the midline or alternatively the examiner can place his thumb in the midline exerting a firm pressure as shown in Figure 4.4.4; this damps any vibrations in the abdominal wall.

Horseshoe-shaped Dullness

- When the amount of ascitic fluid is moderate, the fluid collects in the flanks and the hypogastric region, while the intestines float up in the upper umbilical and epigastric regions.
- On percussion, the flanks and hypogastric regions produce dullness, whereas the epigastric and upper umbilical regions remain tympanitic.

AUSCULTATION

- Auscultation is done by placing a stethoscope (diaphragm) on different areas of the abdomen.
- It is performed to detect the bowel sounds, peristaltic rub and for detecting bruits in the aorta and other abdominal vessels.
- Bowel sounds may be normal, absent or increased.
- Normal bowel sounds are heard every 5–10 sec as intermittent gurgles, low or mediumpitched, with an occasional highpitched noise.

- Normal peristaltic activity of the gut creates characteristic gurgling sound which may be heard from time to time by the unaided ear **(borborygmi).**
- In **_gastrointestinal obstruction_**, these sounds may be greatly exaggerated, increasing in intensity with waves of pain.
- On the other hand, in **_paralytic ileus_** (intestinal paralysis) due to peritonitis or other causes, the sounds are absent a condition called **"silent abdomen"**.
- Auscultate for peristalsis bowel sounds for at least 3 minutes before deciding that they are absent.

Objective Structured Clinical Examination

Aim: To palpate the liver of the subject provided.
Procedural steps: See text above.
Checklist:
1. Ask the subject to lie flat on the bed, relax with knees and hips flexed and to breathe through the mouth. Ask if there is any tenderness or pain. (Y/N)
2. Bend down or kneel beside the subject's right side. Ensure that the hands are warm. (Y/N)
3. Place the right hand flat on the abdomen (with wrist and forearm in the same horizontal plane) and mold it to the abdomen. (Y/N)
4. Starting in the right iliac fossa, with fingers almost straight and slightly flexed at metacarpophalangeal joints, press inward and upward, work up toward costal margin. (Y/N)
5. Ask the subject to take a deep breath and at the height of inspiration, try to feel the liver (does not poke fingers into the subject's abdomen). (Y/N)

QUESTIONS

Q.1. Inspect the abdomen in the subject provided and give your findings.
Q.2. Palpate the abdomen for liver.
Q.3. Palpate the spleen in the subject provided.
Q.4. Palpate the kidneys in the subject provided.
Q.5. Percuss the abdomen and give your findings.
Q.6. Test for the presence of free fluid in the abdominal cavity.
Q.7. Auscultate the abdomen of the subject provided.

OBSERVATION AND RESULT

Examine the GIT system under the following headings:

Inspection

....
....
....
....

Palpation

....
....
....
....

Section 4: Clinical Examination

Auscultation

Percussion

INTERPRETATION

URINE ANALYSIS

Urine is the excretory waste product formed by the kidneys. Urine of a normal healthy person has definite physical and chemical properties. Analysis of urine therefore is important in evaluating kidney functions and also helps in the diagnosis of many other diseases.

Urine Sample Collection (Fig. 4.4.5)

1. **'Midstream morning' sample:** To collect the sample the patient discards initial part of the first voided urine in the morning after getting up. He is then asked to collect 15–20 mL of midstream urine in a clean sterile container. This sample should be analyzed immediately or within a few hours of collection. This is the most commonly used sample for urinary analysis.
2. **24-hour urine sample:** This sample is used for quantitative estimation of constituents like protein, creatinine, calcium, etc. The sample is collected for 24 hours from the time when the subject first voids the urine in the morning.
3. **Random urine sample:** This has limited utility and is generally used for glucose and ketone bodies estimation.

A complete urine analysis includes the following:
1. Physical examination
2. Biochemical examination
3. Microscopic examination
4. Bacteriological examination

Physical Examination

1. **Appearance:** Normal urine is clear and transparent. There is no turbidity or sediment.
2. **Color:** Normally, urine is light yellow or straw colored because of the presence of urobilin. Variation in color can be seen in **jaundice** (deep yellow urine) and **hematuria** (urine is red in color due to presence of RBCs). A dark colored urine may indicate **dehydration.**
3. **Odor:** Odor of urine may provide important information, e.g. urine of diabetics may have fruity odor due to presence of ketone bodies or glucose. Foul smelling odor is seen in infection by bacteria. Normal urine has a slight ammonia like odor.
4. **Volume:** Average daily urine output is 800 mL–2.5 L depending upon the water intake. Variations in urine output may be seen in various diseases. **Polyuria** is defined as increase in urine output more than 2.5–3.0 L/day. **Oliguria** is defined as decrease in urine output less than 300 mL/day. **Anuria** is defined as no urine output in 24 hours. But clinically, it is diagnosed when the urine output is less than 100 mL/day.
5. **Specific gravity:** Normal specific gravity of urine is between 1.010–1.025. It can vary depending on the diet, fluid intake and renal function.
6. **pH:** Normal urine is acidic with pH generally in the range of 4.6–8.0 with a typical average of around 6.0. Much of variations in pH occur due to diet, e.g. a high protein diet results in more acidic urine whereas vegetarian diets result in more alkaline urine (both within the normal range).

Biochemical Examination

For most clinical purposes use of a commercially available **reagent strip test (Fig. 4.4.6)** is sufficient to obtain the necessary diagnostic information.

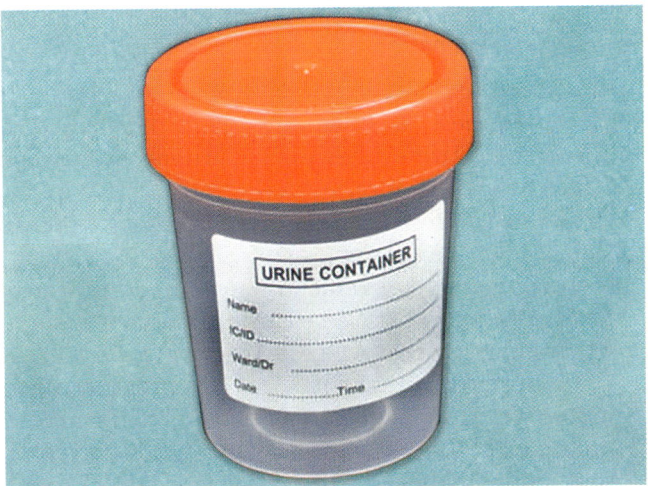

Fig. 4.4.5: Container for urine sample.

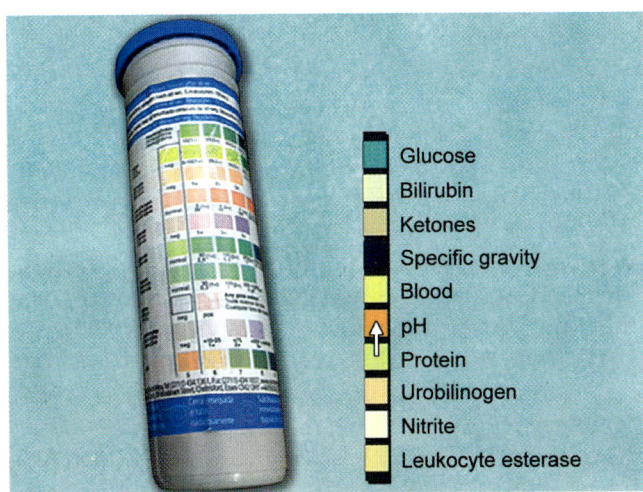

Fig. 4.4.6: Reagent strip test.

Normal Constituents of Urine

Normal urine contains about 15 g of solids dissolve in 1.5 L of urine per day. Urine contains organic and inorganic solids.

1. **Inorganic solids:**
    a. Sodium
    b. Potassium
    c. Chlorides
    d. Smaller amounts of calcium, magnesium, sulfates and phosphates.
    e. Traces of iron, copper, zinc and iodine.
2. **Organic solids:**
    a. *Non-protein nitrogen:* amino acids, ammonia, urea, uric acid and creatinine.
    b. *Organic acids:* Lactic acid, citric acid, oxalic acid and ketone bodies.
    c. *Sugars:* Normally not more than 1 g of sugar is excreted in the urine per day. Very small amounts of glucose not exceeding 150 mg of glucose are normally excreted per day.

Abnormal Constituents of Urine

1. **Reducing sugars:** Normally no glucose is present in the urine. When the venous blood glucose level rises above 180 mg/dL, glucose may appear in the urine, e.g. in diabetes mellitus. Presence of glucose in urine is called as **Glycosuria.** This can also be seen in conditions where there is decreased glucose reabsorption (**renal glycosuria**). Presence of lactose in urine also called **lactosuria,** occurs in infants and in women during late months of pregnancy and during lactation. This is detected by **Benedict's test.**
   False positive results can be due to the presence of excessive substances like creatinine, ascorbic acid, urates and salicylates.
2. **Proteins:** No proteins are present in normal urine. Appearance of turbidity which does not dissolve in glacial acetic acid indicates the presence of proteins. Albumin is the most common and earliest detected protein. **Albuminuria** (Presence of albumin in the urine) occurs when the glomerular membrane is damaged, a condition known as **Glomerulonephritis.** The tests which are usually done to detect the presence of proteins in urine are **Heat coagulation tests, Sulfosalicylic test** and **Heller's test.**
   Bence Jones proteins: These are gamma globulin proteins which are excreted in large amounts in multiple myeloma. It usually consists of immunoglobulin light chains and can be identified in the urine or serum by electrophoresis. This protein disappears on boiling the urine and reappears on cooling.
3. **Ketone bodies:** Ketones are compounds resulting from the breakdown of fatty acids. These are acetone, acetoacetate and beta-hydroxy butyric acid. When produced in excess they can be excreted in urine and this is known as **Ketonuria**. This is detected by **Rothera's test.** This can be seen in patients of diabetes mellitus with ketosis and in prolonged fasting,
4. **Bile salts:** Bile salts are normally not excreted in urine. In conditions like obstructive jaundice bile salts are present in urine. They can be detected by **Hay's Sulfur test.**
5. **Bile pigments:** Bilirubin is the main bile pigment which results from the catabolism of heme. On conjugation with glucuronic acid, it is excreted as bilirubin diglucuronide in the bile. It is converted into urobilinogen in the intestine, majority of which is recirculated. In the urine, traces of urobilinogen are normally excreted. Increased urinary urobilinogen occur in **prehepatic jaundice** and **hepatitis.** It can be detected by **Ehrlich's test**. **Fouchet's** and **Rosenbach's test** are used for detecting bilirubin in urine. The normal level of urinary bilirubin is below the detection limit of this test.
6. **Blood:** RBCs and hemoglobin may enter the urine from the kidney or the lower urinary tract. Normally 2 cells/high power field (HPF) is seen. More than 3 erythrocytes/HPF is considered abnormal. Presence of blood in urine is called **Hematuria** (red color urine) while presence of hemoglobin in urine is known as **Hemoglobinuria** (reddish brown color urine). **Benzidine test** is done to detect the minimal hematuria which may not be seen with naked color.

> **NOTE**
> Care should be taken while handling the benzidine reagent as it is potentially carcinogenic.

Microscopic Examination

For microscopic examination, an adequate sized drop of centrifuged urine is transferred to a clean slide and covered with a cover slip. Urine is then examined under microscope with high power objective.

1. **Crystalluria** is frequently observed in urine specimens stored at room temperature or refrigerated. Such crystals are diagnostically useful when observed in warm, fresh urine by a physician evaluating microhematuria, nephrolithiasis or toxin ingestion.
2. Urine is usually supersaturated in calcium oxalate, often in calcium phosphate and acid urine is often saturated in uric acid. Yet crystalluria is uncommon (in warm, fresh urine) because of the normal presence of crystal inhibitors, the lack of available nidus and the time factor. When properly observed in fresh urine, crystals may

provide a clue to the composition of renal stones even not yet passed, the nidus for such stones or, as such, have been associated with microhematuria.

3. **Leukocytes:** Neutrophils are the most common type of leukocytes found in urine. Normally, less than 5 cells/HPF are present in normal urine. Presence of increased number of leukocytes in urine is known as **Pyuria.** This may indicate inflammatory disease in the genitourinary tract, including bacterial infection, glomerulonephritis, chemical injury, autoimmune diseases or inflammatory disease adjacent to the urinary tract such as appendicitis or diverticulitis.

4. **Casts:**
   a. *White cell casts* indicate the renal origin of leukocytes and are most frequently found in acute pyelonephritis. White cell casts are also found in glomerulonephritis. When nuclei degenerate, such leukocyte casts resemble renal tubular casts.
   b. *Red cell casts* indicate renal origin of hematuria and suggest glomerulonephritis, including lupus nephritis. Red cell casts may also be found in subacute bacterial endocarditis, renal infarct, vasculitis and in malignant hypertension. Degenerated red cell casts may be called **"hemoglobin casts."** Orange to red casts may be found with myoglobinuria as well.
   c. *Hyaline casts* occur in physiologic states (e.g. after exercise) and many types of renal diseases.
   d. *Renal tubular (epithelial) casts* are most suggestive of tubular injury, as in acute tubular necrosis.
   e. *Granular casts:* Very finely granulated casts may be found after exercise and in a variety of glomerular and tubulointerstitial diseases. Coarse granular casts are abnormal and are present in a wide variety of renal diseases. **"Dirty brown" granular casts** are typical of acute tubular necrosis.

> **NOTE**
> **Spermatozoa** may be seen in male urine related to recent or retrograde ejaculation.

Bacteriological Examination

All urine specimens should be examined at once or should be placed in a refrigerator at 4°C until they can be examined. The examination include the following steps:
1. Examination of Gram-stained smear
2. A screening test for bacteriuria
3. A definite culture for urine specimens found to be positive in the screening test and for all specimens obtained by cystoscopy, suprapubic bladder puncture (SBP) or catheterization.
4. Susceptibility tests on clinically significant bacterial isolates.

Preparation and examination of a Gram-stained smear is the first step in laboratory process. This is then examined under the oil immersion lens. One or more bacterial cells/oil immersion field usually implies that there are 10^5 or more bacteria/mL in the specimen. The presence of **one or more leukocytes/oil immersion** field is a further indication of urinary tract infection (UTI). Noninfected urine sample will usually show few or no bacteria and leukocytes in the entire specimen.

A urine specimen that is **Negative** on careful examination of Gram-stained smear does not need to be cultured.

PHYSIOCLINICAL SIGNIFICANCE

Common uses of urinalysis		
Screening	Random	Diabetes mellitus Asymptomatic bacteriuria
	Selective	Antenatal care Hypertensive patients
Diagnosis	Primary renal disease Secondary renal disease Non-renal disorders	Glomerulonephritis Infective endocarditis Jaundice
Monitoring	Disease progression Drug toxicity	Diabetic nephropathy

QUESTIONS

Q.1. How is a urine sample collected?
Q.2. What are the physical properties of a normal urine sample?
Q.3. Name the tests used for chemical analysis of glucose, proteins and ketone bodies in urine.
Q.4. What are Bence Jones proteins?
Q.5. What are the common causes of oliguria and anuria?
   Common causes of **oliguria** are: Shock, severe dehydration due to any cause as in excessive blood loss, excessive vomiting and diarrhea.
   Common causes of **anuria** are: Acute renal failure, shock, post blood transfusion reaction.
Q.6. What is glycosuria? What are its causes?
Q.7. What is pyuria? What are its causes?
Q.8. Name some causes of proteinuria.

STUDY NOTES

CHAPTER 4.5

Clinical Examination of the Nervous System

HISTORY TAKING

In a nervous system examination, taking a careful history of illness is of great importance as the history of progress of disease will provide valuable information about the specific part of the nervous system involved and the nature of underlying pathology.

The diagnosis of a neurology patient depends primarily on correlating the signs and symptoms to the underlying disease process. The anatomical diagnosis depends on the assessment of changes in motor and sensory functions, alteration in reflexes and subjective and objective features of lesions of cranial nerves.

A more focused history may help in formulating a diagnosis and suggest the nature of pathology. In recent years, magnetic resonance imaging (MRI) and computed tomography (CT) scanning have transformed neurological diagnosis and refined clinical approach.

COMMON SIGNS AND SYMPTOMS OF NEUROLOGICAL DISEASE

Some of the common signs and symptoms are:
- Speech and language defects—dysarthria and dysphasia (cognitive disturbance) difficulty in communication.
- Partial unconsciousness with restlessness or coma.
- Altered behavior and emotional state, such as confusion and disorientation.
- Motor defects—such as weakness, paralysis, fits (convulsions), rigidity, tremors, involuntary movements and alterations of gait.
- Sensory disturbances.
- Effects of involvement of cranial nerves, e.g. unilateral visual loss.

The major causes of these signs and symptoms include—vascular insults (hemorrhage and ischemic strokes), head and spinal injuries, degenerative diseases, infections (bacterial and viral) and so on.

EXAMINATION OF NERVOUS SYSTEM

This should proceed along the following lines:
A. Examination of higher functions and speech
B. Examination of cranial nerves
C. Motor system
D. Reflexes
E. Sensory system and evidence of trophic changes.

A: EXAMINATION OF HIGHER FUNCTIONS

Apart from motor and sensory functions and maintenance of vital signs, the brain is concerned with the higher functions of consciousness, intellect, mental state and well-being of the subject. Note the following:

- **Appearance and behavior:** Is the patient wellgroomed or unkempt, disturbed or agitated, whether the attention wanders, any flight of ideas? Note personal hygiene—nails, hands and hair.
- **Emotional state:** Note, if the mood is elevated or depressed or if there is flattening of emotions. Does he appear confused or does he live in a world of his own? Enquire about sleep and dreams.
- **Delusions and hallucinations:** Delusions are false beliefs, which continue to be held despite evidence to the contrary (e.g. believing that "someone is out to kill me"). Hallucinations are false impressions (visual or auditory, e.g. taking a rope to be a snake).
- **Level of consciousness:** Is there any clouding of consciousness? Ask him about events around him. Is there dementia (loss of memory) or coma (a deep state of unconsciousness from which the patient cannot be roused)?
- **Orientation in place and time:** Ask the patient about the date, month and year; and whether he is in a hospital or at his home. Disorientation is an important sign of organic diseases of the brain and in psychiatric disorders.
- **Memory:** Test for recent and past memory by asking pointed questions. In brain injuries, for example, recent memory is affected much more than past memory.
- **General intelligence:** This will be evident during history taking. Ask for educational history and work record. One simple test is to ask her/him to continue deducting 7 from 100. Tests for reasoning and "absurdities" test can give a fair idea of the intelligence.

SPEECH (LANGUAGE) FUNCTIONS

While animals can express their feelings by sounds, gestures and postures (e.g. an angry dog), only man can express his feelings, ideas, thoughts by using symbols (i.e. words) representing ideas, things, etc.

Thus, true speech, i.e. the **ability to understand and express in symbols,** is one of the highest functions of the human brain. For normal speech, not only the cerebral cortex must be intact but the motor mechanisms that control articulation (uttering of words) must also be perfect. Speech has two components:
1. **Receiving** or **sensory part** (vision and hearing)
2. **Expressing or motor part** (spoken and written speech).

Thus, the disorders of speech may be **aphasias** or **dysarthria**.

- **Aphasias,** i.e. loss of the ability to understand and use symbols, may be **sensory** (or **fluent**) that are due to lesions in the Wernicke's area (area for understanding) or **motor** (or **nonfluent**) that are due to lesions in the Broca's area (area 44).
- The third type of aphasia is called **global aphasia** that is due to lesions involving both Wernicke's and Broca's areas.
- **Dysarthria** is simply the inability to utter words though the patient knows what to say.

TESTS

Look for defects of articulation. Test the patient for various types of aphasias. Give him various common objects and ask him to name them and the purpose for which they are used.

B: EXAMINATION OF THE CRANIAL NERVES

AIM

To clinically assess, the functions of the cranial nerves of the given subject.

There are 12 pairs of cranial nerves:

OLFACTORY NERVE (1ST CRANIAL NERVE)

Origin: Olfactory epithelium
Type: Sensory
Function: Sensation of smell (olfaction) (Fig. 4.5.1).

Examination of the olfactory nerve:
- Before testing, ensure that the nasal passages are clear and the person is not suffering from common cold.
- Ask the subject to close his eyes and occlude one of his nostrils.
- Ask him to smell certain familiar objects (oil of cloves, peppermint, asafetida, garlic) and to distinguish the odors of each of the test substances, one by one, in each nostril, separately.
- Irritating substances such as ammonium chloride should not be used as it might stimulate the trigeminal nerve.

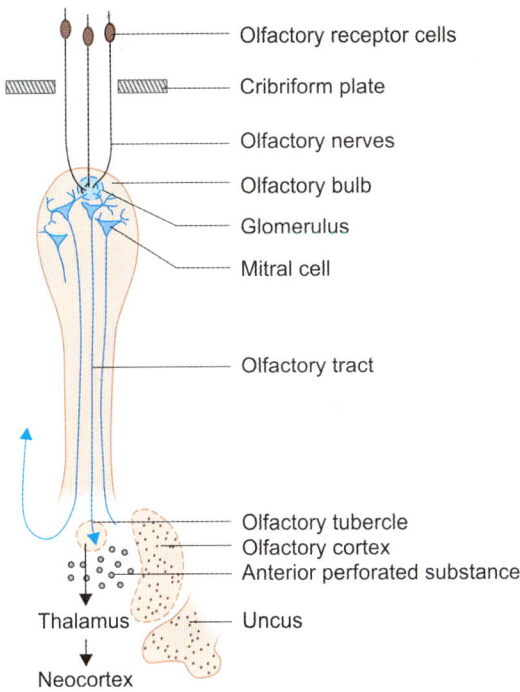

Fig. 4.5.1: Olfactory pathway.

Peculiarities:
1. The olfactory nerve is the only nerve which does not relay in the thalamus.
2. The olfactory mucous membrane is the place where the nervous system is closest to the external environment.
3. The smell receptors adapt rapidly.

Physioclinical significance:
- **Anosmia** refers to complete absence of smell. The most common cause is obstruction of the nasal passage.
- **Parosmia** refers to alterations of smell sensation. It could be psychological also.
- **Hyposmia** is decreased sense of smell.
- The most common neurological cause of the above mentioned conditions is bilateral damage to the olfactory mucosa or the olfactory pathways.
- **Olfactory hallucinations** are characteristic of seizures arising from the temporal lobe.

QUESTIONS

Q.1. What is the pathway for sensation of smell?
Q.2. What are the various abnormalities associated with sense of smell?
Q.3. Test the sense of smell in the subject provided.

OPTIC NERVE (2ND CRANIAL NERVE)

Origin: Retina
Type: Sensory
Function: Transmission of visual sensations to the brain.

Examination of the optic nerve is done under the following headings for each eye:
1. Visual acuity (distant and near vision)
2. Field of vision
3. Color vision
4. Pupillary light reflex
5. Accommodations and near response
6. Examination of fundus.

Visual Acuity

Visual acuity (VA) refers to the degree to which the details and contours of the object are perceived. It is expressed as the minimum separable distance between two points or lines when they can be recognized as two. Visual acuity is tested separately for distant and near vision.
- When perceived as two, they subtend a visual angle of 1 minute (1′) of arc at the nodal point (1° = 60 minutes).
- The nodal point lies at about the middle of the lens and is the optical center of an eye. Any ray passing through this point does not suffer refraction.

Factors Affecting Visual Acuity

1. **Stimulus factors:**
   a. *Illumination:* Bright illumination causes edge enhancement, i.e. the boundary between a bright field and a dark field is emphasized.
   b. Size of the object and its distance from the eye. VA is directly proportional the visual angle.
   c. *Color of the object:* Visual acuity is maximum for the white objects and is less for colored objects.
   d. *Wavelength of light:* The VA is maximum for white light as compared to other colors.
   e. *Brightness and contrast.*
   f. *Time of exposure:* A light flash of very short duration may not be perceived.
2. **Optical factors:** VA is reduced by any error of refraction because the images on the retina are blurred.
3. **Retinal factors (region of the retina stimulated):** The VA is maximal at the fovea centralis where cones are closely packed together.

Testing for Distant Vision

Charts used for testing distant vision:
1. **Snellen's Chart (Fig. 4.5.2)**
   - Snellen's chart has a series of printed black letters of varying sizes on a white background, arranged in 8 lines.
   - The top letter, the largest is visible to the naked eye at a distance of 60 meters and the subsequent letters at distances of 36, 24, 18, 12, 9, 6 and 5 meters, respectively.

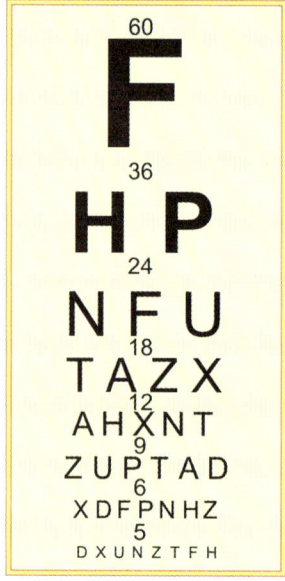

Fig. 4.5.2: Snellen's chart.

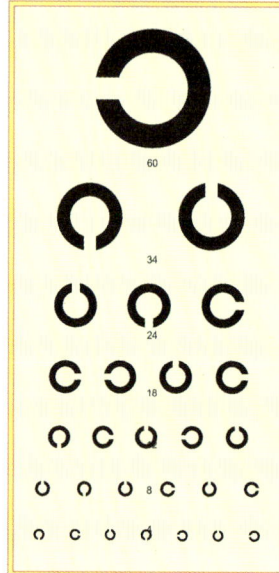

Fig. 4.5.3: Landolt ring chart.

- The distances for each line are indicated above it (or below it in some charts).
- The letters are designed in such a way that from the given distance, the letter as a whole subtends an angle of 5 minutes (5′) of arc at the nodal point.
- The breadth of each line or stroke and the breadth of gaps between two lines or two curves subtend a visual angle of 1 minute (1′) of an arc at the nodal point.
- The distant vision is clinically tested from a distance of 6 meters.

2. **Landolt ring chart (Fig. 4.5.3):** The gap in the ring is positioned at random in the 8 lines. The width of the gap subtends an angle of 1 minute at the nodal point.
3. **E test chart:** The letter E is printed in 8 lines, the "legs" of the letters pointing in different directions. A person (or a child) who cannot read has to indicate the direction in which the legs of each letter are pointing.

Procedure

1. The subject is seated at a distance of 6 meters from the chart and is asked to read down the chart as far as he can.
2. Each eye is to be tested separately. Ensure that the other eye is totally occluded.
3. The VA is recorded according to the formula VA = d/D; where d is the distance at which the letters are read and D is the distance at which the letter should be read by a person with normal vision.
4. Thus, if only the top letter can be read, the VA is 6/60. If the subject can read only the first 4 lines, then the VA is 6/18 and so on.
5. A normal person should be able to read at least the 7th line, i.e. have a VA of 6/6.
6. If the VA is less than 6/60, the subject is moved toward the chart by 1 meter each time until the subject can read the top letter. If the subject can read the top letter from 2 meters the VA is 2/60.
7. If the VA is less than 1/60 other tests can be done in the following order:
   a. **Counting finger test:** The subject can be asked to correctly count fingers held in front of the face.
   b. **Hand movement test:** The subject is asked to identify examiner's hand movements.
   c. **Light perception test:** The subject is asked whether he can appreciate the light shown to him.

Testing for Near Vision

- The subject is asked to read the **Jaeger's chart** held at the reading distance of 9 inches (22.5 centimeters or roughly 25 cm)
- Each eye is to be tested separately. Ensure that the other eye is closed with the palm of his hand.
- This chart has letters of various sizes with the smallest size (J1) at the bottom (Fig. 4.5.4).
- The subject reads down the chart and VA result is expressed as J1, J2, J3, J4, etc. where J1 indicates normal vision.
- These days a modification of the original Jaeger system is used and VA is expressed as N36, N18, N8, N6 instead of J1, J2, etc.; N6 being the smallest type.
- The smallest letter which the subject can read is considered to be the visual acuity for near vision.

Landolt ring chart for near vision is also available. Charts with pictures are used for children for near vision.

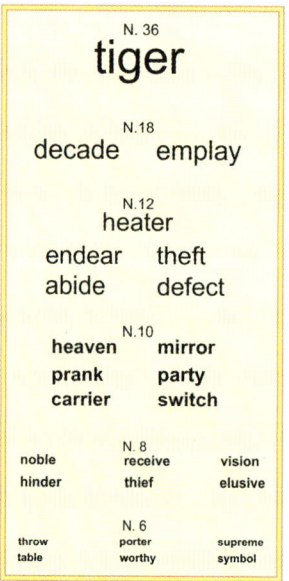

Fig. 4.5.4: Jaeger's chart.

Field of Vision

1. **Confrontation test:** It is a rough test to compare a person's visual fields with the examiner's own (presuming his own to be normal). Only gross changes in the field of vision can be detected with this method. Scotomas (blind areas within the field of vision) are impossible to locate, for which a perimeter is employed.
   Procedure:
   - The subject and the examiner sit facing each other about 1 meters apart (Fig. 4.5.5).
   - While testing the subject's left eye, he is asked to place his right hand over his right eye.
   - Now the subject fixes his gaze on the examiner's right eye, while the examiner closes his left eye.
   - The examiner then holds out his right arm to its full extent out of the patient's visual field.
   - The examiner moves his hand from the periphery toward the center until the examiner can just perceive the movements of the fingers "with the tail of his eye".
   - The subject is now asked whether he sees any movements, telling him meanwhile not to move his gaze.
   - If the subject fails to appreciate the movement of fingers, the hand is moved closer until he is able to see them.
   - The procedure is repeated in all the directions.
2. **Perimetry:** (*Refer* Chapter 3.12).

Color Vision

- The human eye is sensitive to all wavelengths of light from **400–700 nm** which constitute the **visible part of the electromagnetic spectrum.**
- Colors are perceived by cones that are concentrated in fovea and are sensitive to specific wavelengths of light.

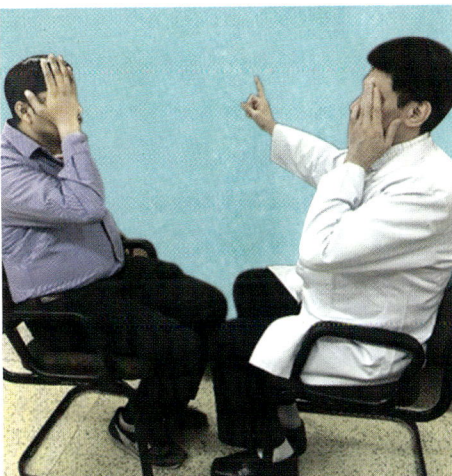

Fig. 4.5.5: Confrontation test.

- There are three **primary colors**—(1) **red**, (2) **green** and (3) **blue**.
- For every color, there is a **complementary** color, which when properly mixed with it produces a sensation of white.
- The sensation of white can be produced by mixing various proportions of primary colors.
- Black is the sensation caused by absence of light. It is probably a positive sensation because the blind eye does not "see black", it "sees nothing".
- Finally, the color perceived depends on the color of other objects in the visual field.
  There are three types of cone pigments:
  1. **Erythrolabe** [red-sensitive or long-wave (723–647 nm) pigment]
  2. **Chlorolabe** [green-sensitive or middle-wave (575–492 nm) pigment]
  3. **Cyanolabe** [blue-sensitive or short-wave (492–417 nm) pigment].

Mechanisms of Color Vision

Two mechanisms are involved:
1. **Retinal mechanism:** The **Young–Helmholtz theory** is based on the existence of three kinds of cones. The ganglion cells of retina add or subtract input from one type of cone to the output of another type. Further processing occurs in lateral geniculate body (LGB) and thalamus and then along specific pathways to the visual cortex.
2. **Cortical mechanism:** The fibers from LGB and thalamus project to clusters of cells (blobs) arranged in a mosaic in layer IV of the primary visual cortex (area 17) which along with visual association area (area 18) is involved in color perception.

Testing of Color Vision

1. **Ishihara charts:** These charts consist of lithographic color plates available in book form. The plates are printed with figures, designs, numbers and wavy lines on a background of differently colored spots of identical size (Fig. 4.5.6).
   Procedure
   - Ask the subject to read the numbers or trace the wavy lines on the given plates.
   - Confirm the status of color vision with the reference key given at the back of the book.
   - For example, the person with normal color vision will read plate 3 in Figure 4.5.6 as 5, while a person with defective color vision will make errors.
2. **Edridge-Green lantern:** In this electrical apparatus, different colored glass pieces (pure red, different intensities of red, yellow, green and signal green) are

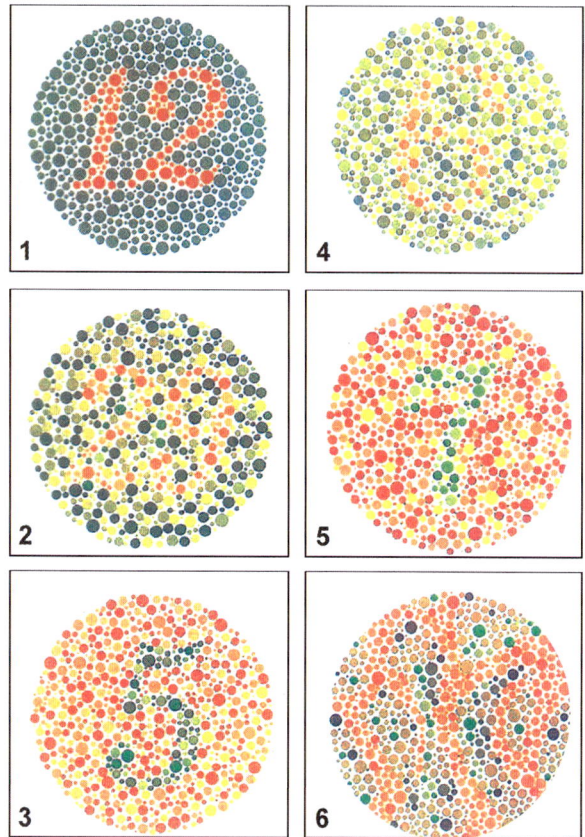

Fig. 4.5.6: Ishihara color plates.

fitted in a rotating disk. These can be brought in front of a small illuminated area, the size of which can be varied. The subject sits in front of the lantern set up in a dimly-lit room and is asked to name the colors as they are brought in front of the aperture.

3. **Holmgren's wools (Yarn matching test):** Small pieces of woolen threads of different colors and hues are placed in a heap on a table. The subject is given a test yarn and is asked to pick out the matching pieces.

Clinical Significance

Color vision is tested mainly in the following groups of people:
1. Drivers of air, sea and road transport vehicles, railway engine drivers, bus and truck drivers, pilots, etc.
2. Workers of textile industry where dyeing of cloth requires a high degree of color perception.
3. Paint and printing industries.
4. Interior decorators and visual artists.

Defects of Color Vision

Abnormal color vision is present as an inherited defect.
- The prefix **"deuter"**—refers to green color, **"trit"**—refers to blue and **"prot"**—refers to red color.
- The suffix—**"anomaly"** refers to color weakness while suffix—**"anopia"** refers to color blindness.

Classification of color blindness

There are various kinds of color blindness:
- **Protanopia** is a severe form of red-green color blindness, in which there is impairment in perception of very long wavelengths, such as reds. Protanomaly is a less severe version.
- **Deuteranopia** consists of impairment in perceiving medium wavelengths, such as greens. Deuteranomaly is a less severe form of deuteranopia.
- A rarer form of color blindness is **tritanopia**, where there exists an inability to perceive short wavelengths, such as blues.

Monochromats are individuals with only one cone system present.

Dichromats have two types of functioning cone system. Dichromacy is hereditary and sex-linked, predominantly affecting males. Physiological dichromatic vision is at the fovea centralis where only red and blue cones are present.

Trichromats have all the three cone systems and require three pure spectral lights to match the colors that they can perceive.

Pupillary Light Reflex

Procedure (Fig. 4.5.7)

1. **Direct Light Reflex**
   - Each eye is tested separately in a shady place.
   - The subject is asked to look at a distance.
   - A bright light from a torch, brought from the side of the eye, is shone into the eye (Fig. 4.5.8).
   - A hand is placed between two eyes so as to prevent the effect of consensual light reflex.
   - The response is a prompt constriction of the pupil of the same eye
   - When the light is switched off, the pupil quickly dilates to its previous size.

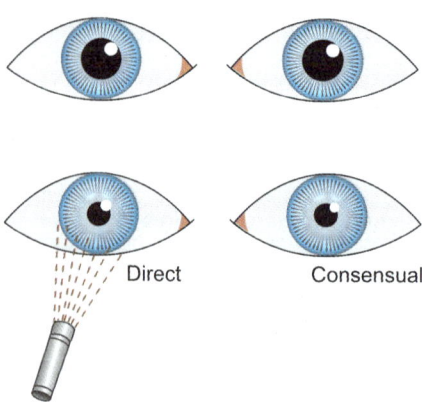

Fig. 4.5.7: Light reflex.

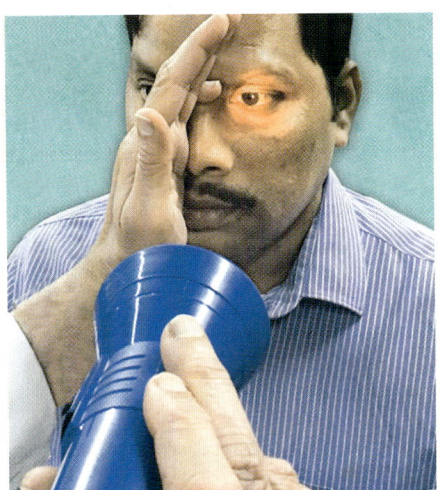

Fig. 4.5.8: Direct light reflex.

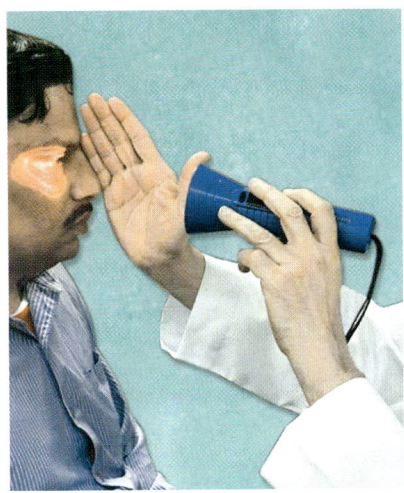

Fig. 4.5.9: Indirect light reflex/consensual light reflex.

2. **Indirect or Consensual Light Reflex**
   - A hand is placed between the two eyes and light is shone into one eye.
   - Observe the effect on the pupil of the opposite (unstimulated) eye (Fig. 4.5.9).
   - The response is constriction of the pupil in the other eye.
   - Thus, the pupils of both eyes constrict when light is thrown into any eye.

Pathway of Light Reflex

Flowchart 4.5.1 shows the pathway of light reflex.

Accommodation and Near Response

Near response consists of three responses (Fig. 4.5.10)
1. Accommodation
2. Convergence of visual axes
3. Pupillary constriction (Miosis).

Procedure

1. Ask the subject to fix his eyes on a distant object.
2. The examiner suddenly brings his finger in front of the subject's eyes close to the nose.
3. Ask the subject to focus his eyes quickly on the finger.

Flowchart 4.5.1: Pathway of light reflex.

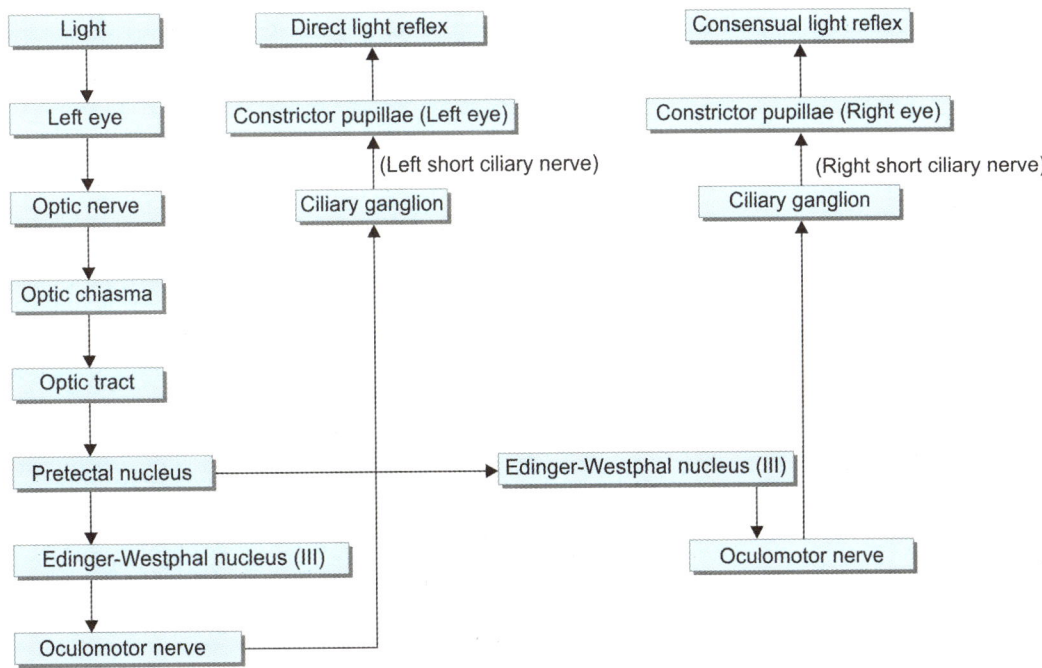

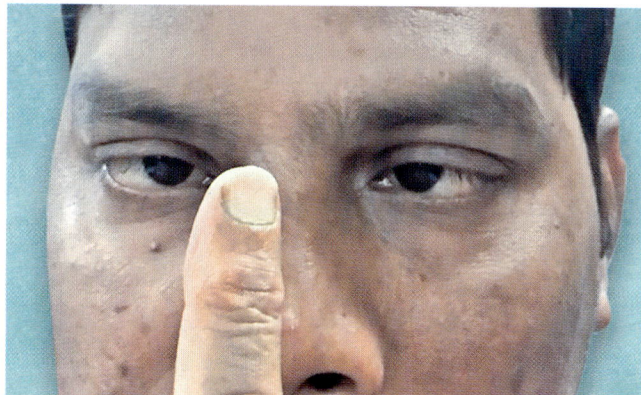

Fig. 4.5.10: Accommodation reflex.

4. There occurs convergence of eyes, constriction of pupil and increase in the curvature of the lens.

These three components or responses are grouped together to be called **the near response**.

When the gaze is suddenly changed from a distant object to a near object—the ciliary muscle contracts. This relaxes the lens ligaments, so that the curvature of the lens increases making it more convex. The change is greatest at the anterior surface of the lens. This is called **accommodation**. In addition, there is convergence of two visual axes and constriction of pupil.

Pathway for Accommodation and Near Response

The pathway is as follows: retina—optic nerve—optic tract—lateral geniculate body—geniculocalcarine tract (optic radiation)—visual cortex (area 17)—frontal eye-field area (area 8)—Edinger-Westphal nucleus of opposite side—oculomotor nerve—ciliary ganglion—ciliary nerves-constrictor pupillae muscle (Fig. 4.5.11).

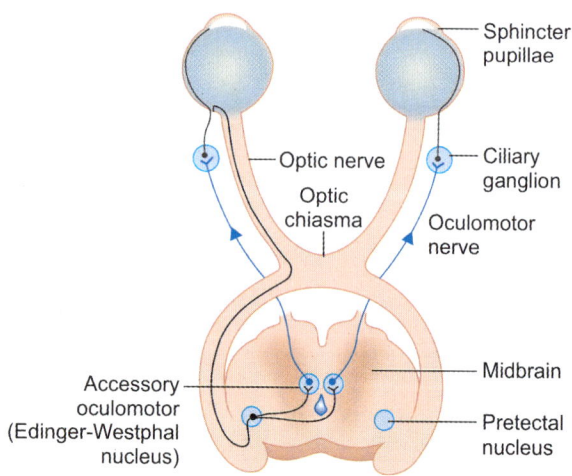

Fig. 4.5.11: Accommodation reflex pathway.

Argyll–Robertson Pupil

A pupil in which the accommodation is present but the light reflex (direct and consensual) is absent is called the **Argyll–Robertson pupil.** It is classically seen in neurosyphilis. The lesion is located in the pretectum of the midbrain behind the optic tract and the 3rd nerve nucleus, thus interrupting the pathway of light reflex while leaving the accommodation pathway intact.

QUESTIONS

Q.1. Define visual acuity? List the factors that affect visual acuity.
Q.2. What is visual angle?
Q.3. How do you test visual acuity for near and distant vision?
Q.4. Describe the theories of color vision.
Q.5. How is color vision tested? What is the principle behind the chart used to test for color blindness?
Q.6. What is color blindness? How is it classified?
Q.7. What is the pathway for color vision?
Q.8. What is near response phenomenon?
Q.9. Test the visual acuity of the subject provided.
Q.10. Test the color vision of the subject provided.
Q.11. Test the peripheral field of vision of the subject provided, using the confrontation test.
Q.12. Test the conjugate movements of the eyes in the subject provided.
Q.13. Demonstrate the light reflex in the subject provided. What is the pathway of this reflex?
Q.14. What is the cause of consensual light reflex?
Q.15. Demonstrate the reaction of the pupil to accommodation for near vision.
Q.16. What is the pathway for accommodation reflex?
Q.17. What is Argyll–Robertson pupil?
Q.18. Demonstrate the corneal reflex.

OCULOMOTOR (3RD), TROCHLEAR (4TH), ABDUCENT (6TH) CRANIAL NERVES

Origin: 3rd and 4th cranial nerve arises from the midbrain while the 6th cranial nerve arises from the pons.
Type: Motor
Function:

- The 3rd, 4th and 6th cranial nerves are examined together because of their close functional interrelationships in the control of the eye movements.
- The 3rd cranial nerve supplies all the external ocular muscles except superior oblique and the lateral rectus muscles. It also sends fibers to the levator palpebrae superioris (LPS) and through the ciliary ganglion it supplies parasympathetic fibers to the sphincter pupillae and the muscle of accommodation, i.e. the ciliary muscle (contraction for near vision).
- The 6th nerve supplies the lateral rectus muscle.
- The 4th nerve innervates the superior oblique.

Before testing these nerves, observe:
- If there is any squint—the patient should also be asked if the subject sees double (diplopia).
- The condition of the pupils—whether they are equal in size and regular in outline, whether they are abnormally dilated or contracted and their reaction to light and accommodation.

Test the conjugate movements of the eyes in the subject provided: Normally, the movement of the eyes is simultaneous and symmetrical, so that the visual axes meet at a point at which the eyes are directed. This is called **conjugate movements of the eyes** (Fig. 4.5.12).

Procedure:
- The head of the subject must be fixed with the left hand.
- The examiner moves his index finger to the right, to the left, upward and downward as far as possible in each direction, i.e. the examiner moves his index finger in the "H-shaped" pathway.
- The subject is asked to follow the examiner's index finger without moving his head.
- Normally, the eyes move 50° outward, 50° downward, 50° inward and 33° upward.
- The rotatory movements should also be tested. Note if there is any limitation of movement in any direction.

The brainstem centers of 3rd, 4th and 6th cranial nerves control reflex movements of the eyes, while conjugate movements of voluntary origin are under the control of higher cortical centers via the corticonuclear tracts.

Physioclinical Significance

Changes in the pupil in cases of head injury and cardiac arrest provide important diagnostic and prognostic information.
- Inequality of the pupils may indicate a rising intracranial tension due to hematoma.
- Dilated and fixed pupils, nonreacting to light, may suggest serious and irreversible brain damage.
- Pupillary responses to light are also watched during anesthesia.

TRIGEMINAL NERVE (5TH CRANIAL NERVE)

Origin: Pons
Type: Mixed (Sensory and Motor).

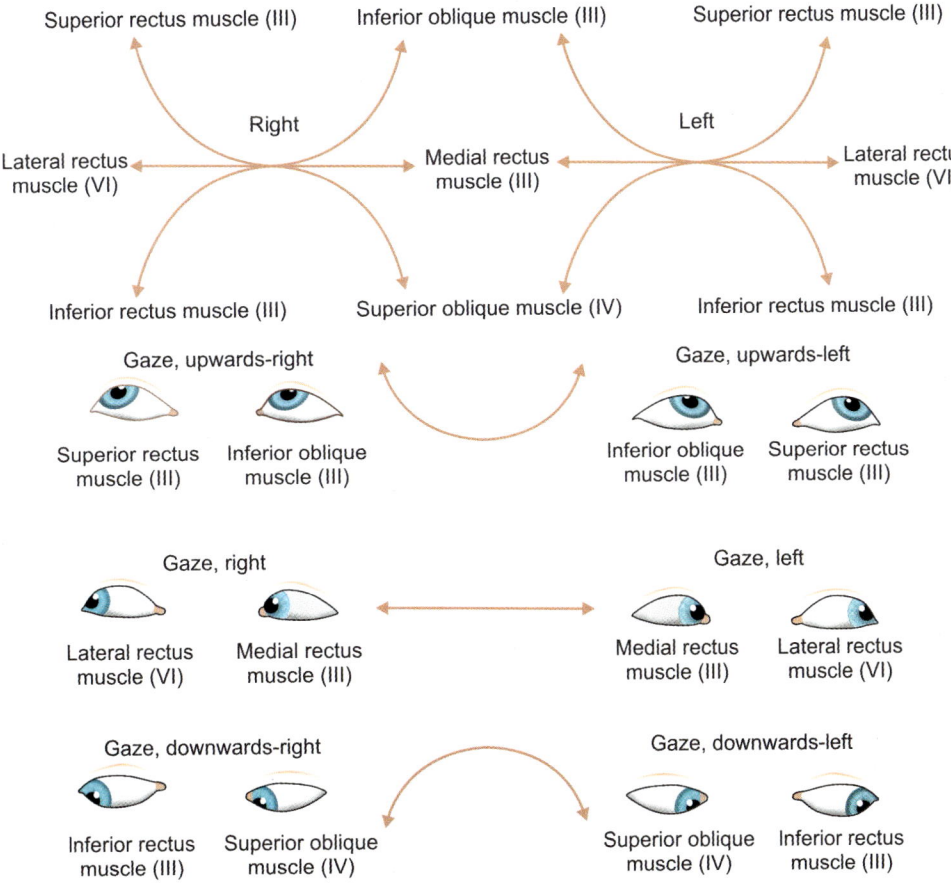

Fig. 4.5.12: Conjugate movement of eyes.

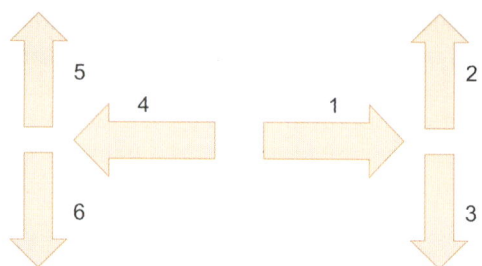

Fig. 4.5.13: Testing the 3rd, 4th, 6th cranial nerves by eye movements.

Testing Sensory Functions (Fig. 4.5.13)

1. **Demonstrate the corneal reflex:**
   - Make a light wisp of absorbent cotton by twisting it into a fine hair.
   - Ask the subject to look at a distant object.
   - Lightly touch *lateral edge of the cornea* with the cotton.
   - The response is bilateral blinking.
   - Compare the reflex in the opposite side also.
   - The afferent pathway of this reflex is ophthalmic division of the 5th nerve, the efferent pathway is 7th nerve, while the center is in the nuclei of these nerves in the pons.

   > **NOTE**
   > The cornea should never be wiped with the cotton and the central cornea should never be touched, because ulceration may occur.

2. **Conjunctival reflex:** It is also a superficial reflex and is elicited in the same manner as the corneal reflex.
   - Touching the conjunctiva with a wisp of cotton causes bilateral blinking (Fig. 4.5.14).

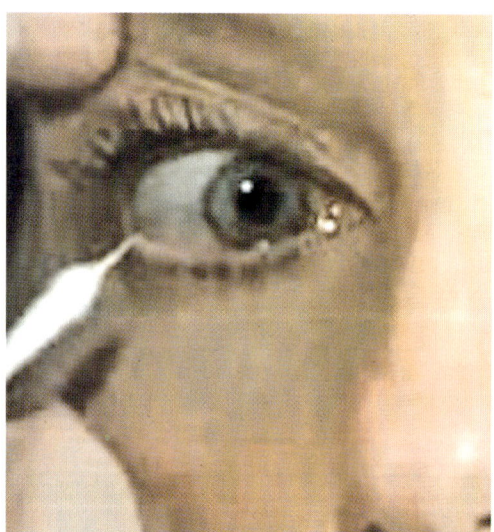

Fig. 4.5.14: Conjunctival reflex.

- The conjunctiva of the lower lid is supplied by maxillary division of the 5th nerve.

> **NOTE**
> **Nasal or sneeze reflex**—sneezing when the nasal mucosa is irritated, also employs 5th nerve as its afferent pathway, while the efferent pathway employs motor components of 5th to 10th cranial and upper cervical nerves.

3. **Test the general sensory functions of the trigeminal nerve:**
   - In addition to the corneal and palpebral conjunctiva, the 5th cranial nerve supplies greater part of the face, forehead, temporal and parietal regions and nasal and buccal mucosa.
   - The sensory fibers arise from unipolar cells in the semilunar or Gasserian ganglion and supply the skin and mucosa described above. The nerve also contains sensory proprioceptive fibers, which innervate muscle spindles in the muscles of mastication and possibly also in the external ocular muscles.
   - The sensations of touch, pain and temperature over the face are tested, with a wisp of cotton, pin pricks and warm and cold objects (*See* Chapter 4.5E).
   - General sensations of touch, pain and temperature are carried from the oral cavity by the 5th cranial nerve.

Testing of Motor Functions

The motor fibers of the 5th nerve, (its nucleus lies at the midpontine level) innervate the muscles of mastication—masseter, temporalis, medial and lateral pterygoids and the tensor tympani of middle ear. The mandibular division of 5th nerve also supplies parasympathetic fibers to the salivary glands.

Procedure

- The subject is asked to open his mouth and show the teeth. Normally, the jaw is symmetrical. If there is paralysis on one side, the jaw deviates to the side of paralysis, the healthy pterygoids pushing it to that side.
- The subject is asked to clench his teeth—the temporalis and masseter muscles contract and become equally prominent on the two sides. The muscles can be palpated to note, if there is any difference in the strength of contraction.
- The subject is asked to open his mouth and move the mandible from side to side.
- The **jaw reflex:** *See* Chapter on Reflexes.

Objective Structured Clinical Examination–I

Aim: To test the 5th cranial nerve in the subject provided.
Procedural steps: See text above.
Checklist:
1. Make the subject sit on a stool and explain the procedure. (Y/N)
2. Ask the subject to look at a distance and touch his/her conjunctiva with a wisp of cotton and note the response. (Y/N)
3. Test the sensations of touch and pain with a wisp of cotton and a pin on identical points on the two sides of the face. (Y/N)
4. Ask the subject to show his/her teeth and then to clench his/her teeth. Watch and feel the masseter and temporalis muscles contracting. (Y/N)
5. Ask the subject to open his/her mouth and move the mandible from side to side then tests the mandibular reflex. (Y/N)

QUESTIONS

Q.1. Test the general sensory functions of the trigeminal nerve.
Q.2. Test the motor functions of the trigeminal nerve in the subject provided.

FACIAL NERVE (7TH CRANIAL NERVE)

Origin: Pons
Type: Mixed

- The facial nerve supplies all the superficial muscles of the face and scalp (except levator palpebrae superioris, which is supplied by 3rd nerve), external ear and the stapedius in the middle ear.
- The parasympathetic fibers from the superior salivatory nucleus innervate the blood vessels and glandular cells of sublingual and submaxillary glands and glands in the mucosa of pharynx, palate, nasal cavity and paranasal sinuses.
- Sensation from a small medial part of the tragus of the pinna, the external auditory meatus and tympanic membrane is relayed by tympanic branch of the facial nerve to the geniculate ganglion.

Test the Motor Functions of the Facial Nerve in the Subject Provided

- Observe the face for any asymmetry, which may be due to the paresis of the facial muscles.
- Observe the symmetry of blinking and eye closure and presence of any ticks or spasms of the facial musculature.
- Observe spontaneous movement of the face, particularly the upper and lower facial musculature during the actions such as smiling.
1. **Testing the upper face:**
   - The subject is asked to raise his eyebrows and look upwards (**occipitofrontalis** muscle is tested). The subject is unable to do so, on the affected side.

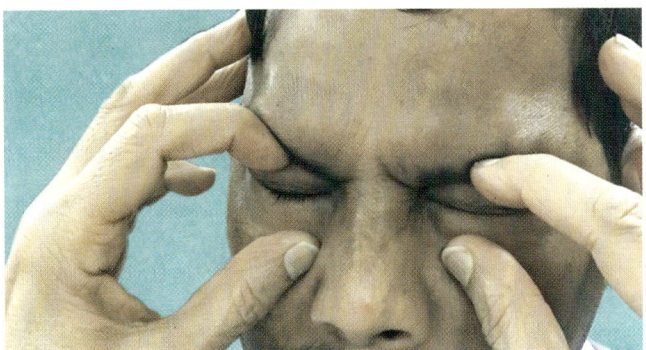

Fig. 4.5.15: Orbicularis oculi muscle testing.

- Ask the subject to frown, the **corrugator supercilii** muscle can be tested by doing this.
- The subject is asked to shut his eyes as tightly as possible. The examiner then tries to open one and then the other eye (Fig. 4.5.15). Normally, it is impossible to do so against the subject's resistance (**orbicularis oculi** muscle is tested).
- The eye can be opened easily on the affected side. In severe cases, the subject may fail to shut his eyes and excessive effort to do the same makes his eye ball rolls upward. This is called **Bell's phenomenon.**

2. **Testing the lower face:**
   - The nasolabial folds on both sides are observed, which are normally symmetrical. Paralysis on one side causes flattening of the folds on that side.
   - The subject is asked to smile or show his upper teeth, he is unable to do so on the affected side (**levator angularis** muscle is tested) and the angle of the mouth is drawn toward the healthy side. This occurs in infranuclear (e.g. **Bell's**) facial palsy (Figs. 4.5.16A to D).
   - Ask the subject to whistle. He is unable to do so.
   - The subject is asked to inflate his mouth with air and blow out his cheeks (**buccinator** is tested) (Fig. 4.5.17). Each inflated cheek is then tapped with a finger. If there is paralysis, the air escapes easily through the angle of the mouth on the paralyzed side.
   - The subject is asked to depress the lower lip (**depressor labii inferioris** and **quadratus labii inferioris** is tested). In case of paralysis, the asymmetry is obvious.

Test the Sensory Function of the Facial Nerve

The patient should always be asked about any abnormal taste sensations if any.

Sensation of Taste

Modalities
There are five basic tastes: (1) **sweet**, (2) **salt**, (3) **bitter**, (4) **sour** and (5) **umami**.

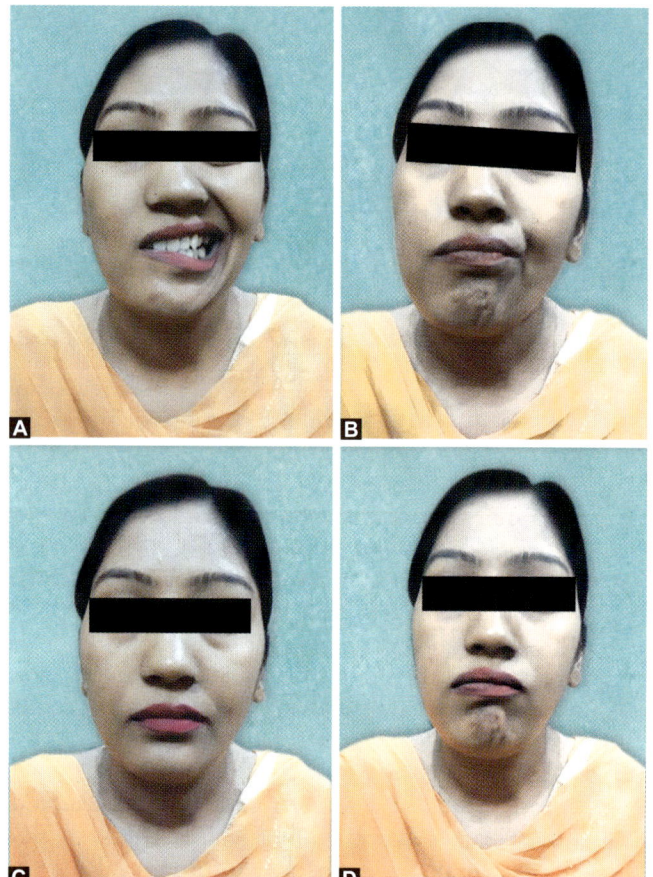

Figs. 4.5.16A to D: Bell's palsy.

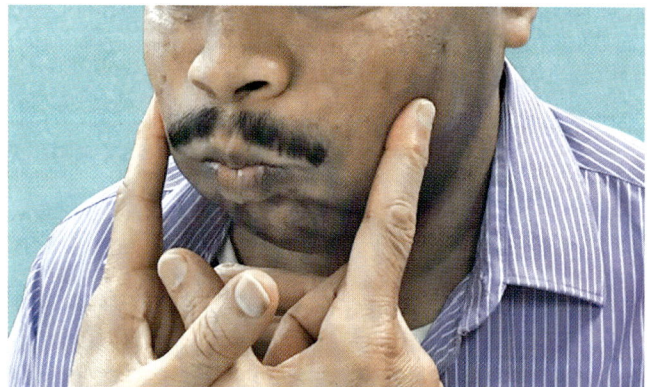

Fig. 4.5.17: Buccinator muscle testing.

Taste Pathway (Fig. 4.5.18)

- Three cranial nerves contain the axons of first-order gustatory neurons that innervate the sensory cells in taste buds—(1) 7th nerve from anterior two-thirds of tongue, (2) 9th nerve from posterior third of tongue and (3) 10th nerve from part of pharynx and epiglottis.

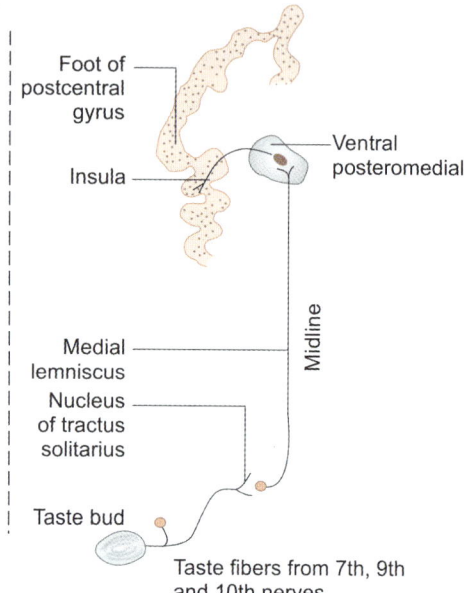

Fig. 4.5.18: The pathway for taste.

- Second-order neurons form nucleus of tractus solitarius travel up in the ipsilateral medial lemniscus to end in nucleus lateralis posterolateralis of the thalamus.
- From thalamus, they are relayed to the taste area I in the postcentral gyrus. Other fibers from thalamus end in taste area II in the insula and to limbic system and hypothalamus.

Abnormalities of Taste

Ageusia (absence of taste)
Hypogeusia (decreased sensitivity to taste)
Dysgeusia (disturbed taste sensation).

Testing the Taste Sensation on Anterior Two-thirds of the Tongue

Apparatus:
- Strong solutions of sucrose (10%), sodium chloride (15%) and weak solutions of acetic acid (1%) and quinine sulfate (0.1%) all kept in drop bottles.
- Small cotton swabs or toothpicks; gauze.
- Four cards with sweet, salt, sour and bitter printed on them.

Procedure:
1. Instruct the subject not to speak during the test. He is asked to indicate the taste felt by him by pointing to an appropriate card as mentioned above.
2. Ask the subject to rinse his mouth; then dry it with gauze.
3. Ask him/her to protrude his tongue and hold it with a swab.
4. Moisten a swab with a few drops of sugar solution, apply it to the tip of the tongue and ask him/her to indicate

without withdrawing the tongue, the taste experienced by him/her.
5. Repeat this procedure with all the four substances on the anterior two-thirds of the tongue in turn.

Physioclinical Significance

Facial paralysis results quite commonly from lesions of upper motor neurons (UMNs) or lower motor neurons (LMNs). To differentiate between these two, it is important to remember that 7th cranial nerve nuclei innervating muscles of upper face are under bilateral cortical motor control, while the facial nuclei supplying the lower face are controlled from the opposite motor cortex only.

- Therefore, in **supranuclear lesion** (UMN paralysis) only the muscles of lower part of face are paralyzed.
- In **infranuclear lesion** (LMN paralysis) as in Bell's palsy, both the upper as well as the lower parts of the face are equally affected. If there is involvement of the fibers of the chorda tympani, the taste sensation from the anterior two-thirds is lost (**taste is not affected in supranuclear lesions**). The sounds on the side of palsy seem unusually loud (**hyperacusis**) because the stapedius muscle is paralyzed.

Objective Structured Clinical Examination–II

Aim: To test the 7th cranial nerve in the subject provided.
Procedural steps: See text above.
Checklist:
1. Explain the procedure to the subject. Look for facial symmetry, furrows on the forehead and the width of the palpebral fissure. (Y/N)
2. Ask the subject to look up and wrinkle his/her forehead and then to shut his/her eyes as tightly as possible against the examiner's resistance. (Y/N)
3. Ask the subject to show his/her upper teeth and to smile. (Y/N)
4. Ask the subject to inflate his/her mouth with air and to blow out his/her cheeks. Then tap his/her cheeks, on either side with his/her finger, to see if air escapes from the angle of the mouth. (Y/N)
5. Ask the subject to depress his/her lower lip. (Y/N)

QUESTIONS

Q.1. Test the motor functions of the facial nerve in the subject provided.
Q.2. Test the taste function of the facial nerve.

VESTIBULOCOCHLEAR NERVE (8TH CRANIAL NERVE)

Origin: Pons (Cerebellopontine angle)
Type: Sensory

The 8th cranial nerve has two components:
1. **Cochlear nerve:** The cochlear nerve supplies the cochlea and subserves hearing.
   The symptoms of cochlear nerve involvement include tinnitus (ringing sensation in the ear); deafness and sensory aphasia in supranuclear lesions.
2. **Vestibular nerve:** The vestibular nerve supplies the semicircular canals and the labyrinth and subserves equilibrium, balance and sensation of bodily displacement.
   The symptoms of vestibular nerve damage include vertigo (a feeling of giddiness); nystagmus (a rhythmic to and fro movement of the eyes); and some general symptoms like nausea, vomiting, tachycardia and low blood pressure.

Mechanism of Hearing

- The sound waves striking the tympanic membrane are magnified by the ossicles and set the basilar membrane to vibrate, which in turn, causes movement of the hair cells of the organ of Corti.
- The bending of the cilia of hair cells transducts mechanical vibrations into action potentials (APs) by releasing a neurotransmitter (probably glutamate) at the bases of hair cells where nerve endings of first-order sensory neurons synapse.
- The APs are carried up the auditory pathway to the primary auditory areas of the cerebral cortex (Brodmann areas 41 and 42).
- Since many fibers cross over from one auditory pathway to the opposite pathway in medulla, the primary auditory areas receive signals from both sides.

Auditory pathway: The **pathway of hearing** (Fig. 4.5.19) from the cochlea to the auditory cortex consists of 4–6 neurons.

- The cell bodies of first-order neurons (bipolar) lie in the spiral ganglion. The peripheral processes end on the hair cells of the organ of Corti, while the central processes which form the auditory nerve enter the upper medulla to synapse on the dorsal and ventral cochlear nuclei.
- The second-order neurons from these nuclei take different routes through the nearby olivary nuclei and the trapezoid bodies of both sides (some fibers end here), cross to the opposite side and turn upward to form the lateral lemniscus.
- The lemniscal fibers synapse on the neurons in the inferior colliculi and medial geniculate bodies from where fresh relays (third-order neurons) spread upward as auditory radiation to terminate in the primary auditory cortex (Brodmann areas 41 and 42).

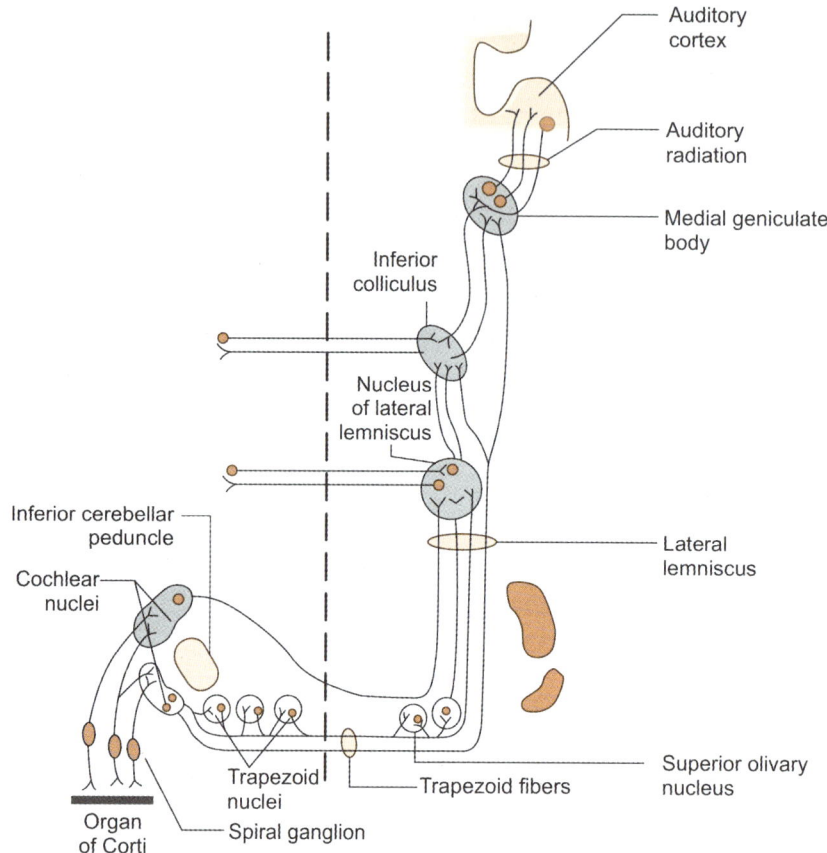

Fig. 4.5.19: Auditory pathway.

Tests of Hearing

Apparatus

- Tuning fork (512 Hz): Avoid using 128 Hz or 256 Hz tuning fork, as these are used to assess the vibration sensation in neurological examination.
- Audiometer
- Ticking watch.

1. **Whisper test:**
- The examiner stands on one side of the subject and closes the subject's opposite ear with his own finger.
- The subject is asked his name by gently whispering into his ear from a distance of 12–14 inches.
- The procedure is repeated on the other side.
2. **Watch test:**
- A ticking watch may be gradually brought toward each ear of the subject, separately.
- The examiner then can compare the subject's hearing with his own.
3. **Tuning fork tests:** These are the most commonly used tests in clinical practice.

Tuning Fork Tests

Air (ossicular) conduction (AC)
Normally, most of the energy of sound waves is transmitted via the outer ear, tympanic membrane and middle ear ossicles to the cochlea where it stimulates the sensory hair cells of the organ of Corti. This mode of conduction of sound is called **ossicular conduction**, though it is commonly and **misleadingly called air conduction.**

Bone Conduction (BC)
Since cochlea is enclosed in a bony cavity (bony cochlea), vibrations of the skull bones themselves can be transmitted to the organ of Corti—a type of sound conduction called bone conduction.

In this case, sound from a vibrating tuning fork directly placed anywhere on the skull can be heard in both ears by bone conduction.

Principles of Tuning Fork Tests
- In *AC hearing*, sound from a vibrating tuning fork held in front of the external ear passes via the external auditory meatus, tympanic membrane and middle ear ossicles to the organ of Corti.
- In *BC hearing*, vibrations from a tuning fork directly placed anywhere on the skull are conducted to the organ of Corti and perceived as sound.
  Normally, AC hearing is better than BC hearing (written as AC > BC).

Conduction (or Conductive) Deafness
Pathology in the outer ear (e.g. wax) or damage to the tympanic membrane (e.g. perforation) or pathology in the middle ear (e.g. loss of mobility or destruction of ossicles), reduces AC hearing without affecting bone conduction (BC hearing), a condition called **conductive deafness**.

Nerve Deafness
Damage to the hair cells in the organ of Corti or auditory pathways will reduce both AC and BC hearing, a condition called **nerve deafness** or **perceptive deafness**. In other words, if BC is normal, the inner ear (cochlea) and auditory pathways must be normal, but if BC is reduced the cochlea or the pathways are at fault.

Procedure
Rinne test (Figs. 4.5.20A and B)
This test compares the subject's AC hearing with his BC hearing in each ear separately.
1. Hold the stem of the tuning fork and set it into vibration by striking one of its prongs on the heel of your hand (the other prong will also start to vibrate).
2. Place its base on the mastoid process (the bony prominence behind the ear). The subject will hear a sound.
3. Ask him to raise his hand when the sound stops. Note the time for which the sound is heard. This part of the test examines the bone conduction of sound.
4. When the sound stops, bring the prongs in front of the ear the sound will become audible once again. Note the time for which it lasts (e.g. for another 10 seconds; total = 45 seconds).
5. Test the other ear and record the timings for BC and AC sounds.

Results:
- *In normal individuals:* AC > BC (Rinne positive).
- *In conduction deafness:* AC < BC (Rinne negative).
- *In nerve deafness (partial):* AC > BC, but duration of both will be decreased as compared to normal.

Weber's test (Fig. 4.5.21)
This test compares the bone conduction of the subject in both the ears.
1. Set the tuning fork into vibration and place its base in the midline on the top of the subject's head or on his forehead.
2. Ask the subject if he hears the sound equally well in both the ears or louder on one side.
   - *In a normal subject:* Bone conducted sounds are heard equally well on the two sides.
   - *In conduction deafness:* Sound is louder/better heard in deaf or deafer ear because of masking effect of environmental noise is absent on diseased side.
   - *In nerve deafness:* The sound is louder/better heard on the healthy side, i.e. the patient lateralizes the sound to healthy side.

Schwabach's test
This test compares the bone conduction of both the subject and examiner. It is assumed that the examiner's hearing is normal.

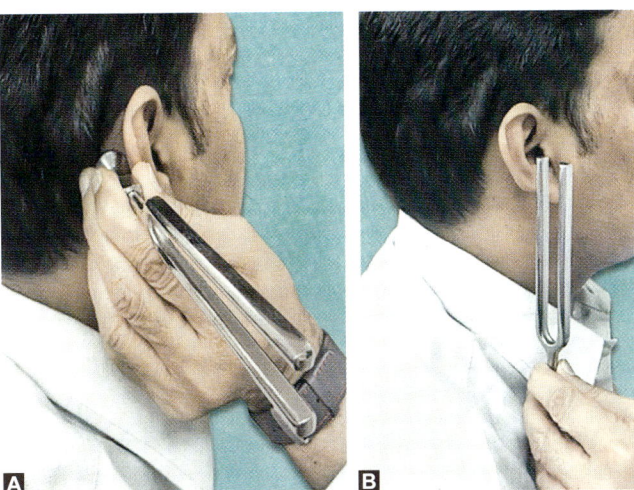

Figs. 4.5.20A and B: Rinne test.

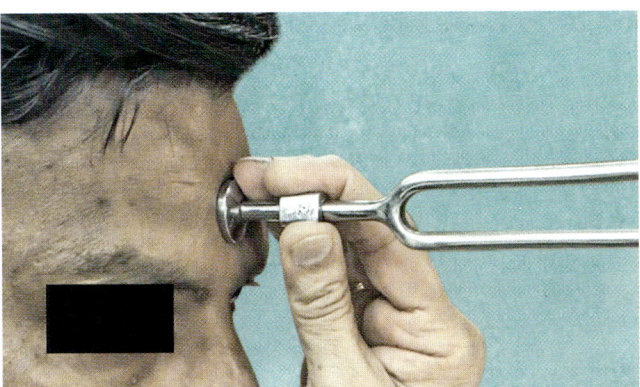

Fig. 4.5.21: Weber's test.

1. Set the tuning fork into vibration as before and place its base on the subject's mastoid process. Ask him to indicate by raising his hand when the sound stops.
2. After the subject stops hearing the sound, place the fork on your own mastoid process.
   - *In a normal person:* BC in the subject is nearly equal to your own.
   - *In conduction deafness:* The subject's bone conduction is better than your bone conduction.
   - *In nerve deafness:* BC in the subject is reduced as compared to your own (this means that you will be able to hear BC after the subject stops hearing this sound).

Brainstem auditory evoked potentials (BAEPs)
The BAEPs recorded from the scalp after applying a suitable auditory stimulus are employed to localize the site of lesion in the central auditory pathways (*Refer* Chapter 3.15).

Audiometry
Audiometry (*audre* means to hear) is an accurate, painless and noninvasive test for hearing that measures a person's ability to hear different sounds, pitches or frequency.
- It is measured with the help of audiometer and the graph obtained is called an audiometer. The test is conducted in a soundproof room.
- Pure tones of different frequencies and different intensities are presented to the ear from an oscillator connected by an amplifier to the earphones. Threshold intensity is the lowest decibel at which the subject hears the tone.
- Hearing loss is determined by increasing the intensity until threshold audibility (intensity) is achieved for each tone tested; the corresponding dB increase on intensity dial is noted.
- In this way audiometric threshold as a function of frequency discrimination is plotted on a graph. This is called an **audiogram.**

Test the Vestibular Function Tests in the Subject Provided

In the **Barany caloric test**, the subject is seated in a special chair, which can be rotated at a definite speed with the subject's head tilted back at 60° and his external auditory meatus is irrigated with 250 mL of water at 30°C (7° below body temperature) for 40 seconds. The test is repeated with water at 44°C (7° above normal). The endolymph in the horizontal canal (which becomes vertical with head tilt) moves due to convection currents, thus stimulating the receptors in the crista ampullaris.

The normal response to caloric stimulation is nausea, horizontal nystagmus, past pointing and falling to stimulated side. In vestibular dysfunction, these reactions to stimulation are diminished.

Objective Structured Clinical Examinations

Task: To demonstrate Rinne test on the subject provided.
Procedural steps: See text above.
Checklist:
1. Explain the test procedure and gives suitable instructions. (Y/N)
2. Select either 216 Hz or 250 Hz tuning fork and strikes one of the prongs on the heel of her hand. (Y/N)
3. Close the external auditory meatus of the subject's other ear with her finger. (Y/N)
4. Place the base of the tuning fork on the patient's mastoid process; when he raises his finger to indicate that the sound can no longer be heard. (Y/N)
5. Quickly transfer the vibrating tuning fork close to the patient's ear. Note if he/she can hear the sound once again. Note down whether air or bone conduction is better. (Y/N)

QUESTIONS

Q.1. Perform the Rinne test on the subject provided.
Q.2. Perform the Weber test on the subject provided.
Q.3. Demonstrate the Schwabach test of hearing.
Q.4. Perform the whisper test in the subject provided.
Q.5. How will you test the vestibular function in the subject provided?
Q.6. What are the limitations of the tuning fork tests?
The tuning fork tests often provide valuable information, but cannot give quantitative estimates about the acuity of hearing. Furthermore, bone-conducted vibrations reach all parts of the skull irrespective of where the fork is placed on the head. Thus, when testing bone conduction in one ear, the patient will also be hearing sound in the other ear, which is likely to confuse him.
Q.7. What is masking and what is deafness?
Masking: It literally means "covering". The auditory system cannot separate the different components of total sound stimulation. For example, in a bus, the low frequency sounds mask (i.e. cover) the high frequency sounds.
Deafness: This refers to the inability of a person to hear either partially or totally. It is of two types: (1) **Conduction deafness** in which there may be wax or a foreign body in the external auditory meatus, thickening or damage to tympanic membrane due to infection (otitis media) and osteosclerosis (stapes gets fixed in oval window) interfere with hearing; and (2) **Nerve deafness** in which there is damage to cochlear hair cells or auditory pathway such as due to prolonged exposure to industrial sounds or very loud music or damage to 8th nerve by drugs.
Q.8. What is audiometry?
Audiometry: An audiometer is an apparatus in which selected pure tones of 125–800 Hz can be fed into each ear separately through headphones. The threshold is determined at each frequency and is then plotted as a percentage of normal hearing. Audiometry is thus the only reliable method to determine the nature and degree of deafness in a patient.

GLOSSOPHARYNGEAL NERVE (9TH CRANIAL NERVE)

Origin: Medulla
Type: Mixed

- The 9th nerve is motor to the middle constrictor of pharynx and stylopharyngeus and sensory for the posterior third of the tongue (both general and taste sensations) and mucous membrane of the pharynx.
- Parasympathetic fibers from inferior salivatory nucleus, after relaying in the otic ganglion, innervate parotid gland. This nerve is rarely involved alone, but generally with the 10th and 11th nerves.

Testing the motor function of 9th cranial nerve:

1. **Gag Reflex (Pharyngeal Reflex):**
   - Touch each side of the pharynx lightly with a wooden spatula.
   - Response is constriction and elevation of the pharynx.
   - The afferent path is 9th nerve; the center is in medulla; and the efferent path is 10th nerve. The reflex is absent when there is damage to its afferent arc.
2. **Palatal Reflex:**
   - A soft touch is applied on the soft palate.
   - The response is elevation of the soft palate.
   - The reflex arc is the same as in the gag reflex described above.

Testing the sensory function of 9th cranial nerve: The sensation of taste over the posterior one-third of the tongue is tested as discussed above for the 7th cranial nerve.

QUESTION

Q.1. How will you test the 9th cranial nerve?

VAGUS NERVE (10TH CRANIAL NERVE)

Origin: Medulla
Type: Mixed Nerve

- The vagus nerve is motor for soft palate, pharynx and intrinsic muscles of the larynx.
- **Somatic sensory fibers** from unipolar cells in jugular ganglion supply external auditory meatus and part of the ear. The **visceral sensory fibers** of unipolar cells in ganglion nodosum innervate pharynx, larynx, trachea and thoracic and abdominal viscera.
- The **parasympathetic fibers** arise from nucleus ambiguous and supply the heart (inhibitory), bronchial muscle and glands, glands and the smooth muscle of most of the gastrointestinal tract and suprarenal gland.

Testing the vagus nerve in the subject provided:

a. The **pharyngeal** and **palate reflexes** are tested as mentioned above.
b. Using a tongue depressor, the subject is asked to open his mouth wide and say "aah". The response is constriction of posterior pharyngeal wall and movement of the uvula backward in the midline. But in vagal paralysis, the uvula is deflected to the normal side.
c. The subject is asked for history of regurgitation of food through the nose, which is due to total paralysis of vagus; a nasal voice may also be noted.

QUESTION

Q.1. How will you test the vagus nerve in the subject provided?

SPINAL ACCESSORY NERVE (11TH CRANIAL NERVE)

Origin:
Cranial part: Arises from the medulla
Spinal part: Arises from spinal cord
Type: Motor nerve.

This purely motor nerve innervates some muscles in the pharynx and larynx as well as sternomastoid and the trapezius.

Test the spinal part of the accessory nerve in the subject provided:

- The examiner presses on the shoulders from behind and asks the subject to shrug his shoulders (this tests the upper part of trapezius) (Fig. 4.5.22). If the 11th nerve is damaged, shrugging is weaker on that side; the shoulder also droops. The subject is asked to approximate his shoulder blades against examiner's resistance (this tests the lower part of the muscle).
- A hand is placed against the right side of the subject's face and he is asked to rotate the head to the right. The left sternomastoid is seen to become prominent. The procedure is repeated on the left side also. In case of a unilateral lesion, the head cannot be rotated to the healthy side.
- The examiner places a hand on the subject's forehead and asks him to bend his head forward against resistance. Normally, both sternomastoids become prominent (Figs. 4.5.23A ad B).

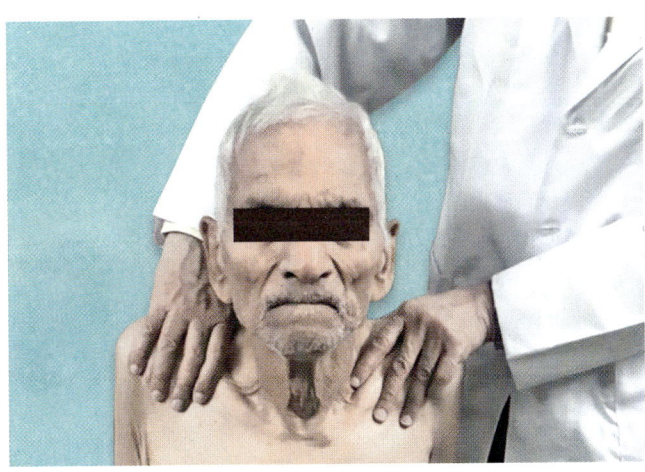

Fig. 4.5.22: Spinal accessory nerve testing.

Section 4: Clinical Examination

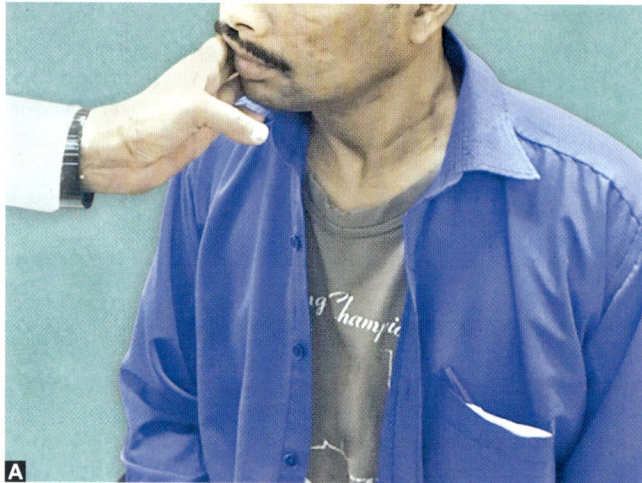

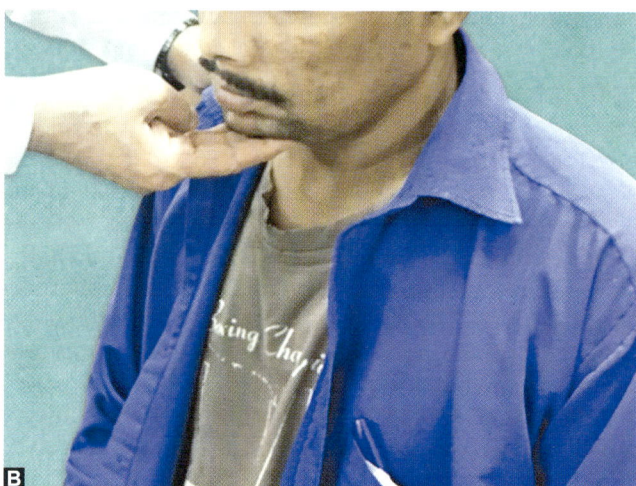

Figs. 4.5.23A and B: Sternomastoid muscle testing.

Objective Structured Clinical Examination–III

Aim: To test the 11th cranial nerve of the subject provided.
Procedural steps: See text above.
Checklist:
1. Ask the subject to sit comfortably and explain the procedure. (Y/N)
2. Stand behind the subject and place his/her hands on his/her shoulders. Then ask him/her to shrug his/her shoulders against his/her resistance. (Y/N)
3. Place his/her hand on the right side of the subject's face and asks him/her to rotate his/her head to the opposite side. Watch the left sternomastoid. (Y/N)
4. Repeat the procedure on the left side and ask him/her to rotate his/her head to the left and watch the right sternomastoid muscle. (Y/N)
5. Place his/her hand on the subject's forehead and ask him/her to bend his/her head forward against resistance. (Y/N)

QUESTION

Q.1. Test the spinal part of the accessory nerve in the subject provided.

HYPOGLOSSAL NERVE (12TH CRANIAL NERVE)

Origin: Medulla
Type: Motor

The motor fibers arise from the hypoglossal nucleus in the lower part of the floor of the 4th ventricle. The fibers innervate the muscles of the tongue and depressors of the hyoid bone. A few proprioceptive fibers from the tongue probably run in this nerve.

Test the hypoglossal nerve in the subject provided (Fig. 4.5.24):

- The subject is asked to push out his tongue as far as possible. Normally, it remains in the midline (genioglossus tested). If the 12th nerve is paralyzed, the tongue is pushed over to the side of the lesion by the healthy muscles on the opposite side. The affected side is also wasted, wrinkled and may show fasciculation, which indicates LMN lesion.
- The subject is asked to move the tongue from side to side over the lips and against the walls of the cheeks (extrinsic and intrinsic muscles of the tongue tested). A finger is placed against the cheek while the subject is asked to press against it with his tongue through the wall of the cheek. The strength of contraction is compared on the two sides.
- The subject is asked to touch the tongue to the palate (palatoglossus tested) and to depress the tongue in the floor of the mouth (hypoglossus tested).

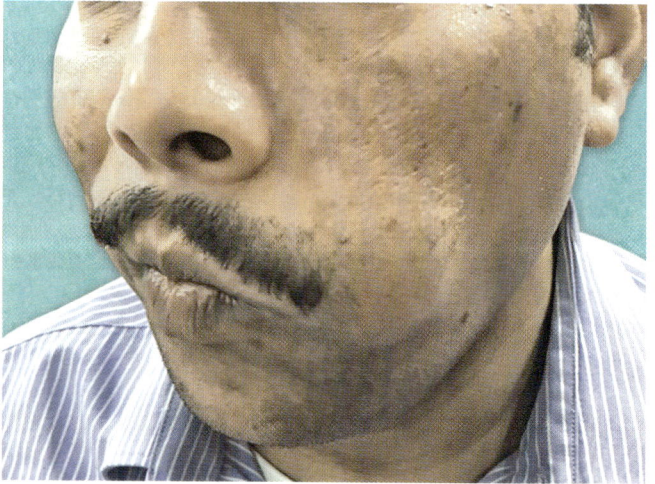

Fig. 4.5.24: Hypoglossal nerve testing.

> **Objective Structured Clinical Examination–IV**
>
> **Aim:** To test the 12th cranial nerve in the subject provides.
> **Procedural steps:** See text above.
> **Checklist:**
> 1. Explain the procedure to the subject. (Y/N)
> 2. Ask the subject to push out his/her tongue as far as possible, then inspect its position, evidence of wasting and fasciculation. (Y/N)
> 3. Ask the subject to move his/her tongue from side to side over the lips and against the walls of the cheeks. (Y/N)
> 4. Place his/her finger over the subject's cheek and ask him/her to push against it. Repeat on the opposite side. (Y/N)
> 5. Ask the subject to touch the tongue to the palate and then to depress it into the floor of the mouth. (Y/N)

QUESTION

Q.1. Test the hypoglossal nerve in the subject provided.

C: EXAMINATION OF THE MOTOR SYSTEM

AIM

To examine the motor system of the subject.

COMPONENTS

The motor system consists of (Fig. 4.5.25):
1. **Motor areas** of cerebral cortex, subcortical structures (basal ganglia, cerebellum, reticular formation, vestibular nuclei, etc.)
2. **Descending motor tracts:** Upper motor neurons (UMNs) and lower motor neurons (LMNs).
3. **Skeletal muscles:** The skeletal muscles can contract only in response to signals received from their motor nerves. The input to the motor neurons is through two sources:
   a. Dorsal nerve root fibers for muscle tone and reflexes.
   b. Descending motor tracts for voluntary movements and postural reflexes.

- During any movement, when the agonists contract the antagonists relax at the same time. This is achieved by **reciprocal innervation,** which is a spinal segmental mechanism.
- Every movement begins in a certain posture and ends in another posture. There is thus a continuous adjustment of posture by changes in muscle tone as movement progress.

Proximal group of muscles consists of axial muscles (hip, trunk and shoulders) and the proximal muscles of the limbs. They are mainly concerned in maintenance of posture, equilibrium and gross movements.

Distal group of muscles includes the muscles of the distal parts of the limbs (fingers, hands and wrists). They are not involved in posture and equilibrium but in voluntary, fine and skilled movements such as those during writing, typing, playing on a musical instrument, etc. (i.e. manipulative behavior).

Lower Motor Neurons

The anterior horn cells of the spinal cord and the motor cranial nuclei in the brainstem that directly innervate the skeletal muscle fibers are called LMN. Their axons leave the CNS via ventral roots (or motor cranial nerves) and eventually become the motor supply to the muscles. In the spinal cord, the most medially located motor neurons **(the medial motor system)** innervate the proximal group of muscles (for posture), while laterally located neurons **(the lateral motor system)** innervate the distal group of muscles (for fine skilled movements). The LMNs constitute the **"final common pathway"** for all motor signals that leave the CNS on their way to skeletal muscles.

Upper Motor Neurons

These fibers arise in the cortex and brainstem. They activate the LMNs. **Traditionally,** the descending motor fibers are classified into **pyramidal** and **extrapyramidal.**

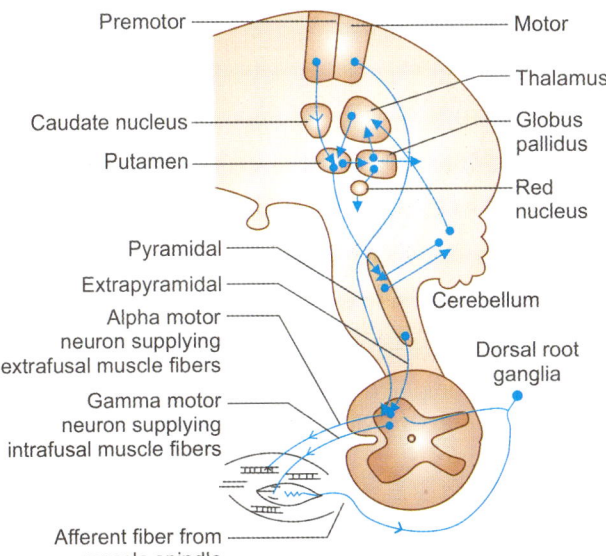

Fig. 4.5.25: Components of the motor system.

Pyramidal Tract

The **pyramidal tract (corticospinal)** includes all fibers (irrespective of their site of origin) descending in the pyramids of the medulla. In lower medulla, majority of the fibers cross over to the other side to descend as the **lateral (crossed) corticospinal–pyramidal system** in the lateral funiculus of the cord to end on the LMN. Only about 3% of the fibers remain on the same side and descend as **the anterior (uncrossed) corticospinal-pyramidal system** to finally end on the LMN.

While the *lesions of LMN* cause flaccid paralysis, muscle atrophy and absence of deep (stretch) reflexes, the *lesions of UMN* cause spastic paralysis and exaggerated deep reflexes without muscle atrophy. However, there are three types of UMN to consider because:

1. Lesions in many of the posture regulating pathways produce spastic paralysis.
2. Lesions in corticospinal and corticobulbar fibers cause weakness (paresis) rather than paralysis and the affected musculature is generally hypotonic.
3. Cerebellar lesions cause incoordination.

"Extrapyramidal" System

It is a widely used term for those tracts (from basal ganglia, etc.) that indirectly control LMN but are not part of direct corticospinal–pyramidal system. This term is now being less frequently used clinically and physiologically.

The motor pathways can also be classified based on their sites of termination in the spinal cord.

1. **The lateral motor system:** The lateral corticospinal (crossed pyramidal) tract plus rubrospinal tract that lies anterior to it, make up the lateral motor system that controls the distal groups of muscles concerned with fine, skilled movement. The red nucleus thus functions in close association with the lateral corticospinal tract. This pathway terminates in the lateral portions of the gray matter of the spinal cord.
2. **The medial motor system:** It includes ventral (anterior) corticospinal (uncrossed pyramidal) tract plus the medially located descending tracts from the brainstem (vestibulo, reticulo, olivo, tectospinal tracts). This system controls the proximal group of muscles (described above) for posture and gross movements. This system ends in the medial ventral horn.

TESTING THE MOTOR FUNCTIONS

This is done under the following headings:
- Bulk of muscle (Fig. 4.5.26)
- Muscle tone
- Power or strength

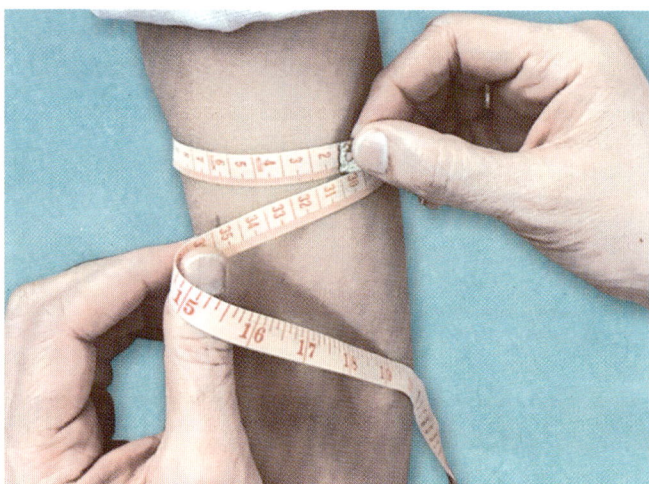

Fig. 4.5.26: Testing bulk of muscle.

- Coordination of muscular activity
- Reflexes
- Presence of involuntary movements
- Gait.

Bulk of Muscles

- This can be easily estimated by inspection and palpation.
- The examination can be done in sitting or lying position after removal of his clothing.
- Inspect the muscle bulk of all parts of the body.
- Note if there is any wasting (atrophy) or increased mass (hypertrophy) in any group of muscles.
- Measure the mid-arm and mid-forearm circumference in the upper limb and mid-thigh and mid-calf circumference in the lower limbs of both sides with a measuring tape.
- Compare the measurements on both the sides.
- The **muscle mass decreases** in muscular atrophy (the muscles are smaller and softer), which may be generalized or localized. It may result from cachexia, disuse (prolonged confinement to bed or when a limb is kept in a plaster cast) or as a consequence of LMN disease. The muscle wasting associated with fibrosis is called contracture.
- The *muscle mass increases* (hypertrophy) with physical exercise and in certain occupations requiring excessive workload. In certain diseases of muscles—dystrophy and pseudohypertrophy, though the muscle bulk is increased, they are weak.

Muscle Tone

Clinically, it is defined as the resistance felt when a joint is moved passively through its range of movement.

Physiologically, it is a state of partial contraction of skeletal muscles due to low frequency asynchronous discharge of motor neuron. This results in continuously maintained state of slight tension or tautness in the healthy muscles even when they appear to be at rest. Though muscle tone is due to a spinal reflex mechanism, it is mainly regulated by supraspinal pathways—the pyramidal (corticospinal) and extrapyramidal tracts. The anterior cerebellum, via the subcortical structures, has a facilitatory effect on muscle tone.

- An increase in tone is called **hypertonia**. This occurs in lesions of UMN.
  - *Spasticity:* The term refers to hypertonia resulting from lesions of the corticospinal system. The increased tone is of **clasp-knife type**, i.e. when the limb is moved, maximum resistance is offered at once, but it suddenly gives way after some effort on the part of the examiner. Spasticity is therefore a form of rigidity, which is sensitive to stretch, i.e. **"stretch-sensitive"**. It is usually maximum in flexors of the arms and extensors of the legs.
  - *Rigidity:* The hypertonia of rigidity results from diseases of the basal ganglia (e.g. Parkinsonism) and is called extrapyramidal rigidity. It may be of **"cogwheel"** type in which the resistance to passive movement decreases in jerky steps (probably a combination of tremor and rigidity) or of **"lead pipe"** type in which resistance is felt throughout the passive movement. The rigidity of Parkinsonism is commonly accompanied by akinesia, i.e. poverty of movement.
- Decrease in tone is called **hypotonia**. It is seen in LMN disease and cerebellar lesions. Passive movement is unusually free and frequently through a greater range than normal.
- Complete loss of muscle tone is known as **atonia**.

> **NOTE**
> From the time of early growth, the bones grow longer at a rate faster than that of muscles. This maintains a slight stretch on the muscles and therefore, on the spindles, throughout the lifetime of an individual, so that the muscles remain in a state of tone.

Procedure

- The examiner holds the forearm of the subject with one hand and alternately flexes and extends the wrist with the other hand.
- Tone at the fingers, elbow and shoulder is tested in a similar manner (Fig. 4.5.27).
- In the lower limbs, passive movements are done at the ankle, knee and hip.
- The ease or difficulty with which a joint can thus be moved is noted and compared with the similar joint on the opposite side.

In hypertonia, the patient's muscles resist the passive movements, while in hypotonia the movements become free and the joints can be hyperextended.

Strength/Power of Muscles

The muscle power is estimated by asking the subject to perform a movement of any part of the body against resistance of the examiner's hand and then compare with same group of muscles on the opposite side (Fig. 4.5.28).

Testing the Muscle Strength in the Upper Limbs of the Subject Provided

- **Abductor pollicis brevis:** The subject is asked to abduct his thumb in a plane at right angles to the palmar aspect of the index finger, against the resistance of the examiner's own thumb. The muscle can be seen and felt to contract. This muscle is supplied by the median

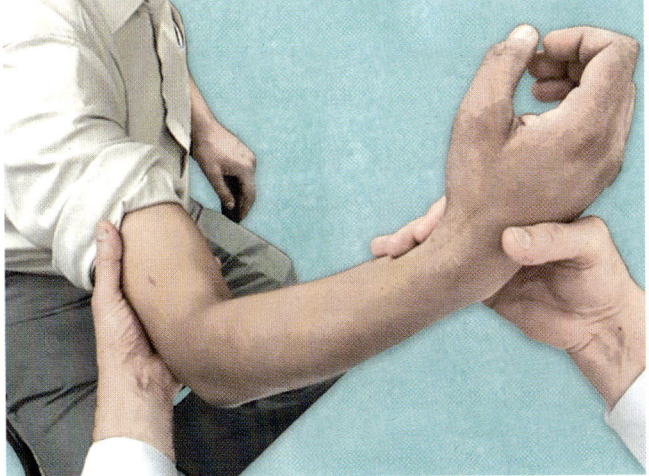

Fig. 4.5.27: Testing for muscle tone in upper limb.

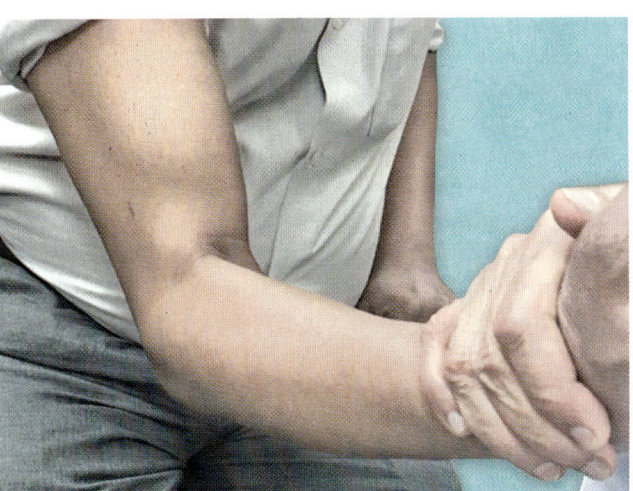

Fig. 4.5.28: Testing of muscle power in upper limb.

nerve, which is sometimes damaged by compression in the carpal tunnel at the wrist (carpal tunnel syndrome).
- **Opponens pollicis:** The subject is asked to touch the tips of all his fingers with the tip of his thumb. The examiner opposes each movement with his index finger or thumb.
- **First dorsal interosseous:** The subject is asked to abduct his index finger against resistance.
- **Other interossei and lumbricals:** The subject's ability to flex his metacarpophalangeal joints and to extend the distal interphalangeal joints is tested. The interossei also adduct and abduct the fingers.
- **Flexors of fingers:** The subject is asked to squeeze the examiner's index and middle fingers to assess the force of grip.
- **Flexors of the wrist:** The subject is asked to bring his fingers toward the front of the forearm, while the examiner opposes this movement with his fingers.
- **Extensors of the wrist:** The subject is asked to make a fist (both flexors and extensors contract), while the examiner tries to flex the wrist against the subject's effort to maintain that position.
- **Brachioradialis:** The subject's arm is placed midway between pronation and supination and then asked to bend the forearm up, while the examiner opposes this movement by grasping the subject's hand. The muscle can be seen and felt to stand out in its upper part.
- **Biceps:** The subject is asked to bend up the forearm against resistance in full supination. The muscle stands out clearly.
- **Triceps:** The subject is asked to straighten out his forearm against resistance.
- **Supraspinatus:** The subject is asked to lift his arm straight out at right angles to his side. The first 30° of this movement is brought about by supraspinatus and the rest 60° is carried out by the deltoid.
- **Deltoid:** The arm is held out, in abduction, straight out.
- The subject offers resistance, while the examiner tries to depress the elbow. The anterior and posterior fibers help to draw the abducted arm forward and backward, which can also be tested against resistance.
- **Infraspinatus:** With the forearm flexed to a right angle, the subject is asked to tuck his elbow into his side. Then he is asked to rotate the limb outward against resistance.
- **Pectorals:** The subject is asked to stretch the arms out in front of him and then to clasp his hands while the examiner tries to hold them apart.
- **Serratus anterior:** The subject is asked to push forward with his hands against resistance, such as a wall. When this muscle is paralyzed, the scapula is "winged".
- **Latissimus dorsi:** The subject is asked to clasp his hands behind his back while the examiner, standing behind the subject offers resistance to downward and backward movement. When the subject is asked to cough, the two posterior axillary folds can be felt by the examiner.

Testing the Muscle Strength in the Lower Limbs

- **Plantar flexion and dorsiflexion of the toes and the ankle:** These are tested by asking the subject to perform these movements against resistance.
- **Extensors of the knee:** The subject's knee is bent and while the examiner presses against his shin, the subject is asked to straighten out the leg again.
- **Flexors of the knee:** The subject's leg is raised up from the bed and while the examiner supports the thigh with one hand and holding the ankle with the other hand, the subject is asked to flex the knee joint.
- **Extensors of the hip:** With his knee extended, the subject lifts the foot from the bed and is asked to push it down against resistance.
- **Flexors of the thigh:** With his leg extended, the subject is asked to raise the leg off the bed against resistance.
- **Abductors of the thigh:** The subject's legs are placed together and he is asked to separate them against resistance.
- **Adductors of the thigh:** The limb is abducted and then the subject is asked to bring it back toward the midline against resistance.
- **Rotators of the thigh:** With the limb extended and resting on the bed, the subject is asked to roll it outward or inward against resistance.

Testing the Muscles of the Trunk

- The subject is asked to sit up in bed from the supine position without the help of his arms (abdominal muscles tested).
- The subject lies on his face and tries to raise his head by extending the neck and back. The muscles can be seen to become prominent (extensors of the back tested).

Grading of Muscle Power

The muscle strength is graded in Table 4.5.1.

Coordination of Muscular Activity

- The term coordination refers to the smooth recruitment, interaction and cooperation of groups of muscles in order to perform a definite motor task.
- The coordination of muscle movement depends on:
  - Intact cerebellum and its tracts
  - The afferent information coming from the joint and muscle receptors
  - Integrity of dorsal column
  - The state of muscle tone
- If coordination of movements becomes impaired, the carrying out of motor activities becomes difficult and sometimes even impossible.

Table 4.5.1: Grading of muscle weakness.	
Grade 0	Complete paralysis
Grade 1	A flicker of contraction only
Grade 2	Muscle power is detected only when gravity is excluded by suitable postural adjustment
Grade 3	The limb can be held against the force of gravity, but not against examiner's resistance
Grade 4	Some degree of weakness is there, which is commonly described as poor, moderate or fair strength, i.e. movements are possible against the examiner's resistance but are weak
Grade 5	The muscle power is normal both without load and against the examiner's resistance

Tests for Coordination

In the upper limbs

1. *"Finger–nose" test:* The subject is asked to extend his arm to the side and then touch the tip of his nose with the tip of his index finger, first with the eyes open and then with the eyes closed. The other limb is tested similarly. A normal subject is able to perform these acts accurately, both slowly and rapidly.
2. The subject is asked to touch his each finger in turn with the tip of the thumb.
3. The subject is asked to draw a large circle in the air with his forefinger.
4. The subject is asked to alternately pronate and supinate his forearms as rapidly as possible. An inability to perform such rapid movements is called **dysdiadochokinesia**. It is an important sign of cerebellar disease where the movements on the affected side become very clumsy or even impossible to carry out.
5. Watching a patient dressing or undressing, picking up pins from a table, handling a book, etc. can provide useful information about muscle coordination.

In the lower limbs

1. The subject is asked to walk along a straight line. The examiner watches carefully as the subject turns to walk back. The subject may also be asked to walk along a line, placing the heel of one foot immediately adjacent to the toes of the foot behind **(tandem walking)**. If incoordination is present, the subject soon deviates to one or the other side and takes a zigzag course like that of a drunk.
2. *"Heel-shin" test:* The subject lies on his back and is asked to lift one foot high in the air, to place its heel on the opposite knee and then to slide the heel down the leg along the shin toward the ankle. The test is done first with the eyes open and then with eyes closed and it is repeated on the other side.
3. The subject is asked to draw a large circle in the air with his toe.

4. **Romberg's sign:** This sign is a test for the **loss of position sense** (sensory ataxia). It is not a test for cerebellar function. The subject is asked to stand with the feet as close together as possible and if he can do it, which a normal person can, he is asked to close his eyes. A normal person can do so with ease.

   However, if the Romberg's sign is present, the patient starts to sway from side to side as soon as he closes his eye. Thus, the patient is more unsteady when his eyes are closed than when his eyes are open.
- In **sensory ataxia** (lesion of dorsal columns of cord or dorsal roots, as in tabes dorsalis) the sensory information from the legs is lacking; therefore, the patient becomes unsteady without the help of vision.
- In **cerebellar ataxia**, the patient is unsteady on his feet whether the eyes are open or closed.

Reflexes

See Chapter 4.5D.

Presence of Involuntary Movements

Note whether the involuntary movements are localized or generalized.

1. **Localized involuntary movements:** These include:
   - *Fibrillation:* They are due to contraction of a single muscle fiber. Usually, they cannot be seen though they can be recorded as electromyography (EMG).
   - *Fasciculation:* These are due to contraction of one or more motor units and are visible on the skin.
   - *Myoclonus:* It is a sudden shocklike contraction of a single muscle or a group of muscles.
   - *Tremor:* It is an involuntary, regular, rhythmic and purposeless movement due to alternate contraction and relaxation of agonists and antagonists. Note whether **they are present at rest or during motor activity.**
     - Fine tremor is seen in anxiety and hyperthyroidism.
     - Coarse tremor is seen in Parkinson's disease, cerebellar lesions, alcoholism, barbiturate and heavy metal poisoning.
2. **Generalized involuntary movements:**
   - *Chorea:* These involuntary movements, seen in degeneration of caudate nucleus, are jerky, rapid, irregular and unpredictable.
   - *Athetosis:* These involuntary movements are relatively slow, writhing contractions of arms. They are sometimes combined with choreiform movements.
   - *Ballism:* These movements are flinging, intense and violent, usually involving peripheral parts of limbs. The lesion is in the nucleus of Luys.
   - *Tics:* These are sudden, rapid, repeated movements, usually in the form of blinking of eyes or wriggling of shoulders.

Section 4: Clinical Examination

- *Epilepsy:* Grand mal epilepsy (generalized) is characterized by tonic-clonic convulsions and loss of consciousness which occur without warning. Any exaggerated and involuntary muscle contraction is referred as **spasm**. If the contraction is continuous, it is called **tonic contraction**. If there is a series of short contractions with partial or complete relaxations in between, it is called **clonic contraction**.

Gait

The term "gait" refers to the manner, style or pattern of walking. Before examination one should ensure that the legs are adequately exposed and the feet are bare. The patient is asked to walk freely across the room and then along a straight line considering the following points:
- Whether the patient is able to walk or not.
- Does he need any assistance?
- Can he walk along the straight line?
- Is there any tendency to fall if yes, in what direction?
- Whether he is able to take a quick turn without unbalancing.

Some forms of abnormal gait are:
1. **Spastic (hemiplegic) gait:** The patient walks on a narrow base. Since the knee cannot be flexed and the foot properly lifted off the ground, he drags his foot on the ground and tends to describe a semicircle with the affected leg, the toes scraping the ground. If spasticity is present on both the sides the patient walks in a typical criss-cross fashion. This is known as **scissor gait.** It is seen in **congenital spastic paraplegia.**
2. **Stamping gait:** The patient raises each foot suddenly and brings it down on the ground with a thump. It is seen in **sensory ataxia** (e.g. tabes dorsalis). He may be quite steady as long as he can see the ground and the position of his feet. **High stepping gait** when there is common peroneal nerve palsy leading to weakness of the extensor
3. **Drunken or reeling gait:** This ataxic gait is seen in **cerebellar lesions**, the patient walks on a broad base, with the feet apart. The gait is clumsy and zigzagging like the gait of a drunkard. The ataxia is equally severe whether the eyes are closed or open.
4. **Festinant gait:** This is seen in **Parkinson's disease**. Walking is usually slow and the patient takes short and shuffling steps. Sometimes, there is an uncontrolled acceleration while walking, a process called festinant gait. When gently pushed forward, the patient may be unable to stop as he chases his own center of gravity (propulsion). Similarly, when pushed back, he is unable to stop (retropulsion).
5. **Waddling Gait:** The patient walks like gait of a duck. The patient sways from side to side, the body is tilted backward with an increase of lumbar lordosis with a protuberant abdomen. Thus, there is difficulty in maintaining trunk and pelvic posture. The feet are plated widely apart and the heels and toes tend to be brought down simultaneously. This is typically seen in patients with proximal pelvic girdle muscular weakness.

Objective Structured Clinical Examination–I

Aim: To assess the muscle tone in the upper limb of the subject provided.
Procedural steps: See text above
Checklist:
1. Explain the procedure to the subject and seat him comfortably. (Y/N)
2. Hold the forearm of the subject and alternately flex and extend his wrist with her other hand. (Y/N)
3. Perform similar passive movements at the fingers, elbow and shoulder. (Y/N)
4. Compare the muscle tone on the opposite side by passive movements. (Y/N)
5. Note down the results. (Y/N)

Objective Structured Clinical Examination–II

Aim: To assess the muscle strength in the right upper limb of the subject provided.
Procedural steps: See text above
Checklist:
1. Explain the procedure to the subject. (Y/N)
2. Ask the subject to shake her hand with full force and then to cause active movements of the fingers and wrist against resistance. (Y/N)
3. Ask the subject to flex and extend the elbow against resistance and watch the prominence of biceps and triceps. (Y/N)
4. Ask the subject to move his shoulder in different directions against resistance. (Y/N)
5. Compare the strength of identical muscles on the opposite side. (Y/N)

QUESTIONS

Q.1. Test the state of nutrition in the upper and lower limbs of the subject provided.
Q.2. Test the tone of the muscles in the upper limbs.
Q.3. Test the muscle strength in the upper limbs of the subject provided.
Q.4. Test the muscle strength in the lower limbs.
Q.5. How is muscle strength graded?
Q.6. Test the muscular coordination in the upper limbs of the subject provided.
Q.7. Test the muscle coordination in the lower limbs.
Q.8. Test the subject provided for Romberg's sign.
Q.9. Perform any three cerebellar function tests in the subject provided.
Q.10. Perform the motor system examination of the given subject and note down the observation in a tabular form.

D: REFLEXES

AIM

To assess the reflexes of the subject.

DEFINITION

A **reflex** or **reflex action** is an involuntary contraction of a muscle or a group of muscles in response to a specific stimulus and which depends on the integrity of the reflex pathway.

Clinically, reflexes are of three types:
1. Superficial reflexes
2. Deep tendon reflexes
3. Visceral reflexes.

SUPERFICIAL REFLEXES

These are polysynaptic reflexes, which are evoked by cutaneous stimulations. These include:
- Superficial reflexes of **spinal origin**: These include plantar reflex, superficial abdominal reflexes, scapular reflex, cremasteric reflex, anal reflex and bulbocavernosus reflex.
- Superficial reflexes of **cranial origin**: These include conjunctival reflex, corneal reflex, papillary light reflex, accommodation reflex and palatal reflex.

Response: In all the superficial reflexes, there is contraction of the underlying muscles when a particular area of the skin is stimulated by touching, scratching, stroking or pinching.

Reflex arcs: The reflex arcs for the skin reflexes are **polysynaptic** as they include a number of interneurons between the sensory and the motor neurons of the reflex arc. The afferent impulses are carried up by dorsal columns and spinothalamic tracts and end in the midbrain, thalamus or cerebral cortex. From here, impulses are carried by corticospinal and extrapyramidal tracts to the anterior horn cells innervating the muscles involved in the reflex. This is the reason why the **superficial reflexes are absent in the upper motor neurons (UMN) lesions**.

Plantar Reflex

Assessment of plantar reflex:
- The subject is asked to relax the muscles of the lower limb.
- A light scratch is given with a key or blunt point of the patellar hammer along the **outer edge of the sole of the foot, from the heel toward the little toe and then medially along the base of the toes up to the 2nd toe** (Fig. 4.5.29).

Response:
- With adequate stimulus, there is plantar flexion and drawing together of the toes, often including the big toe.
- Dorsiflexion and inversion of the ankle and sometimes contraction of the tensor fascia lata also may be seen.
- With stronger stimuli, the limb may be withdrawn (flexed at the knee and hip) and adducted at the hip. This is the normal response in the adults and is called the **flexor plantar reflex**.
- In healthy subjects, the plantar reflex is never completely absent.

Spinal segments involved: L5, S1

Extensor plantar reflex: In lesions of corticospinal tract (UMN lesions), there is **extensor plantar response** in which dorsiflexion (extension) of the great toe precedes all other movement. This is followed by spreading (fanning) out and extension of the other toes, followed by dorsiflexion of the ankle and flexion of the hip and the knee. This is called as **Babinski's sign.**

In some cases with Babinski sign, the reflexogenic area (i.e. the region from which it is obtained) spreads out over a large area so that the same response is obtained by squeezing the calf muscles by a firm downward movement over anterior tibia (**Oppenheim's sign**), by pinching the Achilles tendon (**Gordon's reflex**) or by stroking the lateral malleolus (**Chaddock's sign**). [The clawing movement of the fingers and the thumb upon flicking the terminal phalanx of the index finger is called the **Hoffmann's sign** (the equivalent of Babinski in the upper limb)].

Physioclinical significance: The Babinski's sign is a very important sign in clinical neurology. It has great significance in differentiating between an organic lesion

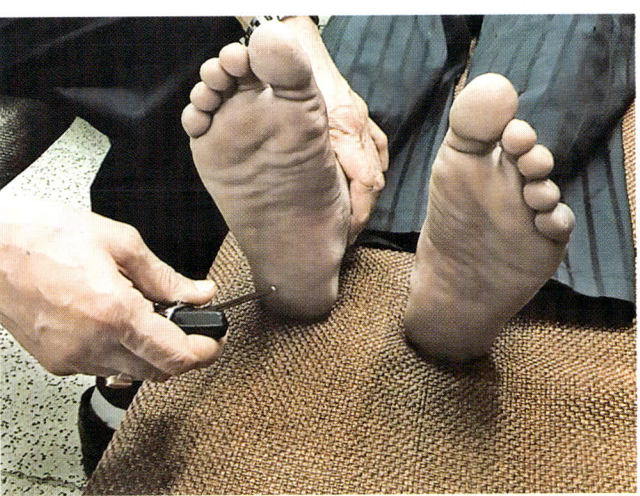

Fig. 4.5.29: Plantar reflex.

and a functional disorder (e.g. psychoneurosis) because it never occurs in the latter conditions.

Babinski's sign is seen in the following:
- Infants below the age of 1 year, i.e. until the corticospinal tracts get myelinated and become functional. The plantar response becomes flexor in the next 6–8 months when the child learns to walk.
- Upper motor neuron (corticospinal or pyramidal) lesions such as cerebral vascular disease (e.g. capsular hemiplegia), disseminated sclerosis, etc.
- Deep narcosis, coma due to any cause and following an attack of grand mal epilepsy when the patient becomes unconscious (It is temporary in some forms of coma and after epileptic fits).
- Biochemical disturbances, such as hypoglycemia, in which convulsions may occur.

Abdominal Reflex

Assessment of the reflex:
- The subject should be relaxed and in supine position with the abdomen uncovered.
- A light but brisk stroke, with a key or blunt point, is given across the abdominal skin, directed toward the umbilicus from the outer aspect, in the upper, middle and lower regions.

Response: The response is a brisk ripple of contraction of the underlying muscles.
Spinal segments involved: T7-T12.
These reflexes are absent in UMN lesions above their segmental level in the spinal cord.

Ciliospinal Reflex

See Table 4.5.2 for description.

> **NOTE**
> Loss of is ciliospinal reflex used as a measure of depth of coma; it is also one of the criteria of brain death.

DEEP TENDON REFLEXES/STRETCH REFLEX

Sudden stretching of the muscle spindles (receptor organ) sends a synchronous volley of impulses from the primary sensory endings into the spinal cord. In the cord, these impulses directly (**monosynaptically**) stimulate the anterior horn cells, which innervate the stretched muscle. Thus these reflexes are monosynaptic stretch reflexes.
Patellar (knee) hammer (Fig. 4.5.30): It has a long metallic handle that bears a triangular rubber piece. The rubber is employed for delivering a sharp blow on the tendon of a slightly stretched muscle. The sudden stretch of the muscle causes a reflex contraction of the muscle.

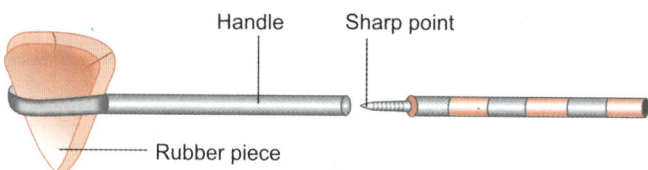

Fig. 4.5.30: Patellar (knee) hammer.

- While using it, the hammer should be held between the thumb and fingers and the **swing should be at the wrist** and not at the elbow or shoulder.
- The upper part of the hammer, which can be unscrewed, has a sharp point for eliciting superficial reflexes.

Biceps Reflex

Assessment of biceps reflex:
- The subject's elbow is flexed to a right angle and the forearm semipronated and supported on the examiner's arm.
- The examiner then places his thumb on the biceps tendon and strikes it with the knee hammer (Fig. 4.5.31).

Response: The response is contraction of the biceps causing flexion and slight pronation of the forearm (if the patient is in bed, his forearm may rest across his chest).
Spinal segments involved: C5, C6.

Triceps Reflex

Assessment of triceps reflex:
- The arm is flexed to a right angle and is supported on the examiner's arm.
- The triceps tendon is then struck with the knee hammer just proximal to the point of the elbow (Fig. 4.5.32).

Response: The response is extension at the elbow.
Spinal segments involved: C6, C7.

Supinator or Brachioradialis Reflex

Assessment of supinator reflex:
- The arm is placed to a right angle and the forearm placed midway between pronation and supination.
- Strike the styloid process of the radius with the help of a knee hammer.

Response: There is flexion at the elbow and supination of the forearm (**Fig. 4.5.33**).
Spinal segments involved: C5/C6.

Knee Reflex

1. **Assessment of knee reflex in supine position:**
   - The subject is asked to relax his legs and is reassured that the patellar hammer will not cause injury. His legs are semiflexed and the observer supports both knees by placing a hand behind them.

Table 4.5.2: Summary of reflexes tested clinically.

Reflexes	How to elicit	Response	Spinal segments involved
1. Superficial reflexes			
a. Superficial reflexes of spinal origin			
• Plantar	Gently scratch using a key or blunt point of the patellar hammer along the outer edge of the sole of the foot, from the heel toward the little toe and then medially along the base of the toes up to the 2nd toe	Plantar flexion of toes (For details see above)	L5, S1
• Abdominal	Scratch on abdominal wall	Contraction of the abdominal muscles	T7-T12
• Scapular	Stroking skin in interscapular region	Contraction of scapular muscles	C5-T1
• Cremasteric	Stroke the skin of the upper medial thigh	Drawing upward of the testicle	L1, L2
• Anal	Scratch on skin near anus	Contraction of anal sphincter	S3, S4
• Bulbocavernosus	Pinching dorsum of glans penis	Contraction of bulbocavernosus	S3, S4
• Ciliospinal	Pinching of skin on back of neck	Dilatation of pupil	T1, T2
b. Superficial reflexes of cranial origin			
• Corneal or conjunctival	Touch lateral edge of cornea or conjunctiva with cotton	Closure of eye	Afferent—V nerve Efferent—VII nerve
• Pharyngeal	Touch on pharynx	Constriction of pharynx	Afferent—IX nerve Efferent—X nerve
• Palatal	Touch on soft palate	Elevation of palate	Afferent—IX nerve Efferent—X nerve
• Pupillary light reflex	Shining of light on retina in one eye	Constriction of pupil on that side	Afferent—II nerve Efferent—III nerve
• Accommodation reflex	Subject looks on finger held in front of one eye	Constriction of pupil in that eye	Afferent—II nerve Efferent—III nerve
2. Deep Tendon Reflexes			
• Biceps reflex	Tapping on biceps tendon with the patellar hammer (pointed end)	Flexion at elbow	C5, C6
• Triceps reflex	Tapping on triceps tendon with the patellar hammer (broad end)	Extension at elbow	C6, C7
• Supinator reflex	Tapping on styloid process of radius	Flexion and supination of forearm	C5/C6
• Knee reflex	Tapping on patellar tendon	Extension at knee	L2, L3, L4
• Ankle reflex	Tapping on Achilles tendon	Planter flexion of foot	S1, S2
• Jaw reflex	Tapping on middle of jaw	Closure of mouth	C5

3. Visceral or Sphincter Reflexes

These reflexes include swallowing, micturition and defecation. They depend upon complex muscular movement excited by increased tension in the wall of the viscera concerned.
- Swallowing: The subject is asked whether he has any difficulty in swallowing (dysphagia). If present, ask him whether he has difficulty in swallowing liquids or solids. As a rule patients with neurological disorders causing dysphagia complain of difficulty in swallowing liquids, whereas in mechanical esophageal obstruction they find difficulty in swallowing solids.
- Defecation: The patient should be asked, if he has any difficulty in passing stools. He should also be asked whether he can feel rectal sensation.
- Micturition: The subject should be asked whether he has any difficulty in controlling or initiating micturition. He should also be questioned for retention and incontinence of urine.

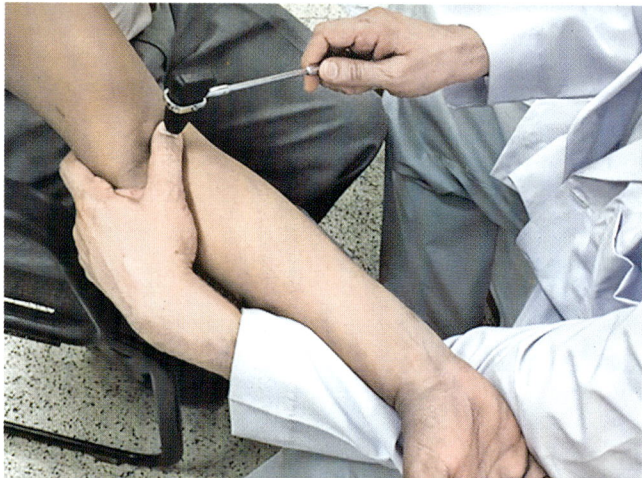

Fig. 4.5.31: Biceps reflex.

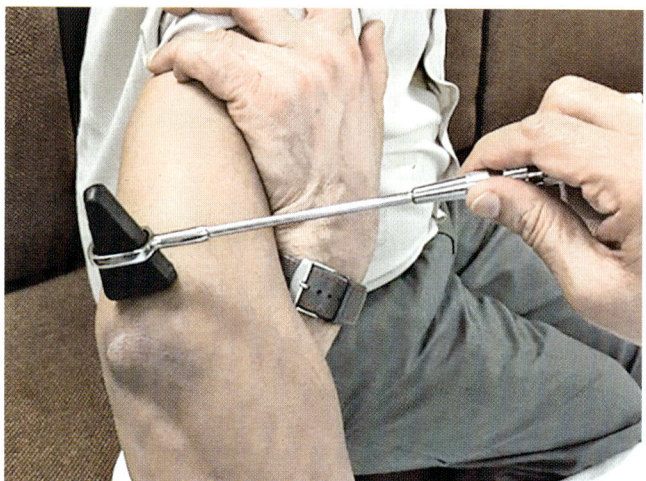

Fig. 4.5.32: Triceps reflex.

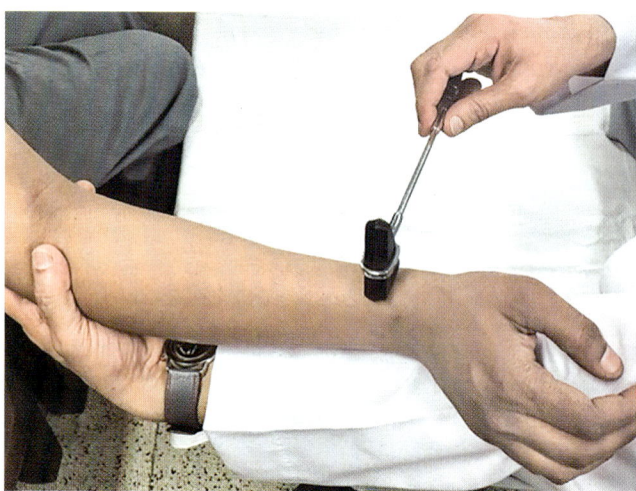

Fig. 4.5.33: Supinator reflex.

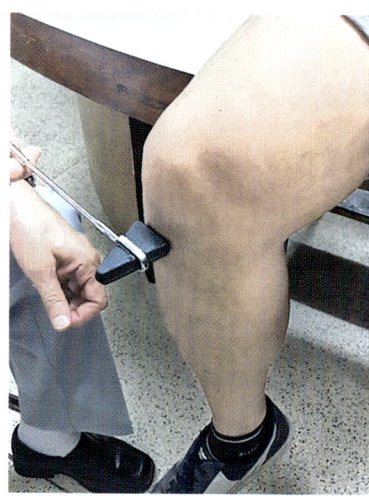

Fig. 4.5.34: Knee reflex in sitting position.

- The patellar tendon is then struck midway between the patella and the insertion of the tendon on the tibial tuberosity (The tendon is located by palpation before striking it).

Response: Extension of the knee due to contraction of the quadriceps femoris muscle.

Spinal segments involved: L2, L3, L4.

2. **Assessment of knee reflex in sitting position:**
    - The subject is seated in a chair and is asked to cross one leg over the other and then the reflex is elicited as discussed above.
    - A better way to elicit this reflex is to ask the subject to sit with both legs swinging loosely over the edge of the chair. It permits a more rapid comparison of the two knee reflexes.

Response: The leg can be seen to kick forward; the muscle can also be felt to contract, if the observer places his hand on the lower front of the thigh (Fig. 4.5.34).

The knee reflex may be pendular in acute cerebellar disease.

Ankle Reflex

Assessment of ankle reflex:
- The subject lies supine, the knee is semiflexed and the hip externally rotated.
- Then with one hand, the examiner slightly dorsiflexes the foot so as to stretch the Achilles tendon (tendo-calcaneus) and with the other hand, the Achilles tendon is struck on its posterior surface by knee hammer.
- Another method is to ask the subject to kneel over a chair, so that he faces the back of the chair and his ankles lie, over its edge. The ankle reflexes are then tested as described above.

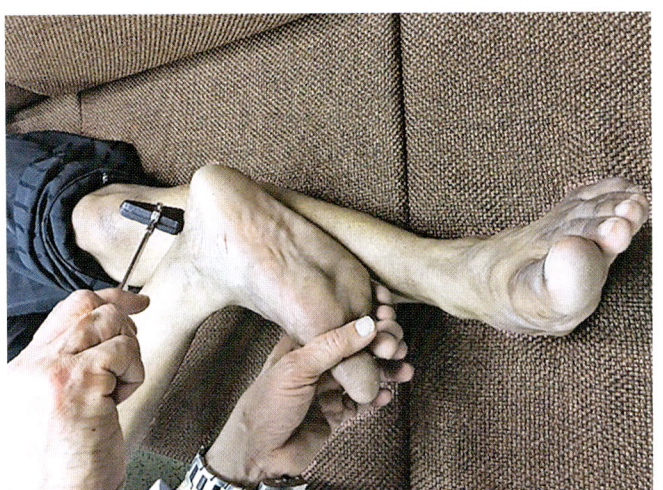

Fig. 4.5.35: Ankle reflex in supine position.

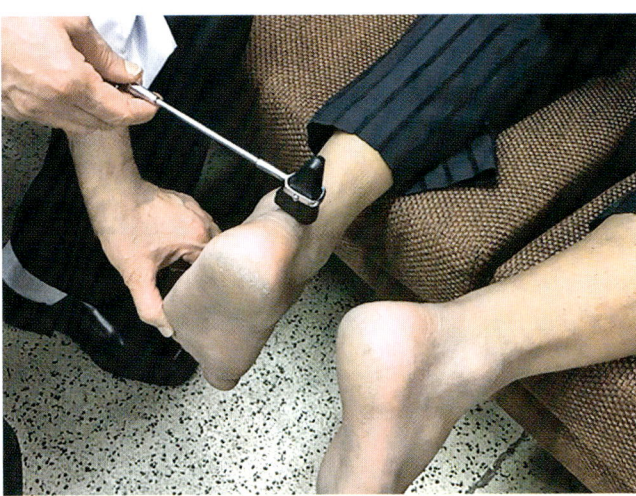

Fig. 4.5.36: Ankle reflex in kneeling down position.

Response: Plantar flexion of the foot due to contraction of the calf muscles (Figs. 4.5.35 and 4.5.36).
Spinal segments involved: S1, S2

Jaw Reflex

Assessment of jaw reflex:
- Place one finger firmly on the chin with the mouth open and tap it suddenly with the other hand as in percussion (Fig. 4.5.37).

Response: Closure of the mouth.

Normally, this reflex is hardly detectable, but it is exaggerated in UMN lesions (as are other deep reflexes).

Both the afferent and efferent paths are along 5th nerve and the center is in the pons.

REINFORCEMENT OF REFLEXES

- The briskness of knee reflex (and other deep reflexes) varies greatly from person to person, but it is hardly ever absent in health. Occasionally, it may be very weak or even appear to be absent. In such cases, **reinforcement (Jendrassik maneuver)** is employed (Fig. 4.5.38).
- This is done by asking the subject to perform some strong muscular effort, such as clenching the teeth or locking the fingers of both hands as hard as possible and then trying to pull them apart while the examiner strikes the patellar tendon. The reflex generally becomes evident.
- Reinforcement acts by increasing the excitability of the anterior horn cells and by increasing the sensitivity of the muscle spindles primary sensor endings to stretch. This is made possible by increasing the gamma motor neuron discharge. It also, perhaps, acts by distracting the subject's attention.

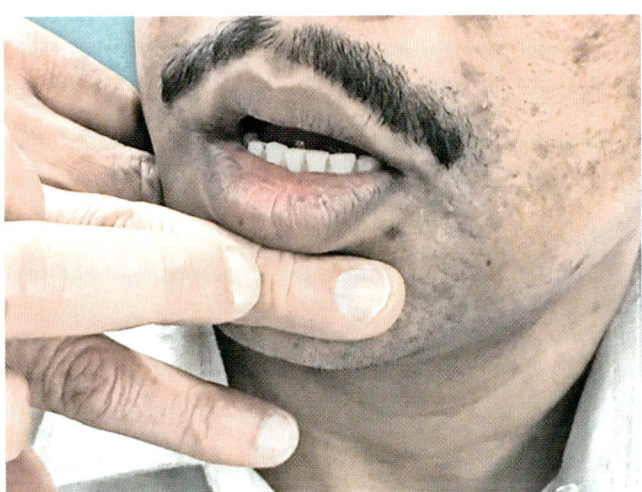

Fig. 4.5.37: Jaw reflex.

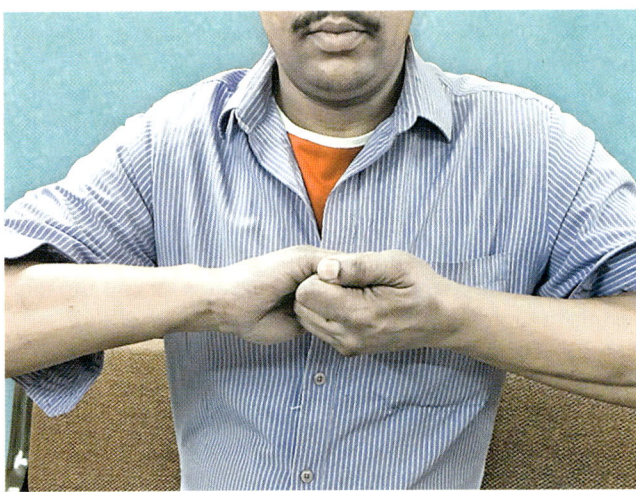

Fig. 4.5.38: Jendrassik's maneuver.

PHYSIOCLINICAL SIGNIFICANCE OF DEEP TENDON REFLEXES

1. **Deep tendon reflexes are diminished or absent in the following conditions:**
   - Lesions involving the afferent pathways (e.g. tabes dorsalis).
   - Lesions of the anterior horn cells (e.g. poliomyelitis) or the efferent pathways.
   - In peripheral neuropathies or peripheral nerve injuries, both sensory and motor fibers are affected.
   - The tendon reflexes are also abolished during spinal shock, e.g. severe injury to the cord (In fact, all motor and sensory functions are lost below the site of lesion for the duration of the spinal shock).
   - Tendon reflexes are also lost bilaterally in coma.

   As mentioned earlier, the deep reflexes may be sluggish or appear to be abolished in some healthy individuals; reinforcement is employed in these cases.

2. **Deep tendon reflexes are exaggerated (hyperreflexia) in the following conditions:**
   - Upper motor neurons lesion.
   - Anxiety or nervousness.
   - Hyperexcitability of the nervous system, as in hyperthyroidism and tetanus.

   The cause of exaggeration of deep reflexes in lesions of corticospinal system is the hypertonia (spasticity) resulting from overactivity of the stretch reflexes; this system keeps these reflexes under check. When this inhibition is lost, the deep reflexes are more easily elicited. Exaggeration of reflexes is thus a "release" phenomenon—as is the Babinski response.

Clonus: It is a rhythmic series of involuntary muscle contractions. The stretch reflex—inverse stretch reflex sequence may contribute to clonus. However, it can occur on the basis of synchronized motor neuron discharge without golgi tendon organ discharge. **Sustained clonus is abnormal** and is seen in UMNs lesion. It is always associated with increased tendon reflexes and an extensor planter response. Unsustained clonus is seen in healthy persons, especially those who are very tense or anxious.

Ankle clonus: The subject's knee is slightly flexed and the leg is held up by supporting it with a hand placed behind the knee. Then the examiner suddenly dorsiflexes the foot after grasping its forepart. The sudden stretch of calf muscles results in their alternate contraction and relaxation.

Patellar clonus: The subject's leg is placed in extension. The examiner holds the patella from its sides with his thumb and fingers and then presses it sharply and firmly downward. If clonus is present, the patella shows a rapid up and down movement, which continues as long as the stretch is maintained.

Grading of tendon reflexes: Tendon or deep reflexes are usually graded as follows:
- Grade 0—Absent
- Grade 1—Present (as a normal ankle reflex)
- Grade 2—Brisk (as a normal knee reflex)
- Grade 3—Very brisk
- Grade 4—Clonus.

MOTOR NEURON LESIONS

The pathophysiological responses to damage to lower and upper motor neurons are very distinctive (Table 4.5.3).

VISCERAL REFLEXES

The visceral reflexes include—pupillary reflexes, reflexes from the heart and lungs (sinoaortic, Hering-Breuer, etc.), deglutition, vomiting, defecation, micturition and sexual reflexes. Those which are tested clinically are—pupillary, oculocardiac, carotid sinus reflex, bulbocavernosus and sphincter reflexes. The tests employed for assessing autonomic function are based on some visceral reflexes. They depend upon complex muscular movement excited by increased tension in the wall of the viscera concerned.

- **Swallowing:** The subject is asked whether he has any difficulty in swallowing (dysphasia). If present, ask him whether he has difficulty in swallowing liquids or solids. As a rule patients with neurological disorders causing dysphasia complain of difficulty in swallowing liquids, whereas in mechanical esophageal obstruction they find difficulty in swallowing solids.
- **Defecation:** The patient should be asked, if he has any difficulty in passing stools. He should also be asked whether he can feel rectal sensation.
- **Micturition:** The subject should be asked whether he has any difficulty in controlling or initiating micturition. He should also be questioned for retention and incontinence of urine.
- **Pupillary reflexes:** The light reflex, accommodation reflex and ciliospinal reflexes may be demonstrated.
- **Oculocardiac reflex:** While the examiner feels the pulse of the subject with one hand, a gentle pressure is applied on the eyeball with the thumb of the other hand. The response is a slowing of the heart. Afferent—trigeminal nerve; center—medulla; efferent—vagus nerve.
- **Carotid sinus reflex:** Pressure with the thumb on the carotid sinus in the neck (on one side only, never on both sides) causes slowing of the heart. **Afferent**—glossopharyngeal; **center**—medulla; **efferent**—vagus. This reflex is hyperactive in some persons with marked vasomotor instability; slight stimulation of this type may cause fainting (carotid sinus syncope).

Table 4.5.3: Differences between upper and lower motor neuron lesions.

		Upper motor neuron (pyramidal and extrapyramidal)	Lower motor neuron (anterior horn cell type including peripheral nerve injuries)
1.	Loss of power	Incomplete	Complete
2.	Extent of paralysis	More extensive and equal involvement of muscles of a limb	Less extensive and unequal involvement
3.	Atrophy and wasting	None or slight; generalized; due to disuse	Marked, focal. May involve 70–80% of muscle mass
4.	Muscle tone	Increased (rigidity)	Decreased (flaccidity)
5.	Reflexes: a. Deep b. Superficial	Exaggerated Absent or diminished on the side of involvement	Absent or diminished Unaffected unless thoracic anterior horn cells are affected
6.	Pathological reflexes: a. Babinski b. Gordon's c. Oppenheim's d. Hoffman's sign	All are present	All are absent
7.	Muscle fasciculation and fibrillation	Absent	Often present
8.	Electrical changes in muscle	Normal reactions to galvanic and faradic current	Partial or complete reaction of degeneration in the involved muscles
9.	Vasomotor phenomena	Mild	Marked
10.	Associated movement, e.g. Strümpell's sign	Present	Absent

---

Objective Structured Clinical Examination-III

Aim: To elicit the knee reflex in the subject provided.
Procedural steps: See text above
Checklist:
1. Seat the subject on a stool and ask him to cross one leg over the other. (Y/N)
2. Give instructions about the procedure and assure him that the hammer will not cause any pain. (Y/N)
3. Place her hand on the subject's quadriceps muscle. (Y/N)
4. Locate the patellar tendon and then strike it between the patella and the tibial tuberosity, holding the hammer between thumb and fingers and swinging it from the wrist. (Y/N)
5. Watch/feel the contraction of quadriceps muscle and the kicking forward of the leg. Compare the response with the opposite side. (Y/N)

Objective Structured Clinical Examination-IV

Aim: To elicit the ankle reflex in the supine position in the subject provided.
Procedural steps: See text above
Checklist:
1. Give instructions about the procedure and assure that the hammer will not cause pain. (Y/N)
2. Ask him to lie supine on the examination couch and place the right knee semiflexed and externally rotated. (Y/N)
3. Slightly dorsiflex the foot with her hand to stretch the Achilles tendon. Holding the patellar hammer between the thumb and fingers, strike the tendon with a movement at the wrist. (Y/N)
4. Watch the plantar flexion of the foot, toes and ankle with contraction of calf muscles. (Y/N)
5. Elicit the ankle reflex on the other side for comparison. (Y/N)

Section 4: Clinical Examination

> **Objective Structured Clinical Examination-V**
>
> **Aim:** To elicit the right plantar reflex on the subject provided.
> **Procedural steps:** See text above
> **Checklist:**
> 1. Explain the procedure and ask the subject lie supine on the examination couch. (Y/N)
> 2. Stand on the subject's right side, ask him to relax the leg and foot and flex the knee slightly. (Y/N)
> 3. Support the foot by placing her hand on the medial malleolus. (Y/N)
> 4. Give a light scratch with the blunt point of the patellar hammer along the outer edge of the sole of the foot, starting from the heel toward the little toe and then medially along the base of the toes. (Y/N)
> 5. Watch the response carefully. Repeat once more, if required. (Y/N)

QUESTIONS

- Q.1. Elicit the flexor plantar reflex in the subject provided.
- Q.2. Why does Babinski sign appear in corticospinal tract lesions?
- Q.3. Demonstrate abdominal reflexes in the subject provided.
- Q.4. Elicit the ciliospinal reflex.
- Q.5. Demonstrate any three superficial reflexes.
- Q.6. Demonstrate the knee reflex in the subject provided.
- Q.7. Elicit the ankle reflex.
- Q.8. Test the biceps reflex in the subject provided.
- Q.9. Elicit the triceps reflex.
- Q.10. Test the radial supinator and wrist reflexes.
- Q.11. What is reinforcement of reflexes and when is it required?
- Q.12. When are the deep reflexes diminished or absent?
- Q.13. When are the deep reflexes exaggerated?
- Q.14. What is clonus? Demonstrate this phenomenon in the subject provided.
- Q.15. Demonstrate some visceral reflexes in the subject provided.
- Q.16. What is meant by the terms upper motor neurons and lower motor neurons? What are the chief distinguishing features of the lesions of these neurons?

OBSERVATION AND RESULT

Test the various reflexes in the subject provided and note down your observations in a tabular form.

INTERPRETATION

E: EXAMINATION OF THE SENSORY SYSTEM

AIM
To clinically assess the sensory system of the given subject.

COMPONENTS

- Sensory impulses arise in the receptors or end organs. The cells of origin of peripheral sensory fibers lie in the dorsal root ganglion. The impulse passes along the first order neurons (peripheral process of ganglion cell) and enters the spinal cord.
- The first order neurons (the center process of ganglion cell) carrying the sensation of pain, temperature and crude touch, synapse with the second order neurons in the posterior horn of the spinal cord.
- The second order neurons then cross over to the opposite side of the spinal cord and ascend in the contralateral spinothalamic tracts.
- The fibers carrying crude touch travel in the ventral spinothalamic tract while the fibers carrying pain and temperature ascend in the lateral spinothalamic tract.
- The fibers subserving the proprioception, fine touch and vibration sense synapse in the posterior horn, thence the secondorder neurons ascend up in the posterior column of the same side to synapse in the nucleus gracilis and nucleus cuneatus.
- From there, the second order neurons cross to the opposite side at the level of the upper part of the medulla to ascend in the medial meniscus to relay in the thalamus.
- Third order neurons originating from the thalamus convey all the sensations to the somatosensory cortex (Fig. 4.5.39).

The most common symptoms related to the sensory system include the following:

- ***Hypoalgesia*** is decreased sensations especially of temperature, pain or light touch.
- ***Analgesia*** refers to loss of pain sensation.
- ***Hyperalgesia*** is exaggerated sensitivity to pain, so that a mild stimulus that was painless before now evokes pain.
- ***Hyperesthesia*** refers to increased sensitivity to cutaneous sensations.
- ***Paresthesia*** refers to abnormal sensations, e.g. pricking, numbness, sense of insects crawling on the skin (esthesia = perception).
- ***Anesthesia*** is complete loss of touch sensation.

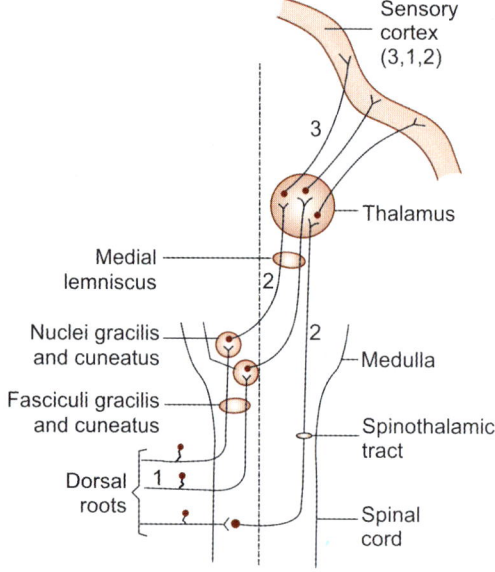

Fig. 4.5.39: Dorsal column-medial lemniscal system and the anterolateral spinothalamic system for the general sensations.

CLINICAL TESTING OF SENSORY MODALITIES

Before starting the sensory examination:
1. Ensure that the subject has been informed about the test.
2. The subject should close his eyes or turn his face to the other side during the test.
3. Always compare the corresponding dermatomes on both the sides.

The clinically tested general sensations include:
- *Tactile (Touch) sensibility includes*—light touch, pressure, tactile localization and two point discrimination
- *Proprioception*
- *Vibration sense*
- *Pain*
- *Temperature:* Cold and hot
- *Stereognosis.*

Apparatus
- Pins, cotton
- Hot and cold water in test tubes
- Weber's compass
- Von Frey's hair esthesiometer

1. **Touch (Tactile) Sensation:**
    - The subject is asked to close his eyes and to respond verbally to each touch.

- A wisp of cotton wool (Fig. 4.5.40) or Von Frey's hair esthesiometer (Fig. 4.5.41) is used to examine the dermatomes sequentially, e.g. in the upper limb start on the outer border of the arm (C5), then proceed downward to the lateral border of the forearm and thumb (C6), index finger (C7), etc.
- Ask the subject to raise his finger or say "yes" when he feels the sensation of touch.
- The subject is asked from time to time for the sensation without the stimulus also so that the subject does not anticipate the test.

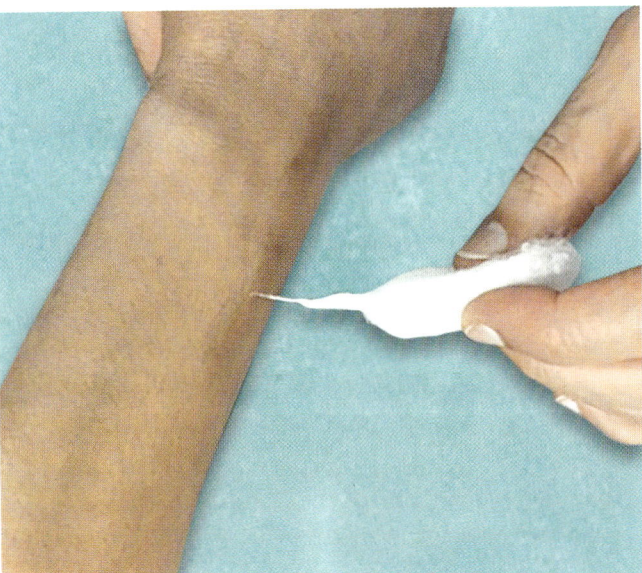

Fig. 4.5.40: Testing for fine touch.

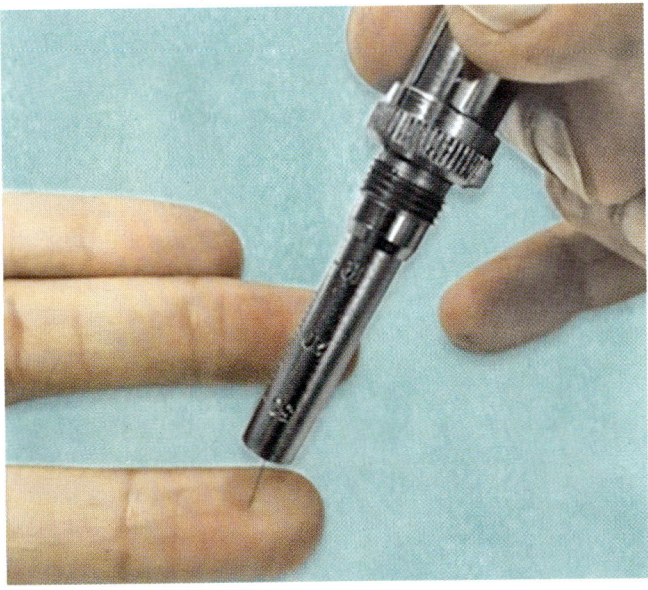

Fig. 4.5.41: Von Frey's esthesiometer.

- Compare sensations in the corresponding area on the opposite side.

Von Frey's esthesiometer: Von Frey's hair esthesiometer is used for touch perception. It has a sliding graduated tube bearing a hair that fits into an outer barrel. It can record the pressure at which the hair will bend to produce a perception of touch.

2. **Tactile localization**: The ability to tell precisely the part of the body touched.
    - Ask the subject to close his eyes.
    - Lightly touch with a blunt pencil or pen on different areas on fingers, arms and back one at a time.
    - Ask him to open the eyes and then localize the site of touch.
    - Compare sensations in the corresponding area on the opposite side.
3. **Pressure:** Pressure is sustained touch. The instrument used to measure the pressure applied is called **algometer.**
    - Ask the subject to close his eyes.
    - Repeat the procedure as mentioned above by applying firm pressure over the skin in different regions with a fingertip or blunt object such as pencil.
    - Compare sensations in the corresponding area on the opposite side.
4. **Two-point discrimination:** The ability to distinguish two simultaneously applied touch stimuli as two separate. It can be tested with a Weber's compass (Fig. 4.5.42) or compass esthesiometer (Fig. 4.5.43). It has two sharp points and two blunt points and a scale to read the distance between the two points (Fig. 4.5.44).
    - Perform the test with the subject's eyes closed.
    - This sensory modality is generally tested on fingertips, back of hands, forearms, leg and the back of the subject.

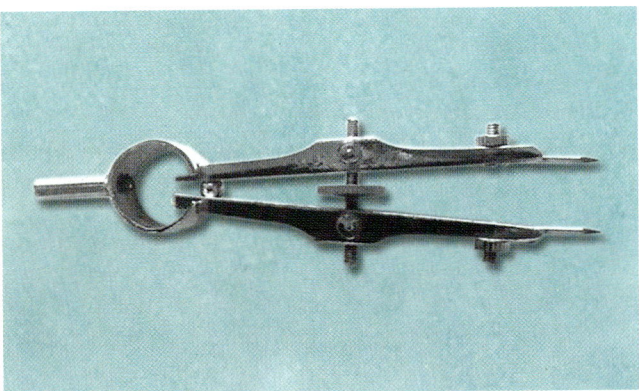

Fig. 4.5.42: Weber's compass.

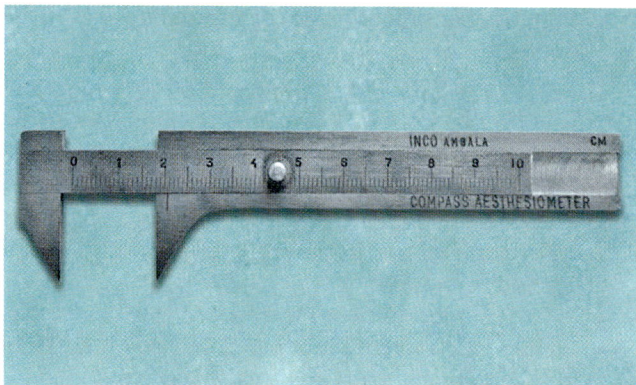

Fig. 4.5.43: Compass esthesiometer.

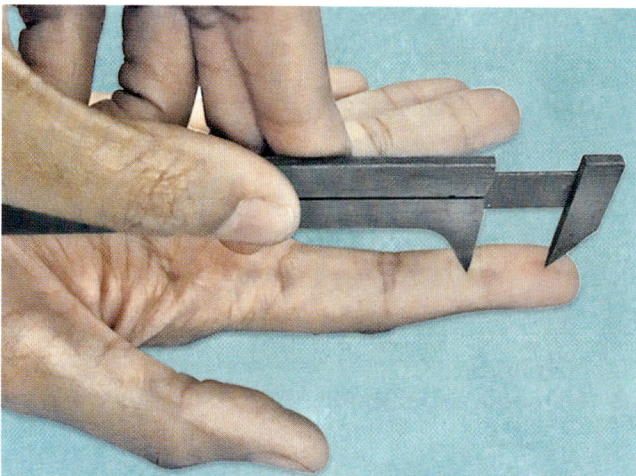

Fig. 4.5.44: Testing two-point discrimination.

- Ask the subject to say "one" or "do not know" or "two", every time the examiner touches the test areas using the compass.
- Determine the minimum distance at which two points are perceived as separate.

The distance varies at different points—2 mm at fingertips, a few mm on fore-arms, legs and many centimeters at the back. It is related to the density of the touch receptors.

5. **Proprioception:** Joint position sense.
   - The subject is shown the intended movements of the joint and name them (e.g. "up" and "down" movements)
   - Ask the subject to close his eyes to avoid guessing.
   - Test the sensation initially at the most distal parts of the limb, e.g. the first test done in the upper limb is at the distal interphalangeal joint of the index finger.
   - The examiner gently moves the terminal phalanx of a finger or toe in one or the other direction.
   - Ask the subject to identify the direction of movement. A normal person is able to appreciate displacement of only a few degrees at various joints.
   - When a limb is placed in a certain position, the subject should be able to place his opposite limb in a similar position.
   - The test is repeated on the contralateral side also.

6. **Vibration sense:** Vibration is a phasic sensation caused by repeated mechanical simulation of touch receptors and Pacinian corpuscles. Vibration sense is lost in peripheral neuropathies (diabetes mellitus), tabes dorsalis and dorsal column disease.
   - Ask the subject to close his eyes.
   - The base of a vibrating low frequency tuning fork (128 Hz) is placed over bony prominences, such as knuckles, head of radius, elbow, patella, malleoli, iliac crest, etc. (Figs. 4.5.45A and B). The subject is normally conscious of a vibrations and not just the sensation of touch.
   - The subject is asked to tell when the feeling of vibration stops.
   - Compare it on the opposite side.
   - If the examiner can still appreciate the sense of vibration after the subject has stopped feeling, it indicates that the subject's perception of vibration is impaired.

7. **Pain:** This sensation is tested either with a cutaneous stimulus, such as the prick of a pin (superficial pain) or by pressure on deeper tissues, such as muscles and bones (deep pain).

Testing the superficial pain in the subject provided (Fig. 4.5.46):
- The subject is asked to close his eyes and to respond verbally to each prick.
- Test by pricking on each limb and over the trunk in different dermatomes sequentially.
- Ask the subject to say "yes" when he feels the sensation of pain and if there is any change in the quality of sensation (e.g. hypoesthesia, hyperesthesia).
- The subject is asked from time to time for the sensation without the stimulus also so that the subject does not anticipate the test.
- Map out the boundaries of abnormal area if any.
- Compare sensations in the corresponding area on the opposite side.

Testing the deep pain in the subject provided:
- Squeeze the muscle bellies (e.g. calf muscle, biceps or triceps) or apply firm pressure on Achilles tendon in the lower limbs.
- Ask the subject to report as soon as the sensation becomes painful.

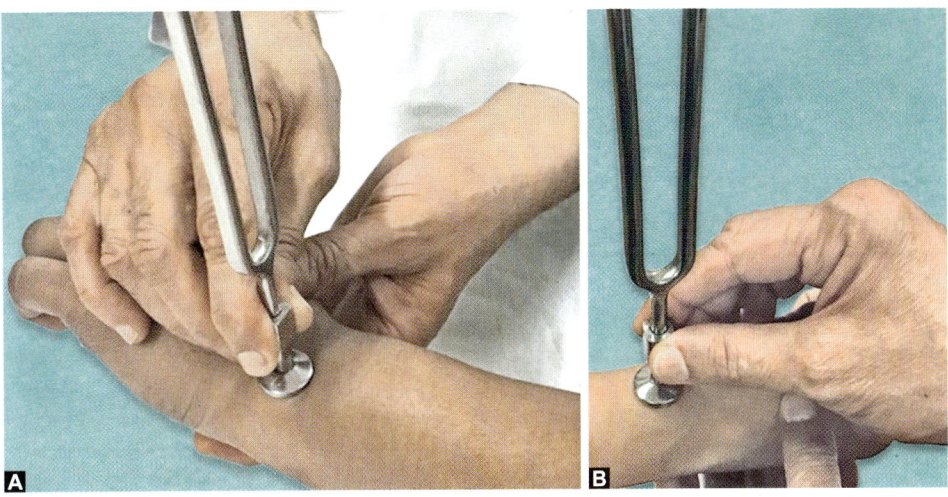

Figs. 4.5.45A and B: Testing for vibration sense.

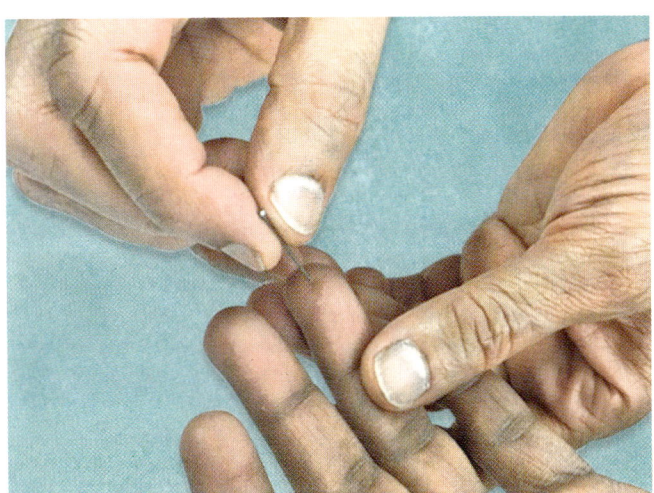

Fig. 4.5.46: Testing superficial pain sensation.

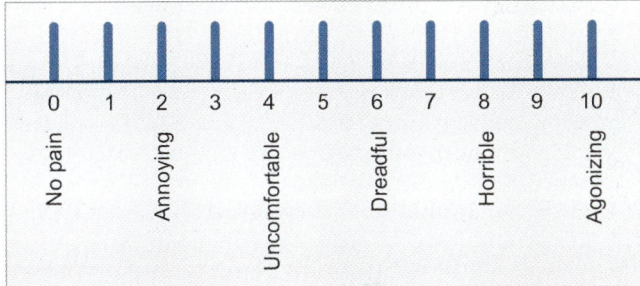

Fig. 4.5.47: The visual analog scale of pain. The patient is asked to point out a number on the scale to indicate the intensity of pain.

> **NOTE**
> **Visual analog scale of pain:** The intensity of pain is difficult to describe and assess. However, one can use the visual analog scale (VAS) for pain. The patient is asked to point out a number on a 10 cm scale, with 0 (no pain) on its left end and 10 (intolerable pain) at its right end, with annoying, uncomfortable, dreadful and horrible pain in between these two ends (Fig. 4.5.47).

8. **Temperature (Figs. 4.5.48A and B):**
   - The subject is asked to keep the eyes closed.
   - Touch the subject by using two test tubes containing cold and warm (not hot) water.
   - The test is performed on face, forearms, hands, trunk and legs.
   - The tubes should be interchanged at random.
   - The patient is asked to report "cold" or "warm".
9. **Stereognosis:** It is the ability to identify common objects by feeling them with the eyes closed. It is a cortical

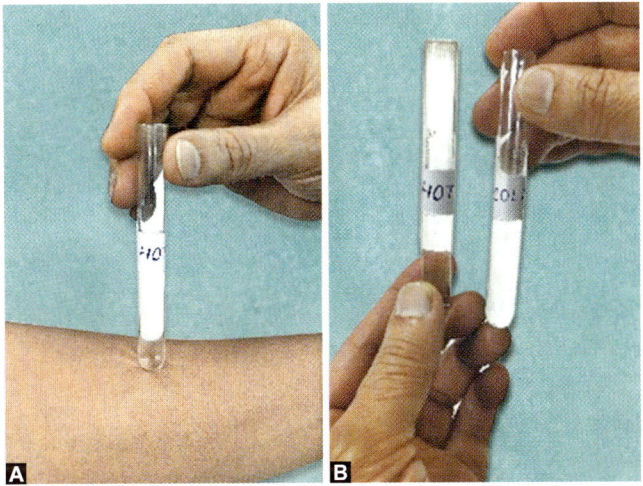

Figs. 4.5.48A and B: Testing for temperature sense.

sensation which depends upon the integrity of the dorsal column and the cerebral cortex (parietal lobe). Certain features of an object—its size, shape, form, weight softness or hardness, roughness or smoothness (e.g.

the milled edge of a coin), dryness or wetness—help in identifying an object.
- The subject is asked to close his eyes.
- Place some common objects like a coin, pencil, keys, matchstick, etc. in the subject's hand, one after the other.
- The subject is asked to identify and describe the shape, size and weight of the object.

> **NOTE**
> Loss of stereognosis is known as astereognosis and it may result from lesions of the parietal lobe or of the dorsal columns of spinal cord.

Objective Structured Clinical Examination–I

Aim: To test the sensation of fine touch on the frontal aspect of the subject's left forearm.
Procedural steps: See text above
Checklist:
1. Make the subject sit on a stool and explain the procedure. (Y/N)
2. Ask him to bare his forearms and put them on the table in front. Tell him to close his eyes. (Y/N)
3. Take a piece of cotton and twist it into a pointed "wisp". Then lightly touch the skin on the fingertips, palms and forearm and ask "now?" and the subject responds with a "yes", "no" or "do not know". (Y/N)
4. Check the responses occasionally without the stimulus. (Y/N)
5. Compare the responses on the opposite forearm. (Y/N)

Objective Structured Clinical Examination–II

Aim: To test two-point discrimination on the anterior forearm of the right side.
Procedural steps: See text above
Checklist:
1. Explain the procedure to the subject and ask him to respond "one", "two" or "do not know" when his skin is touched with the compass points. (Y/N)
2. Ask him to close his eyes. Open the compass a little and lightly touch the fingertips, palm, back of fingers and hand, front and back of forearm, one after another. (Y/N)
3. If the response is "one" at any place, open the compass points and tests again, till he responds with "two". (Y/N)
4. In this way, note the discrimination of two points at various places. (Y/N)
5. Compare the responses on the opposite side. (Y/N)

Objective Structured Clinical Examination–III

Aim: To test the sensation of vibration in the left leg and arm of the subject provided.
Procedural steps: See text above
Checklist:
1. Explain the procedure and assure him that no pain will be caused. (Y/N)
2. Select a tuning fork of 128 Hz, strike one prong against the edge of your hand to set it into vibration. Then place its base on his knuckle to familiarize him with the "vibrating tremor". (Y/N)
3. Test the vibration sense on his knuckles, head of radius, elbow, patella and medial malleolus. (Y/N)
4. Note the response in each case with a "yes", "no" or "do not know", if the response is "no" or "do not know", test on another bony prominence. (Y/N)
5. Compare the responses on the other side. (Y/N)

OBSERVATION AND RESULT

Test the following sensations in the subject provided and note down your observations in the following table:

A. Examination of higher functions
1. Mental state
2. Memory
3. Speech

Contd...

Contd...

B. *Examination of cranial nerves*		
	Right side	**Left side**
I. Olfactory nerve: Smell		
II. Optic nerve		
1. Visual acuity		
a. Distant vision		
b. Near vision		
2. Field of vision		
3. Color vision		
4. Light reflex		
a. Direct light reflex		
b. Indirect light reflex		
5. Accomodation and near response		
III. Oculomotor nerve		
IV. Trochlear nerve		
VI. Abducent nerve		
1. Ptosis		
2. Squint		
3. Nystagmus		
4. Ocular movement		
a. Upward gaze		
b. Downward gaze		
c. Medial/Nasal		
d. Lateral/Temporal		
5. Pupil: Size, shape		

Contd...

Contd...

- V. Trigeminal nerve
  1. Sensory function
  2. Motor function
  3. Corneal reflex

- VII. Facial nerve
  1. Tests for taste sensation
     a. Sweet
     b. Salt
     c. Sour
     d. Bitter
  2. Secretomotor function: Test for lacrimation
  3. Motor function

- VIII. Vestibulocochlear nerve
  1. Tests for vestibular functions
  2. Tests for cochlear function.

- IX. Glossopharyngeal nerve
  1. Taste sensations in posterior 1/3rd of tongue
  2. Palatal reflex

- X. Vagus nerve
  1. History of regurgitation of fluids through nose
  2. Nasal twang
  3. Palatal reflex
  4. Soft palate movements

- XI. Spinal nerve

- XII. Hypoglossal nerve

Contd...

Contd...

C. *Examination of motor system*			
1. Bulk of motor system			
2. Tone of motor system			
3. Coordination			
4. Power of motor system			
5. Gait			
6. Involuntary movements			
D. *Reflexes*			
1. Superficial reflexes			
2. Deep reflexes			
E. *Examination of sensory system*			
Sensation			
Fine touch, touch localization and two-point discrimination			
Proprioception			
Vibration			
Pain			
Temperature			
Stereognosis			

STUDY NOTES

Teacher's Signature

APPENDIX

Units and Measures Employed in Physiology

INTRODUCTION

The most widely used system of measurement is the International System of Units [SI, abbreviated from the French Système International (d'unités)].

Examples of basic SI units (Table A1):

Table A1: Characteristics of basic SI units.

Physical quantity	Name of SI unit	Symbol of SI unit
Length	meter	m
Mass	kilogram	kg
Amount of substance	mole	mol
Energy	joule	J
Pressure	pascal	Pa
Time	second	s (or sec)
Electric current	ampere	A
Thermodynamic temperature	kelvin	K
Luminous intensity	candela	cd

DECIMAL, MULTIPLES AND SUBMULTIPLES OF THE SI UNITS (TABLE A2)

These are formed by the use of prefixes. The Greek prefixes (deca, hecto, kilo, myria) denote multiplication. The Latin prefixes (deci, centi, milli) denote division. [The METER (Fr, METRE), the unit of length is the ten-millionth part of a line drawn from the pole to the equator].

Unit of volume: The SI unit of volume is the *cubic meter* (m^3). But because of its inconvenience the *liter*

Table A2: Decimal, multiples and submultiples of the SI units.

Multiple	Prefix	Symbol	Submultiple	Prefix	Symbol
10^1	deca	da	10^{-1}	deci	d
10^2	hecto	h	10^{-2}	centi	c
10^3	kilo	k	10^{-3}	milli	m
10^6	mega	M	10^{-6}	micro	µ
10^9	giga	G	10^{-9}	nano	n
10^{12}	tera	T	10^{-12}	pico	p
10^{15}	peta	P	10^{-15}	femto	f
10^{18}	exa	E	10^{-18}	atto	a

(L) and *deciliter (dL)* are used as the units of volume for most applications in physiology and biochemistry. The equivalents of *metric, United States* and *English (Imperial)* measures are also shown.

- $1 m^3$ = 1,000 liters
- 1 dL = 100 mL
- 1 cubic inch = 16.39 mL
- 1 fl oz = 29.57 mL
- 1 mL = 0.0352 oz
- $1 mm^3$ (1 cu. mm) = 1 µL (microliter)
- 1 liter = 1.76 pints
- 1 pint = 568 mL = 20 fl oz
- 1 liter = 1.06 US liq quart
- $1 m^3$ = 1.31 $yard^3$
- 1 US = 32 fl oz = 0.951 liq quart
- 1 US = 0.83 English
- 1 gallon = 4.55 liters
- $1 m^3$ = 275 bus (bushel)
- 1 bus = 0.0364 m^3.

Unit of amount of substance: The "Molar" (e.g. mol/L; mmol/L) is used for substances of defined chemical composition. It replaces the equivalent concentration (mEq/L) which is not part of the SI system for measurements of sodium, potassium, chloride and bicarbonate (the numerical value of these four measurements is unchanged because these ions are univalent).

Unit of weight (mass concentration): The SI unit is the *kilogram* (kg).
- 1 kg = 1,000 g (grams)
- 1 kg = 2.20 pounds (lb; avoirdupois) = 2.68 pounds (apothecaries')
- 1 lb = 453.6 g = 16 oz
- 1 oz = 28.35 g
- 1 grain = 65 mg
- 1 tonne = 1,000 kg = 0.984 ton = 2,204 lb
- 1 ton = 1,016 kg = 1.02 tonne = 2,244 lb.

Unit of length: The SI unit is the *meter (m)*.
- 1 Angstrom unit (Å) = 10-10 m = 0.1 nm
- 1 micrometer (μm) = 10-6 m (micron, μ, is obsolete and in its place, the unit μm is used).
- 1 inch = 2.54 cm
- 1 cm = 0.394 inch
- 1 yard = 0.9144 m
- 1 meter = 39.37 inch
- 1 meter = 1.09144 yard
- 1 meter = 3.28 ft (feet)
- 1 km = 0.621 mile
- 1 mile = 1.609 km
- 1 mile = 1,760 yard
- 1 nautical mile = 1.852 km = 1.14 mile = 6,080 ft
- Knot = Nautical miles per hour.

Unit of area: The SI unit of area is the *square meter (m^2)*.
- 1 cm^2 = 0.155 $inch^2$
- 1 $inch^2$ = 6.452 cm^2
- 1 ft^2 = 929 cm^2
- 1 m^2 = 10.8 ft^2
- 1 m^2 = 1.20 $yard^2$
- 1 $yard^2$ = 0.836 m^2
- 1 acre = 4,840 $yard^2$ = 4,047 m^2 = 0.4047 hectare
- 1 hectare = 2.471 acres
- 1 sq mile = 2.59 km^2 = 640 acres.

Unit of pressure: The SI unit of pressure is the *Pascal (Pa)*. This is the pressure exerted by 1 Newton force on an area of a square meter (1 Pa = 1 N m^{-2}).
- 1 cm water = 98.1 Pa
- 1 mm Hg = 1 torr = 133.3 Pa = 0.1333 kPa
- 1 kPa = 7.60 mm Hg = 10.1 cm H_2O
- 1 lb/$inch^2$ = 6.894 kPa
- 1 millibar (mb) = 0.1 kPa
- 1 dyne/cm = 10^{-4} kPa
- 1 normal atmosphere = 1 bar = 760 mm Hg = 101.3 kPa.

Temperature: The SI temperature scale is the kelvin scale (K), but it is inconvenient to use in medicine. The *Celsius* (formerly centigrade) scale (°C) has been retained.
- To convert Celsius degrees to Fahrenheit, multiply with 9/5 and add 32.
- To convert Fahrenheit degrees to Celsius, substract 32 and multiply by 5/9.

°C	−40	−10	0	10	20	30	35	37	40	45	100
°F	−40	14	32	50	68	86	95	98.6	104	113	212

LABORATORY VALUES OF CLINICAL IMPORTANCE

The following laboratory values are some of those which have frequent clinical relevance. Values in SI units are shown in brackets after the values in traditional units.

Body Fluids and other Mass Data

Body fluid, total volume: 50% (in obese) to 70% (lean) of body weight.
- Intracellular: 30–40% of body weight
- Extracellular: 20–30% of body weight.

    (Of about 40 liters of water in a 70 kg man, 14 liters are in ECF (3.5 liters in vascular and 10.5 liters in interstitial fluid compartments) and 26 liters in ICF).

Blood (Total Volume)

- Males: 70 mL/kg body weight
- Females: 65 mL/kg body weight (7.5–8% bw).

Plasma Volume

- Males: 39 mL/kg body weight
- Females: 40 mL/kg body weight.

RBC Volume

- Males: 30 mL/kg body weight
- Females: 25 mL/kg body weight.

Blood—Reference Intervals

Arterial Gases

- $PaCO_2$: 35–45 mm Hg
- PaO_2: 80–100 mm Hg at sea level.

Arterial Oxygen Saturation (At Rest)

- Sea level: 97%
- 5,000 ft: 90%
- 15,000 ft: 75%.

Adult blood contains 0.3 mL O_2 in physical solution and about 19 mL/dL in chemical combination with hemoglobin.

Carbon Dioxide Content, Plasma (Sea Level): 50-70 volumes/dL (21-28 mmol/liter).

Carboxyhemoglobin

- Nonsmokers: 0-2.3%
- Smokers: 2.1-4.2%.

Bleeding Time

- Duke method (finger, ear lobe): <5 minutes
- Ivy method (5-mm wound): <9 minutes
- Simplate: <7 minutes.

Coagulation Time

- Capillary blood: 2-5 min
- Venous blood (Lee and White): 5-15 min.

Erythrocyte sedimentation rate (ESR), mm 1st hour:
Westergren:
- Males: 0-15
- Females: 0-20.

Wintrobe:
- Males: 0-9
- Females: 0-20 (Increases with age).

Fragility of red cells: Hemolysis begins at 0.45% NaCl; complete at 0.35% NaCl solution.

Hematocrit [Hct; packed cell volume, (PCV)]
- Men: 40-52%
- Women: 37-47%
  [(SI: Men: 0.4-0.52 L/L, Women: 0.37-0.47 L/L)].

Mean corpuscular (cell) volume (MCV): 75-94 μm^3 (75-94 fl).

Mean corpuscular hemoglobin (MCH): **27-32 pg**

Mean corpuscular hemoglobin concentration (MCHC): 30-36% (SI: 30-36 g/L).

Osmolality (serum): 275-295 mOsm/kg water.

Red cell count:
- Males: 4.5-6.5 million/mm3 (SI: 4.5-6.5 × 1012/L)
- Females: 4.0-5.5 million/mm3 (SI: 4.0-5.5 × 1012/L)

Hemoglobin

- Males: 13.5-18 g/dL
- Females: 11.5-16 g/dL.

White cell count (WCC): 4,000-11,000/mm³ (SI: 4.0-11.0 × 10^9/L)
- Neutrophils: 40-75% WCC (2.0-7.5 × 10^9/L)
- Eosinophils: 1-6% WCC (0.04-0.44 × 10^9/L)
- Lymphocytes: 20-45% WCC (1.3-3.5 × 10^9/L)
- Basophils: 0-1% WCC (0-0.10 × 10^9/L)
- Monocytes: 2-10% WCC (0.2-0.8 × 10^9/L).

Platelet count: 150,000-400,000/mm³ (SI: 150.0-400.0 × 10^9/L).

Lifespan: 8-10 days.

CARDIOVASCULAR SYSTEM

Cardiac output (Fick): 4.5-6 liters/min (cardiac index: 2.5-3.6 liters/min/m² BSA).

Capillary pressure (systemic):
- Arterial end: 32 mm Hg
- Venous end: 12 mm Hg
- Mean: 20 mm Hg.

Pulmonary capillaries (mean):
8 mm Hg (osmotic pressure of blood: 25 mm Hg; no tissue fluid formed).
Cardiac output (Fick): 4.5 liters/min.
(Cardiac index: 2.5-3.6 liters/min/m² BSA).

Coronary Artery blood flow: 50-120 mL/100 g left ventricle (Represents total left ventricular flow of about 115 mL/min in a 70 kg man).

Cerebral artery blood flow (total): 750 mL/min (50-60 mL/100 g tissue/min).
Cardiac rate:
- Infants: 130 beats/min
- Men: 70-72 beats/min
- Women: 78-80 beats/min.

Renal blood flow: 1,300 mL/min.

Hepatic (mean flow), total: 1.0 L/min.

BRAIN

Nerve cells (neurons): Total number in human nervous system: >100 billion. **Growth:** Rate of growth reaches maximum early in life. By 6 months, the brain doubles in size; by 3 years, it triples; at 6 years, the brain is 95% of mature size with remaining growth achieved in about equal yearly increments of 10 g until age 20. Some replacement of damaged neurons continues later in life.

BIOCHEMISTRY

Reference Values (S: Serum; P: Plasma)
(Values in SI units are given in brackets after the values in traditional units)

Aminotransferases (S):
- Aspartate-aminotransferase (AST, SGOT): 10–14 Karmen units/mL; 6–18 IU/L (100–300 mmol/L).
- Alanine-aminotransferase (ALT, SGPT): 10–40 Karmen units/mL; 3–26 IU/L (50–430 mmol/L).

Amylase (S): 60–180 Somogyi units/dL (13–53 nmol/L).

Ammonia (whole blood): 80–110 mg/dL (45–65 mmol/L).

Bicarbonate (S or P): 24–30 mEq/L (24–30 mmol/L).

Bilirubin (total, S or P): 0.3–1 mg/dL (5–17 mmol/L) (About half is direct).

Calcium, total (S): 8.5–10.5 mg/dL (2.12–2.62 mmol/L) (varies with protein concentration).

Chloride (S): 350–375 mg/dL; 95–105 mEq/L (95–105 mmol/L).

Cholesterol (S): 140–300 mg/dL (3.6–7.8 mmol/L).

Fibrinogen (P): 150–400 mg/dL (1.5–4 g/L).

Glucose, normal, fasting (P): 80–90 mg/dL (4.4–4.9 mmol/L), Upper limit: 110 mg/dL (6 mmol/L).

2-hour postprandial (or after drinking 75 g glucose (50 g in children under 14 years of age).

Normal: 140 mg/dL (7.8 mmol/L). No value exceeds in renal threshold of 180 mg/dL (9.9 mmol/L).

Impaired glucose tolerance: 140–200 mg/dL (7.8–11.1 mmol/L).

Diabetes mellitus: >200 mg/dL (>11.1 mmol/L on more than one occasion).

- Two fasting levels >145 mg/dL confirm the diagnosis of diabetes mellitus.

Immunoglobulins (S):
- **IgA:** 90–350 mg/dL
- **IgD:** 0–8 mg/dL
- **IgE:** <0.025 mg/dL
- **IgG:** 800–1,500 mg/dL
- **IgM:** 45–150 mg/dL (SI units in g/L).

Magnesium (S or P): 2–3 mg/dL (0.75–1.05 mmol/L).

Nonprotein nitrogen (NPN) (S): 20–30 mg/dL (14–21 mmol/L).

Osmolality (P): 285–295 mOsm/kg of serum water.

Phosphate (as inorganic P) (P): 2.5–4.5 mg/dL (0.8–1.45 mmol/L).

Phosphatase, acid, serum: 0.2–1.8 IU (3–30 nmol/L).

Phosphatase, alkaline, serum: 21 × 91 IU at 37°C (0.4 × 1.5 mmol/L).

Potassium (S): 14–20 mg/dL (3.5–5.0 mmol/L).

Proteins, total, serum: 5.5–8.0 g/dL (55–80 g/L).

Protein fractions:
- **Albumin:** 3.5–5 g/dL
- **Globulin:** 2–3.5 g/dL
- **Alpha$_1$:** 0.2–0.4 g/dL
- **Alpha$_2$:** 0.5–0.9 g/dL
- **Beta:** 0.6–1.1 g/dL
- **Gamma:** 0.7–1.7 g/dL.

SGOT, SGPT: See aminotransferases.

Sodium (S): 310–340 mg/dL (136–145 mEq/L) (135–145 mmol/L).

Triglycerides, as triolin (S): 25–150 mg/dL (0.28–1.69 mmol/L).

Thyroid binding globulin (TBG) (P): 7–17 mg/L.

Thyroxine (T$_4$) (P): 70–140 nmol/L.

Thyroxine (free) plasma: 9–22 pmol/L.

Triiodothyronine (T$_3$), plasma: 1.2–3.0 nmol/L.

Urea (urea nitrogen) (S): 10–20 mg/dL (3.6–7.1 mmol/L).

Uric acid (urate) (S or P): 2–7 mg/dL (0.15–0.48 mmol/L) (slightly less in females).

Xylose (B): 5–50 mg/dL (0.33–3.33 mmol/L).

Zinc (S): 50–150 mg/dL (7.65–22.95 umol/L).

Figure A1 shows the nomogram for determination of body surface area from height and weight (Adults).

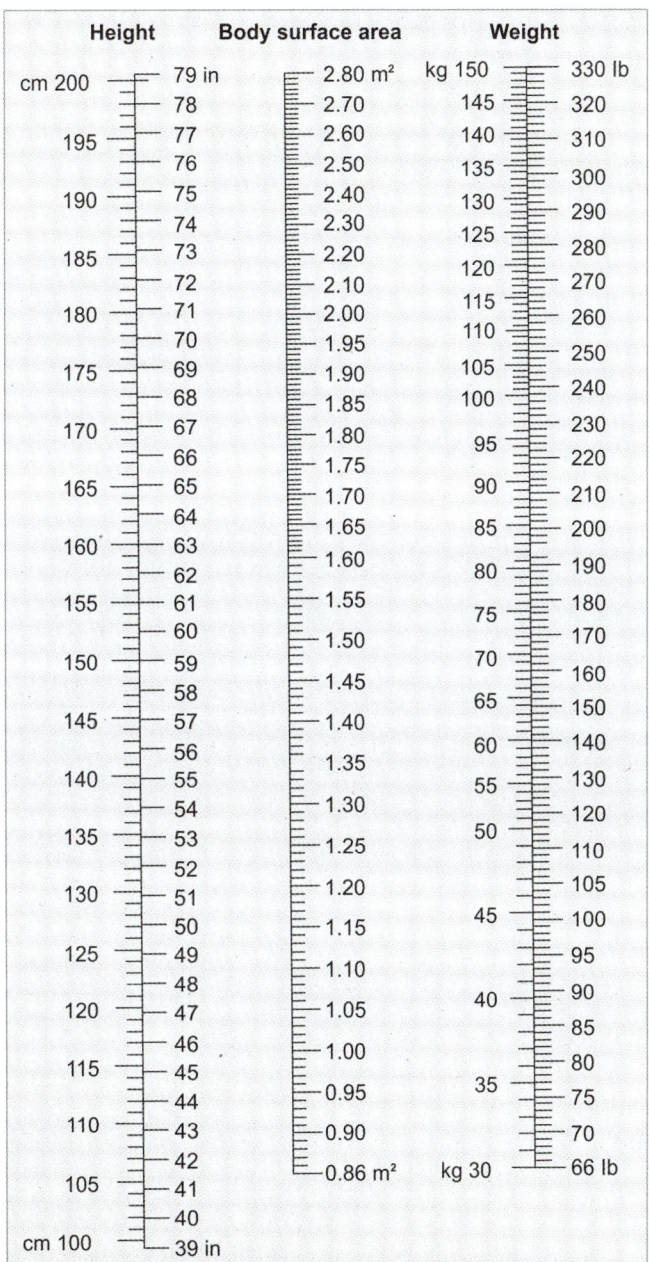

Fig. A1: Nomogram for determination of body surface area from height and weight (adults).

Figure A2 shows the basal metabolism per day (Du Bois Nomogram).

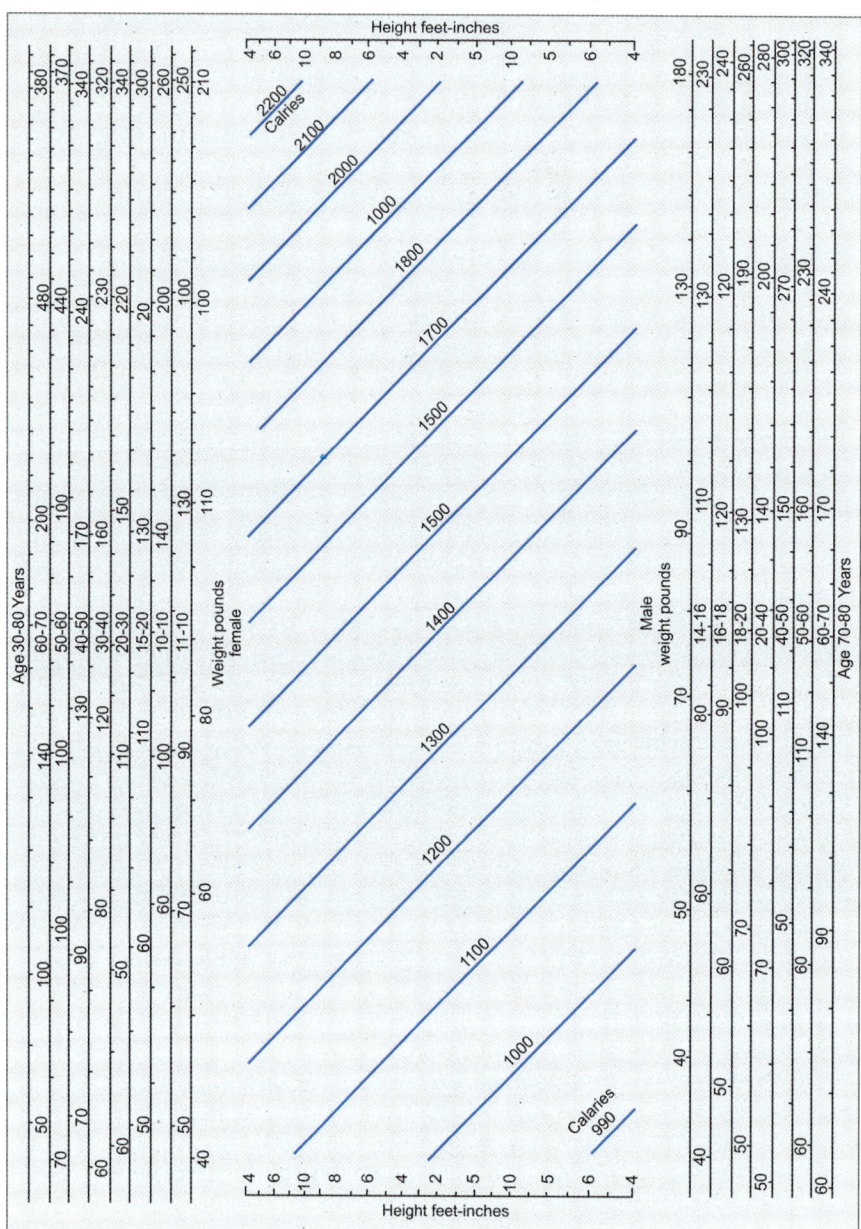

Fig. A2: Basal metabolism per day (Du Bois Nomogram).

Figure A3 shows the body mass index (BMI) chart as per WHO Guidelines.

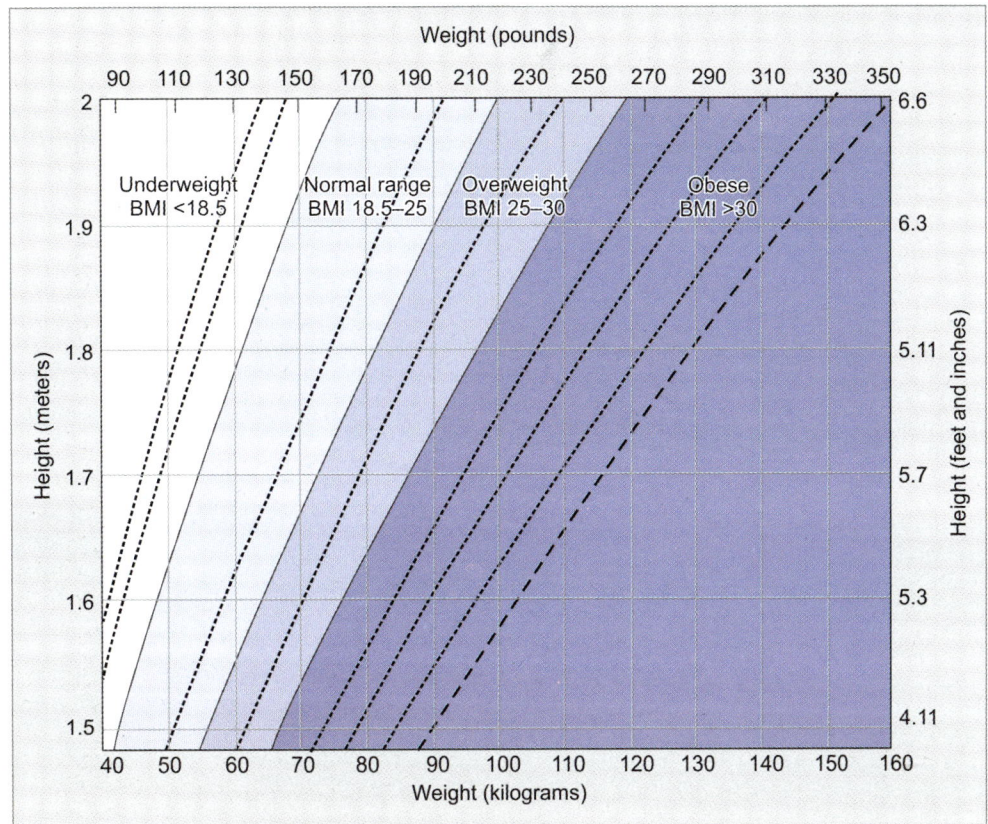

Fig. A3: Body mass index (BMI) chart: WHO guidelines.

Index

Page numbers followed by *f* refer to figure and *t* refer to table.

A

Abdomen 282
    clinical examination of 305
    distension of 305
    examination of 305
    flat 306
    round 306
    scaphoid 306
    silent 309
    tenderness of 305
Abdominal reflex 340
Abdominal ultrasound 271
Abdominal walls, movements of 306
Abducent nerve 322, 353
Abductor pollicis brevis 335
ABO
    antibodies 54*t*
    blood group 53
    system antibodies 54
Absolute eosinophil count 80
    normal 80
Absolute leukocyte count 44, 44*t*
Absolute refractory period 125, 149
Absolute reticulocyte count 84
Accessory nerve, test spinal part of 331
Accommodation 321, 322
    reflex 322*f*
        pathway 322*f*
Acetone-free and water-free methyl
    alcohol 39
Acetylcholine 158-160, 162, 163
    depletion of 155
    effect of 159, 159*f*
Acetylcholinesterase 160
Acid 360
    citrate-dextrose 12
    hematin 16
Acquired coagulation disorders 62
Acquired immunodeficiency
    syndrome 45, 220, 274
Adenine 12

Adenosine triphosphate 267
Adrenal medulla, tumor of 178
Adrenaline 158, 160, 162, 163
    effect of 159, 159*f*
Adrenocorticotropic hormone 81
    treatment 45
Adventitious sounds 292
Aerobic exercises 186
Afibrinogenemia 62
Ageusia 326
Agglutination 53
Agglutinins 53
Agglutinogens 53
Agranulocytes 43
Air
    conduction 328
    pump 174
Airway 220
Airway resistance
    measurement of 213
    resistance, total 213
Alanine 360
Albumin 360
    loss of 94
Albuminuria 312
Alcohol 251
Algometer 349
Alkaline 360
    hematin method 19
Allergic conditions 45, 81
Allergic diseases 45
Allergic reactions 58
Alpha rhythm 241
Alveolar ventilation 207
Ambient pressure 229
Ambulatory electrocardiogram
    monitoring 195
American Heart Association
    Guidelines 174
Aminotransferase 360
Ammonia 360
Ammonium oxalate method 76

Amphibia 155
Amphibian
    experiments 97
    Ringer's solution 111, 145
    Ringer-Locke solution 162
        composition of 162
Amylase 360
Anacrotic limb 169
Anacrotic pulse 169
Anaerobic exercise 186
Anaerobic mechanisms 186
Analgesia 348
Anaphylactic shock 221
Anatomical dead space 213
Androgens stimulate erythropoiesis 30
Anemia 17, 20, 94, 168
    morphological classification of 74*t*
Aneroid blood pressure apparatus 180
Aneroid manometer 174
Aneroid sphygmomanometer 174*f*
Anesthesia 348
Angina 194
Ankle
    clonus 344
    reflex 342
        assessment of 342
Ankylosing 208
Anopia 320
Anosmia 317
Antibodies 53, 56
Anticholinesterases 160
Anticoagulants therapy 62
Antidromic conduction 248
Antigens 53, 56
Antihypertensive medication 181
Anti-Rh
    antibodies 57
    gamma globulin 57
Anti-serum
    A 56
    B 56
    Rh 56

Anuria 311, 313
Anxiety 152
Aortic area 296f, 300
Aortic regurgitation 169
Aortic stenosis 169, 169f
Apex beat 290, 298, 299f
　character of 299
　position of 290, 299
Aphasias 316
Apical percussion 291
Aplasia 36
Aplastic anemia 20, 81
Apnea, deglutition 201
Apparatus 10, 11, 15, 28
　study of 102
Appetite, loss of 305
Argyll-Robertson pupil 322
Arm circumference, two-thirds of 173
Arneth count 49
Arneth curve 50f
Arrhythmias 195
Arterial blood 11
　flow 257
Arterial gases 358
Arterial occlusion, effect of 257
Arterial oxygen saturation 358
Arterial pressure, mean 172, 176, 182, 186
Arterial pulse 167
　abnormal character of 169
　absent 221
　examination of 167, 296
　normal character of 169
　peripheral 169
　tracing 169f
　weak 221
Aschheim-Zondek test 270
Ascites 308
Asepsis 9
Aspartate aminotransferase 360
Aspiration, vacuum 276
Asthma, severe 169
Athetosis 337
Athrombocytopenic purpura 63
Atonia 335
Atrial rhythm 150
Atropine 158, 159, 160
　effect of 159, 159f
Audio amplifier with speaker 250
Audio signals 251
Audiogram 330
Audiometer 328
Audiometry 330
Auditory pathway 327, 328f
Auditory reaction time 237, 238
Auscultate chest 291
Auscultatory areas 296f
Auscultatory gap 177

Auscultatory method 173, 175, 178
Autoimmune
　disease 45
　hemolytic anemia 89
Autonomic function tests 260
　classification of 260
Autonomic nervous system 260
　divisions of 260
　efferent pathways of 261f
　integrity of 181
Autorhythmicity 149

B

Babinski's sign 339, 340
Back-pressure arm-lift method 222
Bacterial endocarditis, subacute 45
Bacteriuria, screening test for 313
Ballism 337
Barany caloric test 330
Barrier methods 274
Basal body temperature 275
Basal metabolic rate 228
Basal metabolism
　measurement of 228
　per day 362f
Basal percussion 291
Basal pulse rate, record 197
Basic life support 220
Basic SI units, characteristics of 357t
Basopenia 45
Basophilia 45
Basophils 43–45
Bell's facial palsy 325
Bell's palsy 326f
Bell's phenomenon 325
Bence Jones proteins 312
Benedict's test 312
Benzidine test 312
Beta rhythm 241
Bicarbonate 360
Biceps reflex 340, 342f
　assessment of 340
Bile pigments 312
Bile salts 312
Bilirubin 360
Binasal hemianopia 235
Binocular microscope 3, 3f
Binocular vision 231
Biochemistry 360
Biological tests 270
Biot's breathing, 203
Biphasic muscle potential 247
Bipolar leads 189
Bipolar limb leads 189
Birth control 274
　methods 274

Bitemporal hemianopia 235
Bladder length 174
Blast cells, immature 37
Bleeding time 9, 60, 61f, 359
　physioclinical significance of 61
Blind spot 234
　physiological 234
　position 234
Blood 12, 92, 312, 358
　and tissue perfusion, circulation of 177
　cells 22
　　faded appearance of 42
　　types of 44f
　centrifugation of 69f
　clot, formation of 60
　coagulation 78
　drop, position of 93f
　film 9
　　head end of 42
　gravity of 93t
　group 53, 56
　　determination of 53, 54, 55f
　　physioclinical significance of 55
　　reaction of different 56t
　　systems 53
　indices, absolute values of 73
　lancet 10, 34
　loss 181
　　excessive 20
　osmotic pressure of 89
　peripheral 9
　pressure 61, 172, 177, 180-182, 184, 197, 285, 260
　　apparatus 264
　　classification 172
　　diastolic 172, 182, 186, 262
　　recording of 174f
　　regulation of 177
　　regulatory 177
　　short-term regulation of 177
　　sudden fall in 178
　reference intervals 358
　sample 34
　　collection of 9
　smear
　　features of ideal 41
　　fixing of 40, 41
　　peripheral 42, 84f
　　preparation of 40
　　preparation of peripheral 39
　　uses of peripheral 45
　specific gravity of 92
　transfusion, incompatible 89
　vessels, contraction of injured 60
　whole 360
Blowing out, repeat cycle of 223

Blue appearance, excessively 41
Body fluid 358
    total volume 358
Body mass index 363
    chart 363f
Body surface area 228
Body temperature 229, 285
Bone
    conduction 328
    marrow
        depression of 45
        hyperactive 50
        proliferation 84
        reserve 36
Brachioradialis reflex 336, 340
Bradycardia 168, 195
Bragg-Paul pulsator 224
Brain 359
    attack 178
    tumors 243
Brainstem auditory evoked potential 251, 252, 252f, 330
    waveforms, measurement of 252
Breath curve, single 213
Breath holding
    effect of 201
    time, duration of 201
Breath sounds 292
    bronchial 292, 292t
    character of 292
    intensity of 292
    reduced 292
    type of 292, 292f
Breathing 220, 221
    capacity, maximum 207
    closed circuit 228
    reserve 209
    test, deep 263
    type of 290
    voluntary stoppage of 203
Bright-field microscopy 7
Bronchophony 292
Bronchoscopy 214
Buccinator muscle testing 326f
Bulbus arteriosus 146
Burns 36

C

Cabrera system 193
Calcium 312, 360
    chloride 111, 162
Calibrated scale 212f
Capillary blood 9, 10, 10t
Capillary fragility test 60, 77
Capillary pressure 359
Carbaminohemoglobin 19
Carbon dioxide 359

Carboxyhemoglobin 19, 359
Cardiac axis 193
Cardiac cycle, electrical events of 191f
Cardiac efficiency
    index 197
    tests 197
Cardiac index 359
Cardiac massage
    external 224, 224f
    internal 225
    open 225
Cardiac muscle
    cells, individual 188
    properties of 149
Cardiac output 186, 359
Cardiac reserve 198
Cardiac resuscitation 224, 224f
Cardiac vagal effect 262
Cardiac vector 193
    calculation of 193f
Cardiogram 145
    normal 145
    recording of normal 146
Cardiopulmonary arrest 220
    causes of 221
    signs of 221
    symptoms of 221
Cardiopulmonary resuscitation 220, 224, 225
Cardiovascular disease
    signs of 296
    symptoms of 296
Cardiovascular system 167, 296, 359
    clinical examination of 296
    examination of 296
Cardioversion 225
Carotid arterial pulse 297, 297t
Carotid sinus reflex 344
Carpal tunnel syndrome 248
Catacrotic limb 169
Catecholamines 178
Cathode ray oscilloscope 125, 245, 247, 250, 251, 253, 264
Cell
    counting 25, 25f, 29, 35
        sources of error in 25
    membrane 56
    type 43
Central cyanosis 283
Central fixation point 234
Central nervous system 245, 258
Central venous pressure 297
Cerebellar ataxia 337
Cerebellar lesions 338
Cerebral artery blood flow 359
Cervical secretions, examination of 275
Chaddock's sign 339

Chart drive 107
Chart paper 211
Chart reverse knob 211
Chelation 11
Chemical stimuli 203
Chest 282
    abnormal forms of 289
    barrel-shaped 289
    compression 224f
    expansion of 290, 290f
    leads 189
        unipolar 190
    normal 289
    pain 296
    plain X-ray 214
    shape of 289, 289f, 298
Cheyne-Stokes breathing 203
Chickenpox 45
Chin rest 233
Chloride 312, 360
Cholesterol 360
Chorea 337
Christmas disease 63
Chronic diseases 20
Ciliospinal reflex 340
Citrate 12
Clasp-knife type 335
Clonic contraction 338
Clonus 344
    sustained 344
Clot
    dissolution of 60
    lysis time 60
    retraction 78
        time 60
Clotting time 9, 60, 61, 63
    physioclinical significance of 62
Clutch lever 104
Coagulation time 62, 359
Coarctation of aorta 168, 178
Cobra, venom of 89
Cochlear function, tests for 354
Cochlear nerve 327
Cogwheel type 335
Cold pressure response 261
Collagen diseases 45
Collapsing pulse 169
Color blindness, classification of 320
Color index 74
Color of object 234
Color vision 317, 319, 353
    defects of 320
    mechanism of 319
    testing of 319
Compass esthesiometer 350f
Compound microscope 3f, 4t, 5, 34, 39
    parts of 3
    ray diagram of 5f

Compound muscle action potential 247, 248f
   amplitude of 248
   duration of 248
Concentric needle electrode 246
Condenser 4
   position of 4
Condom 274
Conduction deafness 329, 330
Confrontation test 235, 319, 319f
Conjunctival reflex 324, 324f
Consciousness, level of 316
Consensual light reflex 321f
Constipation 305
Contraception, emergency 275
Contraction period 114, 115, 115f, 138
Contraction phase 126
Cooke-Arneth count 49, 50f
Copper
   T 275
   traces of 312
Copper sulphate
   falling drop method 19
   stock solution of 92
Cornea, lateral edge of 324
Corneal reflex 354
   demonstrate 324
Coronary artery
   blood flow 359
   disease 194
Corrigan's water hammer 169
Corrugator supercilii muscle 325
Corticospinal-pyramidal system
   anterior 334
   lateral 334
Cough 202, 288
Counting, rules of 25, 29, 29f
Coupler housing 108
Cranial nerve 324f
   eighth 327
   examination of 316, 353
   first 316
   nineth 331
   seventh 325
   sixth 322
   tenth 331
   twelfth 332
Cranial origin 339
   superficial reflexes of 341
Crystalluria 312
Current, types of 99
Cushing's syndrome 45, 81, 178
Cutaneous blood vessels 185
Cyanmethemoglobin 19
   method 19
Cyanolabe 319
Cyanosis 282, 283
   peripheral 283
Cylindrical chamber 216
   double walled 210
Cytoplasm 43
Cytoplasmic granules 43, 44f

D

Dacie's solution 29
Dark-field microscope 7
Dead space
   measurement of 213
   physiological 213
Deafness 330
Deep tendon reflexes, physioclinical significance of 344
Deflections
   direction of 194
   magnitude of 194
   sequence of 194
Deglutition apnea, physiological significance of 203
Dehydration 181, 311
Delta rhythm 241
Deltoid 336
Delusions 316
Desynchronization 241
Deuteranopia 320
Dextrocardia 299
Dextrose 12, 89
Diabetes mellitus 45, 360
Diapedesis 28
Diaphragm 274, 291
Diarrhea 305
Dichromats 320
Dicoumarol 13
Dicrotic notch 169f
   and wave 169
Dicrotic pulse 169
Dicrotic wave 169f
Diffusion, tests of 213
Digitalis overdose 152
Diluting fluid 268
Diluting pipettes 23
Diphtheria 221
Direct light reflex 320, 321f, 353
Disodium phosphate 162
Dissection 112
   apparatus 145
   microscope 7
Distant vision 353
   testing for 317
Distilled water 39, 87
Diurnal variations 177
Dizziness 296
Dorsal column-medial lemniscal system 348f
Dorsalis pedis 169
Double oxalate mixture 12
Drinker's tank respirator 223
Drowning 221
Drum, speed of 114, 118, 121, 124, 128, 133, 136, 140, 145, 149
Dry sounds 292
Du Bois nomogram 362f
Du Bois-Reymond induction coil 103, 103f, 104f, 114
Dual electric contact arms 104
Dudgeon's sphygmograph 169
Duke's method 60, 61
Dullness 291
Dunger's diluting fluid 81
Dynamometer 256f
Dysarthria 315, 316
Dysdiadochokinesia 337
Dysfibrinogenemia 62
Dysgeusia 326
Dyspepsia 305
Dysphagia 305
Dysphasia 315
Dyspnea 288, 296
Dyspneic index 209

E

E test chart 318
Ear frame 173
Earlobe prick 10
Edema 282, 284, 296
Edinger-Westphal nucleus 232
Edridge-Green lantern 319
Ehrlich's test 312
Einthoven's law 190
Einthoven's triangle 190, 190f
Ejection clicks 301
Electric kymograph 104f
Electric motor 104
Electrical potentials 251
Electrical stimulators 245
Electrocardiogram 108, 188, 190, 221
   common abnormalities of 195
   components 192t
   interpretation of 188
   leads, classification of 189
   machine 188, 188f, 264
   normal 192f
   paper 188, 189
   physiological basis of 191
   recording of 188
   systematic analysis of 194
   uses of 195
Electrocardiograph 188
Electrocardiographic leads 189
Electrocardiography 188
Electrocorticogram 240

Electrode 188, 189, 241, 246, 264
  jelly 188, 189, 247
  paste 241, 250, 251
  placement 242
    system of 243f
Electroencephalogram 108, 240, 243f
  clinical applications of 243
  interpretation of 243
  machine 241
  paper 242
  waves
    features of 240
    rhythm of 240t
Electroencephalograph 240
Electroencephalography 240
  electrodes 251
Electrograph 188
Electrolyte
  imbalance 152
  paste 248
Electromagnetic spectrum, part of 319
Electromyogram 108
Electromyography 249
  machine and preamplifier 264
Electroneurodiagnostic tests 245
Electronic stimulator 245, 247, 248, 253, 264
Electronystagmogram 108
Electroshock defibrillation 225
Emotional stress 177
Endocrine diseases 178
Endosmosis 89
Enzyme-linked immunosorbent assay 270, 271
Eosinopenia 45, 81
Eosinophil, differential count of 80
Eosinophilia 45, 81
Eosinophils 43–45, 81f
Epigastrium 305
Epilepsy 243, 338
Equilibrium length 142
Equipment, sterilization of 9
Ergograph 255
Erythremia 31
Erythroblastosis fetalis 56
Erythrocyte sedimentation rate 12, 66, 69, 359
  clinical significance of 69
  determination of 66
  estimation of 66
Erythrolabe 319
Erythropoietin 31
Ethylenediamine tetraacetic acid 11
Eve's rocking method 224
Exercise
  effect of 184, 202
  electrocardiogram 195
  intensity of 184
  test, two-step 185f
  tolerance test 197
    purpose of 198
    type of 184
Exhaled-air ventilation 222
Exosmosis 89
Expectoration 288
Expiratory flow
  rate 212f
  volume curve, maximum 208f, 209
Expiratory reserve volume 206, 207, 216
Expiratory spirogram 208, 208f
Extensor plantar
  reflex 339
  response 339
Extra-amniotic ethacridine lactate 276
Extracellular fluid 163
Extrapyramidal system 334
Extrasystole 149, 150
Eye
  effect of opening 242
  movements of 108, 324f
Eyepiece, focus of 5f

F

Facial nerve 325, 354
  test sensory function of 325
False negative tests 270
False positive
  reaction 55
  results 312
  tests 270
Faradic current 99
Fasciculation 337
Fast-speed pipette 24
Fatigue 136, 137, 255
  causes of 136
  genesis of 136
  phenomenon of 137f
  site of 137
Festinant gait 338
Fetal abnormalities, congenital 271
Fetal hemoglobin 18, 19
Fever 168, 305
Fiber type 247
Fibrillation 337
Fibrin thread formation 62
Fibrinogen 360
Fibrinolysis 60
Field error 30
Field of vision 231, 317, 319, 353
  normal extent of 231
Filling pipette 24, 24f, 29, 34
Finger
  flexors of 336
  percussing 284, 291
  test, counting 318

Finger-nose test 337
First expiratory volume 208
Fixation point 232
Fixation time 41
Flatulence 305
Flexor plantar reflex 339
Flow-volume loop 213
  normal 213f
Fluctuation test 283
Fluid thrill 308
  detection of 308f
Fluorescence microscope 7
Focusing under high power 6
Focusing under
  low power 6
  oil immersion 6
Folic acid 74
Follicle stimulating hormone 275
Forced expiratory
  flow 209
  volume 208
Forced vital capacity 207, 209, 216
Fouchet's and Rosenbach's test 312
Fragility 88
Frank-Starling law 142
Frequency domain analysis 264
Friction sound 292
Friedman test 270
Frog's cardiogram 147, 154
  temperature on 146
Frog's experiments 97
Frog's gastrocnemius muscle 115
Frog's heart 145, 146f, 158, 159, 162, 163t
  exposure of 145
  normal cardiogram of 145, 145f
  perfusion of 162, 163f
  preparation 163f
  properties of 149
Frog's nerve muscle preparation 124
Functional disorders, electroencephalogram organic and 243
Functional platelet defects 61
Functional residual capacity 207, 214
Functional syncytium 150
Fundus, examination of 317
Funnel shaped chest 289

G

Gag reflex 331
Gait 282, 338, 355
Galli-Mainini test 270
Galvanic current 99
Galvanic skin response 261
Gas exchange function
  tests of 213
  tests to assess 206

Gastrocnemius nerve muscle
    preparation, dissection of 111
Gastrointestinal obstruction 309
Gastrointestinal tract
  disease
    signs of 305
    symptoms of 305
    examination of 305
Gauze swab 34, 87
General physical examination 281
Gestational age 271
Glass dropper 39, 87
Glass marking pencil 87
Globin deficiency 74
Globular abdomen 306
Globulin 360
Glomerulonephritis 312
Glossopharyngeal nerve 331, 354
Glucocorticoid treatment 45
Glucose 89
  normal, fasting 360
  tolerance, impaired 360
Glucose-6-phosphate dehydrogenase,
    deficiency of 89
Glycosuria 312
Gold-plated disks 240
Gordon's reflex 339
Gram-stained smear, examination of 313
Grand mal epilepsy 243
Granular casts 313
  dirty brown 313
Granulocytes 43
Grave jaundice 56
Gravindex test 270
Growth 359

H

Haldane's carboxyhemoglobin
    method 19
Hammerschlag's method 92
Hand movement test 318
Handgrip
  dynamometer 255, 257f, 258
  spring dynamometer 257
  test 262
Harvard step test 185, 197
Hay's sulfur test 312
Hayem's fluid 28, 29
  composition of 28
Head injuries 221
Headphones 251
Hearing
  mechanism of 327
  pathway of 327
  tests of 328

Heart
  attack 178, 194
  beating 149
    sequence of 146
  block 152, 168
  electrical axis of 193
  enlargement of 298
Heart rate 146, 151, 160, 163, 180-182,
    184, 186, 194, 195, 197, 260
  factors affecting 168
  variability 264, 264f
    analysis 264, 264f
    recording 265
Heart sounds 300, 300f
  absence of 221
  deviations of 300
  splitting of 300
Heat coagulation tests 312
Heat rigor 119
Heel-Shin test 337
Heimlich maneuver 225
Helium dilution method 207
Heller's test 312
Hematemesis 305
Hematocrit 70, 359
Hematuria 311, 312
Hemiplegic gait 338
Hemoconcentration 31
Hemocytometer 22
Hemocytometry 22
Hemodilution 94
Hemofluidity 63
Hemoglobin 15, 359
  abnormal 18
  adult 18, 19
  basic values of 73
  casts 313
  embryonic 18
  estimation of 15
  normal 18
  reduced 19
Hemoglobinometer
  pipette 15, 16f
  tube 15
    graduated 16f
Hemoglobinuria 312
Hemolysis 16, 88
Hemolytic anemias 20, 74
  chronic 84
Hemolytic disease 56
Hemophilias 62
Hemoptysis 288
Hemorrhage 84
  acute 36, 74
Hemostasis 60
  tests for 60
Hemostatic plug formation 78

Heparin 12, 13
Hepatojugular reflux 297
Hereditary spherocytosis 84, 89
Hernial sites 306
Heteronymous hemianopia 235
Hexaxial system 193f
Hip, extensors of 336
Hoffmann's reflex 253
Hoffmann's sign 253, 339
Hogben test 270
Holger Nielsen method 222, 222f, 226
Holmgren's wools test 320
Homonymous hemianopia 235
Homonymous quadrantanopia 235
Hormonal methods 275
Hormones 31
Horn cell, anterior 345
Horseshoe-shaped dullness 308
H-reflex, recording of 253f
Human chorionic gonadotropin 270
Human experiments 165
Human fatigue, study of 255
Hutchinson's index 289
Hyaline casts 313
Hydrops fetalis 56
Hyperacusis 327
Hyperaldosteronism 178
Hyperalgesia 348
Hyperesthesia 348
Hyperreflexia 344
Hyperresonance 291
Hypersensitivity, denervation 264
Hypertension 172
  classification of 178
  complications of 178
  essential 178
  malignant 178
  secondary 178
Hyperthyroidism 152, 178
Hypertonia 335
Hypertonic saline 89
Hypertrophy 334
Hyperventilation
  effect of 242
  harmful effects of 203
  time clock 241
Hypoactive bone marrow 50
Hypoalgesia 348
Hypogeusia 326
Hypoglossal nerve 332, 354
  testing 332f
Hypoplasia 36
Hypoproteinemia 74
Hyposmia 317
Hypotension
  chronic primary 178
  postural 178, 265

Hypothermia 221
Hypotonia 335
Hypotonic saline 89
Hypoxia 152

I

Icterus 282
　gravis neonatorum 56
Idioventricular rhythm 150, 155, 155*f*
Immunoglobulins 360
Immunological tests 270
Impulses, synchronization of 129
Infection
　acute 36
　chronic 74
　severe 89
Infectious mononucleosis 45
Infranuclear lesion 327
In-hospital electrocardiogram
　　monitoring 195
Ink-writing stylus 105
Inorganic solids 312
Inspiratory reserve volume 206, 207, 216
Interference-contrast microscope 7
Interosseous, first dorsal 336
Intestinal obstruction 308
Intra-amniotic hypertonic saline
　　solution 276
Intrauterine
　contraceptive devices 275
　devices 275
Intravenous injection 225
Intrinsic pathway 62
Iodine, traces of 312
Iris diaphragm 4
Iron
　deficiency anemia 74
　lung 223
　overload 58
　traces of 312
Ishihara charts 319
Ishihara color plates 320*f*
Isometric contractions 257
Isometric exercise 184, 186, 262
　effect of 255
Isometric lever 106
Isometric tension, maximum 262
Isotonic contractions 255
Isotonic exercise 184-186
　effect of 184
　　acute 186
　　long-term 186
Isotonic muscle lever 105, 105*f*
Ivy's method 60, 61

J

Jaeger's chart 318, 318*f*
Jaundice 282, 305, 311
Jaw reflex 324, 343, 343*f*
　assessment of 343
Jendrassik's maneuver 343, 343*f*
Joint National Committee 172
Jugular vein, internal 297
Jugular venous
　pressure 282, 297, 297*f*
　pulse 297, 297*t*
　　tracing, normal 298*f*
　waveform 298

K

Kala-azar 45
Karmen units 360
Kernicterus 56
Ketone bodies 312
Ketonuria 312
Kidney
　disease 94
　palpation of 307
Kinetic energy 172
Kiss of life 222
Knee
　extensors of 336
　flexors of 336
　hammer 340
　reflex 340, 342*f*, 343*f*
　　assessment of 340, 342
Korotkoff sounds 175
　phases of 175*f*
Krebs cycle 267
Kuppermann test 270
Kymograph 104, 114, 210, 255
　with drum 145, 237
Kyphoscoliosis 208
Kyphosis 289, 298

L

Labii inferioris, depressor 325
Lacrimation, test for 264
Lactosuria 312
Landolt ring chart 318, 318*f*
Landsteiner law 53
Language functions 316
Latent period 114, 115, 126, 138
Lateral motor system 333, 334
Lateral pressure 172
Latissimus dorsi 336
Lead selector switch 189
Lee and White test tube method 61, 62
Left ventricular failure 169
Leishman stain 39, 44*f*, 77
Lenses, objective 4*f*
Leukemia 36, 37, 45,
Leukemoid reaction 37
Leukocyte 42, 313
　count, differential 39, 49
　differential count of 43
　largest 43
　types of 42
Leukocytosis 36, 37
Leukopenia 36
Levator angularis muscle 325
Lig*ht*
　perception test 318
　source of 5
Light reflex 232, 320*f*, 353
　indirect 321, 321*f*, 353
　pathway of 321
Limb 282
　leads
　　augmented 189, 190
　　classical 189
　　unipolar 190
Lipoprotein
　high density 185
　low density 185
Liver
　disease 62, 74
　palpation of 307, 307*f*
Living cells 85
Living tissue 99
Local blood flow regulation 78
Lower face, testing 325
Lower limbs 337
　testing muscle strength in 336
Lower meniscus 17
Lower motor neurons 327, 333, 345
Lucas chamber 105, 105*f*, 145, 146
Lung
　auscultation of 291
　capacity, total 207, 208, 213
　diffusion of 206
　perfusion of 206
　scan 214
　tests to assess perfusion of 206
Lung disease 208*f*, 209*t*
　evidence of 214
　restrictive 208*f*
Lung volumes 206, 212*f*
　and capacities 206
　　determination of 206
　　dynamic 207
　　measurement of 206
Luteal supplementation pill 275
Luteinizing hormone 275

Lymph nodes, presence of 290
Lymphadenopathy 282, 283
Lymphocyte 43-45
Lymphocytopenia 45
Lymphocytosis 45
   relative 45

M

Macular region, except 234
Magnesium 312, 360
   sulfate 89
Magnifying system 4
Malaria 45
Malnutrition 36
Mammalian myelinated nerve fiber, thick 125f
Mapping blind spot 234
Marey's or Brodie's tambour 200
Mariotte bottle 162
Master's step 185
   test 198
Master's two step test 185, 187
Mean arterial pressure, significance of 176
Mean cardiac
   axis 193
   vector 194
Mean corpuscular
   hemoglobin 73, 359
      concentration 73, 359
   volume 73, 359
Mean electrical axis 193
   of heart 193
Mean vector, direction of 193
Mechanical respirators 223
Mechanical ventilation 223
Medial motor system 333, 334
Median nerve 247, 247f, 252
Membrane potential, resting 163
Memory 316, 352
Menstrual regulator syringe 276
Menstruation 84
Mental state 352
Mercuric chloride 29
Mercury manometer 173
Metabolic equivalent of task 184
Metal
   arc 232
   trace of 31
Methemoglobin 19
Methylene blue 39, 83
Metronome 255, 256, 256f
Microchemical tests 9
Microscopes, types of 7
Microscopy, physical basis of 5
Micturition 344
Midstream morning sample 311

Mid-systolic clicks 301
Mini Wright's peak flow meter 212f
Minute ventilation 207
Mismatched transfusion reactions 57
Mitral area 296f, 300
Moist sounds 292
Monochromats 320
Monoclonal antibodies 57
Monocular microscope 3, 3f
Monocular vision, white object for 231
Monocyte 43-45
   macrophage system 45
Monocytopenia 45
Monocytosis 45
Mosso's ergograph 255, 256f, 258
   parts of 255
Motor cerebral cortex 203
Motor evoked potentials 251, 252
Motor function 354
   testing 324, 331, 334
Motor nerve conduction 247
   velocity 108, 247f
Motor neuron lesions 344
   absent in upper 339
   lower 345t
   upper 345t
Motor system
   bulk of 355
   components of 333f
   examination of 333, 355
   power of 355
   tone of 355
Motor tracts, descending 333
Motor unit 249
   number of 129
   potential 249
      characteristics of 249
      factors affecting 250
      normal 250f
Mouth-to-mouth
   method 222
   respiration 222, 223f
      advantages of 223
      disadvantages of 223
Multichannel polygraph 264
Multifunctional spirometers, computerized 214
Multiple pregnancy 272
Murmurs 301
Muscarinic receptors 158
Muscle 245
   blood flow 186
   bulk of 334
   contraction 125f, 140f, 141f
      temperature on 118
   distal group of 333
   fibers, initial length of 129

force transducer 109
   lengthening 186
   mass decreases 334
   power of 335
      grading of 336
   proximal group of 333
   pump 181
   shortening 186
   testing bulk of 334f
   tone 334
      testing for 335f
   trough 105, 105f
   twitch, simple 114, 114f, 115f, 115t, 118, 118f, 119
   type of 134
   weakness, grading of 337t
Muscular activity
   coordination of 336
   gradation of 129
Muscular exercise 168, 177
   types of 184t
Myelin sheath, presence of 122
Myocardial damage 152
Myocardial infarction 36
   acute 221
Myoclonus 337
Myograph board 114, 145
Myxedema 168

N

Nails, curving of 283
Nasal twang 354
Nausea 305
Near vision 317, 353
   testing for 318
Needle electromyography 250, 250f
Neef's hammer 104, 133
Nerve
   cells 359
   conduction
      studies 245
      velocity of 121, 121f, 122
   deafness 329, 330
   fiber
      diameter of 121, 122
      type 247t
   impulses, frequency of 129
   injuries, peripheral 345
   muscle preparation 111f, 136
   myelination of 121
   near muscle end 121f
   peripheral 245
Nervous system 237
   clinical examination of 315
   examination of 315
Neubauer's chamber 22, 22t, 23f, 25, 28, 29f, 84, 268

Neubauer's counting chamber 28, 76
Neurological disease
    signs of 315
    symptoms of 315
Neuromuscular junction 137
Neurons 359
Neutropenia 45
Neutrophilia 45
Neutrophils 43-45
Nicotine 158-160
    effect of 159, 159*f*
Nicotinic receptors 158
Nitric oxide 178
Nitrogen washout method 207
Non-pitting edema 284
Nonprotein nitrogen 312, 360
Nonpyogenic organisms 36
Normal semen, characteristics of 267
Nose clip 211
Nutritional anemias 20
Nystagmus 353

O

O_2 consumption 184
Obstructive lung disease 208*f*
    chronic 208*f*
Occipitofrontalis muscle 325
Ocular movement 353
Oculocardiac reflex 344
Oculomotor nerve 322, 353
Odor 311
Olfactory hallucinations 317
Olfactory nerve 316, 353
    examination of 316
Olfactory pathway 317*f*
Oliguria 311, 313
Open circuit method 228
Oppenheim's sign 339
Opponens pollicis 336
Optic chiasma 231
Optic nerve 353
    fibers 231
Optic radiations 232
Optic tract 231
Optical factors 317
Optical system 4
Optimal length 142
Oral contraceptives 275
Orbicularis oculi muscle 325
    testing 325*f*
Organic acids 312
Organic solids 312
Orthodromic conduction 248
Orthopnea 296
Orthostatic hypotension 181, 265
Oscillatory method 173, 175

Osmolality 359, 360
Osmosis 88
Osmotic fragility
    normal range of 88
    test 88*f*
Ossicular conduction 328
Ovum, normal paths of 275
Oxygen consumption 184
    multiples of basal 184
    per minute, calculation of 229
Oxyhemoglobin 19
    method 19
Oxytocin 276

P

Packed cell volume 66, 73
    measurement of 68
Pain 288, 350, 355
    intensity of 351*f*
    visual analog scale of 351, 351*f*
Palatal reflex 331, 354
Pallor 282
Palpating apex beat, significance of 299
Palpation 290, 307
    protocol for 307
Palpatory method 173, 174, 178
    advantages of 175
    disadvantages of 175
Palpitation 296
Paralysis
    ascending 221
    complete 337
Paralytic ileus 309
Parasitic infections 45
Parasitic infestations 81
Parasternal heave 299, 299*f*
Parasympathetic fibers 331
Parasympathetic functions, tests for 262
Parasympathetic nervous system 260
Paratyphoid infections 45
Paresthesia 348
Parfocal system 4
Parkinson's disease 338
Parosmia 317
Pasteur pipette 66, 67*f*, 68
Patellar clonus 344
Patellar hammer 340, 340*f*
Peak expiratory flow rate 211, 214
Pectorals 336
Pectus carinatum 289
Pectus excavatum 289
Pen recording system 107, 242
Perceptive deafness 329
Percussion 291*f*, 299, 308
    wave 169, 169*f*
Perfusion functions, tests for 214

Pericardial effusion, large 169
Pericardial friction 301
Perimeter chart 233*f*
Perimetry 231, 319
Periodic abstinence 274
Peripheral blood smear, examination of 41
Peritoneum, free fluid in 308
Petit mal epilepsy 243
Phagocytosis 78
Pharyngeal reflexes 331
Phase-contrast microscope 7
Phenol solution 268
Pheochromocytoma 178
Phosphatase 360
Phosphate 12, 312, 360
Photic stimulation 241, 242
Physical and mental rest, complete 228
Physiography, use of 109
Pigeon-shaped chest 289
Pill
    classical 275
    morning-after 275
    sequential 275
Pilot's diluting fluid 80
Pilot's fluid, composition of 80
Pipette
    high speed 25
    slow-speed 24, 25
Pitocin 276
Pitting edema 284
Placenta
    benign tumor of 272
    malignant tumor of 272
    position of 272
Plantar flexion 336
Plantar reflex 339, 339*f*
    assessment of 339
Plasma 92, 92*t*, 360
    volume 358
Plasticine 268
Platelet 42
    count 60, 63, 76, 359
        low 61
        normal 77
    diluting fluid 76
    plug formation 60
Pleural rub 292
Poisons 89
Polarizing microscope 7
Poliomyelitis 221
Polycythemia 31
    physiological 31
    primary 31
    secondary 31
    vera 31
Polygraph 250
Polyuria 311

Position sense, loss of 337
Postganglionic neurons 261f
Potassium 312, 360
    chloride 111, 162
Precordial leads 189
Precordium 296
    bulging of 298
    examination of 296, 298
Preganglionic neurons 261f
Pregnancy 56, 218
    diagnostic test 270
        ELISA for 271f
    exercise 168
    laboratory tests of 270
    toxemias of 178
Prehepatic jaundice 312
Premature beat 150
Pressure 175, 349
    unit of 358
    volume transducer 108
Pricking apparatus 39, 54, 60, 61, 80
Pricking heel 10
Pricking needle 10, 34
Priestley Smith perimeter 231, 232, 232f
Prominent veins, presence of 306
Prostaglandins 276
Prostate specific antigen 267
Protanopia 320
Protein 31, 312, 360
    fractions 360
Prothrombin time 13, 60
Psychic stimuli 203
Ptosis 353
Pulmonary area 296f, 300
Pulmonary capillaries 359
Pulmonary eosinophilia 81
Pulmonary function tests 206
    classification of 206
    physioclinical significance of 214
Pulmonary reserve 209
Pulmonary resuscitation 222
Pulmonary vascular pressures,
    determination of 214
Pulmonary ventilation 207
Pulse 167, 285
    deficit 167, 170
    high volume 168
    pressure 172, 182, 186
    rate of 167, 168, 180
    respiration coupler 108
    slow-rising 169
    tracing, normal 169f
    transducer 109
Pulsus alternans 169
Pulsus paradoxus 169
Pulsus parvus 169
Pupillary constriction 321
Pupillary function, test for 263
Pupillary light reflex 317, 320
Pupillary reflexes 344
Purpura
    causes of 78
    drug induced 63
    primary 78
    secondary 78
Pus forming bacteria 36
Pyogenic bacteria 36
Pyogenic infections, acute 45, 81
Pyramidal tract 334
Pyrogenic reactions 58
Pyuria 313

Q

Quadratus labii inferioris 325
Quiescent heart 149

R

Racking microscope 6
Radial artery 167
Radial pulse, examination of 167f
Radiofemoral delay 168
Radioimmunoassay 270, 271
Randolph's diluting fluid 81
Reaction time 237
    actual recording of 238f
Reagent strip test 311, 311f
Recording device 99, 100
Recording electrodes 246, 248, 250
Recording time tracing 115
Rectal bleeding 305
Red blood cell 22, 28, 42, 66, 73, 83
    count 28
        total 28
    indices 73
        determination of 73
    osmotic fragility of 87
    pipette 24, 28, 28f, 76
    volume 358
Red cell 42, 89, 92
    casts 313
    clumping of 55f
    count 17, 359
        calculation of 30
        high 17
    dimensions 28
    fragility of 89, 359
    sedimentation of 66
    suspension, preparation of 54, 54f
    testing osmotic fragility of 88t
Reddish appearance, excessively 42
Rees-Ecker method 77
Reflex 337, 339, 341, 355
    assessment of 340
    deep 355
    reinforcement of 343
    superficial 339, 341, 355
    tested clinically 341t
Refractory period 149
    relative 125, 149
Relative load index 184
Relaxation period 114, 115, 115f, 138
Renal blood flow 359
Renal body fluids volume system 178
Renal disease 74, 178
Renal glycosuria 312
Renal tubular casts 313
Renin-angiotensin-aldosterone 178
    system 180
Repolarization positive, T wave of 193
Reproductive system 267
Rescue breath 222
Residual volume 206-208
Resolving power 5
Respiration
    artificial 220, 222f
    transducer 109
Respiratory disease
    signs of 288
    symptoms of 288
Respiratory movements 289
    effect of modified 202
    recording 201
Respiratory muscles, strength of 218
Respiratory rate 285
Respiratory system 200, 288
    clinical examination of 288
    examination of 289
    pressure volume curve of 213
Reticulocyte 84f
    count 83
    identification of 84
    number of 85
    response 84
    staining 83
Reticulocytopenia 84
Reticulocytosis 84
Reticuloendothelial system 45
Retina stimulated, region of 317
Retinal factors 317
Retinal mechanism 319
Rh
    antibodies 54, 54t
    blood group 53
Rheumatoid arthritis 45
Rhonchi 292
Rhythm 168, 194, 290
    method 274
Right kidney, palpation of 307

Rigor mortis 119
Ringer's solution 105, 112, 114, 118, 119, 137, 159
Ringer-Locke solution 162, 162*t*
Rinne test 329, 329*f*
Romberg's sign 337
Rosenbach's test 312
Rothera's test 312
Rubber tube 23
Rules of percussion 284, 291

S

Safe period 274
Sahli's acid hematin method 15
Sahli's hemoglobinometer 15, 16*f*
Sahli's method
    advantages of 17
    disadvantages of 17
Sahlin's jacket model 224
Saline
    normal 29
    solutions, preparation of 88*t*
Scanning electron microscope 7
Schafer's prone position 222
Schaff cell 49
Schamroth's sign 283
Schirmer's test 264
Schwabach's test 329
Sciatic nerve 121
    of frog, conduction velocity of 121
Scissor gait 338
Scotoma 234
    physiological 234
Secretomotor function 354
Semen 267
    analysis 267
Sensation 355
Sensitive galvanometer 188
Sensitivity control 241
Sensory
    ataxia 337, 338
    function 354
        testing 324, 331
    modalities, clinical testing of 348
    nerve action potential 248
        duration of 249*f*
    nerve conduction 248
    system, examination of 348, 355
Serratus anterior 336
Serum 56, 92
    specific gravity of 92*t*
Sexually transmitted diseases 274
Sherrington's recording drum 105
Shock 168, 169
    electric 221
Short circuiting key 102, 237

SI units, submultiples of 357*t*
Sickle cell anemia 84
Silent killer 178
Silver cup electrodes, recording 248
Simple muscle twitch
    correlation of 115, 115*f*
    temperature on 118
Single channel recording 188*f*
Sinoatrial node 149
Sinus
    arrhythmia 168, 263
    venosus 145, 146
Skeletal muscle 333
    contraction 124, 128, 129*f*, 132, 140
Skin 282
    state of 306
    sterilization of 9
Sleep, lack of 152
Smallpox 45
Smoking 106, 152
Snake venom 89
Sneeze reflex 324
Sneezing 202
Snellen's chart 317, 318*f*
Soda lime tower 210
Sodium 312, 360
    bicarbonate 89, 111, 162, 225, 268
    bromide 89
    chloride 28, 89, 111, 162
        solution 87
    fluoride 12
    nitrate 89
    sulfate 29
Soft palate movements 354
Somatic sensory fibers 331
Somatosensory evoked potentials 251, 252
Sound
    intensity of 300
    produced, character of 291
    sudden muffling of 175*f*
Spasm 338
Spastic gait 338
Spastic paraplegia, congenital 338
Special senses 231
Specific gravity 92, 311
Spectrophotometric methods 19
Speech 282, 352
    and language defects 315
    functions 316
Sperm
    counting 268
        principle of 268
    motility, assessing 268
    normal paths of 275
Spermatic fluid 267
Spermatozoa 313

Spermicidal agents, use of 274
Sphincter reflexes 341
Sphygmogram 169*f*
Sphygmomanometer 173, 173*f*, 180, 185, 255
Spinal accessory nerve 331
    testing 331*f*
Spinal nerve 354
Spinal origin 339
    superficial reflexes of 341
Spinal segments 343
Spinothalamic system, anterolateral 348*f*
Spirit swabs 247, 248
Spirogram 210
    normal 212*f*
Spirometer
    computerized 209, 211, 212*f*, 216
    parts of 210*f*
    recording 209, 210, 210, 211*f*, 216
    simple 216
    working of 210*f*
Spirometry 206, 209
Spleen, palpation of 307, 307*f*
Splenomegaly 307
Spondylitis 208
Spontaneous activity 250
Spring time marker 106
Sputum 288
Squint 353
Stab cell 49
Stain granules, presence of 41
Stained blood
    film 43*t*
    smear 41, 41*f*
Staining defects 41
Stains, Romanowsky group of 39
Staircase phenomenon 132, 150, 151*f*
Standard copper sulfate solutions, preparation of 93*t*
Stannius ligatures 149, 150
    effect of 150, 151*f*
    first 150
    second 150
Staphylococcus 36
Starling's heart 146
    lever 105, 105*f*, 145, 162
Starling's law 142
Static capacities 207
Static lung
    capacities 206, 207*t*
    volumes 206, 207*t*
Static volume 207
Stem 23
Stereognosis 351
Sterile cotton 34
Sternomastoid muscle testing 332*f*
Steroids, excess 45

Stethograph 200
Stethography 200, 201f
   recording 202f
Stethoscope 173, 173f, 180, 185
   bell of 291
Stimulating electrodes 106, 106f, 114, 246, 248, 253
Stimulating silver ring electrodes 248
Stimulation
   mark point of 105
   point of 114, 118, 115f
Stimulator 108, 245
Stimulus 99
   artifact 246
   factors 317
   frequency of 132
   maximal 128
   strength of 99, 114, 121, 124, 128, 129, 133, 136, 140
Stony dullness 291
Strain gage coupler 108
Streptococcus 36
Stress testing 197
Stretch reflex 340
Student physiograph 107, 108f, 109, 194
Student stimulator 106
Student's perimeter 233f, 234
Submaximal stimulus 128
Subminimal stimuli, summation of 150
Substance, unit of amount of 358
Subthreshold stimulus 128
Sucrose 89
Sugars, reducing 312
Sulfates 312
Sulfhemoglobin 19
Sulfosalicylic test 312
Superficial pain sensation, testing 350, 351f
Supinator reflex 342f
   assessment of 340
Supramaximal stimulus 128
Supranuclear lesion 327
Supraspinatus 336
Supravital staining 83, 85
Surface electrodes 246
Surface electromyography 250
Surgical sterilization 275
Swabs moist 253
Sweat glands 261
Sylvester's supine position 222
Syme's cannula 162
Sympathetic functions, tests for 260
Sympathetic nervous system 260
Sympathetic skin response 261
Syncope 296
Systemic arterial blood pressure 172
   record of 172, 178
Systemic examination 281
Systemic physical examination 284
Systolic blood pressure 172, 182, 186, 257
Systolic pressure 175f
   criterion of 176

T

Tachycardia 168, 195, 296
   ratio 263
Tactile localization 349
Tallquist method 19
Tally bar method 44
Tandem walking 337
Taste
   abnormalities of 326
   pathway 326
   sensation of 325, 354
   testing 326
Temperature sense, testing for 351f
Temperature transducer 109
Temporal lobe epilepsy 243
Tendon reflexes
   deep 339, 340, 341, 344
   grading of 344
Test tube
   method, single 62
   number 88
   rack 87
Tetanizing frequency 133
Tetanus 132
   complete 132
   genesis of 132, 132f
Tetany 58
Thalassemia 74, 84
Theta rhythm 241
Thigh
   abductors of 336
   flexors of 336
   rotators of 336
Thomson's hip-lift chest pressure methods 222
Thorn's test 81
Thready pulse 169
Threshold stimulus 128
Thromboasthenic purpura 63
Thrombocytopenia 61, 78
Thrombocytopenic purpura, idiopathic 63
Thrombocytosis 78
Thromboxane A2 77
Thumb rule 173
Thump chest 221
Thyroid binding globulin 360
Thyrotoxicosis 168
Thyroxine 360
   plasma 360

Tibial nerve, posterior 252
Ticking watch 328
Tics 337
Tidal volume 206, 207, 216
Tidal wave 169, 169f
Timed vital capacity, physioclinical significance of 208
Toes and ankle, dorsiflexion of 336
Tomography, computerized axial 214
Tongue
   anterior two-thirds of 326
   posterior 1/3rd of 354
Tonic contraction 338
Total leukocyte count 34, 39
Total magnification, calculation of 5
Touch sensation 348
Tourniquet test 60, 77
Toxic chemicals 89
Trachea
   auscultation of 291
   position of 290, 298
Transmission electron microscope 7
Transvaginal ultrasound 271
Treadmill test 195, 198
Tremor 337
Triceps reflex 340, 342f
   assessment of 340
Trichromats 320
Tricuspid area 296f, 300
Trigeminal nerve 354
   sensory functions of 324
Triiodothyronine 360
Triple rhythm 301
Trisodium citrate 12
Tritanopia 320
Trochlear nerve 322, 353
Trunk, testing muscles of 336
Tube
   external 4
   inner draw 4
Tuning fork 106, 114, 115f, 328
   tests 328
      principles of 329
Turk's fluid, composition of 34
Typhoid infection 45

U

Ulnar nerve 248
Umbilicus, state of 306
Universal donor 57
Upper face, testing 325
Upper limb 337
   testing of muscle
      power in 335f
      strength in 335
Upper motor neuron 327, 333, 345

Urate 360
Urea 360
   nitrogen 360
   solution 89
Uric acid 360
Urinalysis, common uses of 313
Urine 89
   abnormal constituents of 312
   analysis 311
   normal constituents of 312
   sample
      collection 311
      container for 311f
      random 311
      twenty-four-hour 311

V

Vagal escape 154, 155
   phenomenon of 155f
Vagal inhibition 154
Vagal stimulation 155f, 156
Vagal tone 155
Vagosympathetic trunk
   exposure of 154
   stimulation of 154, 155f
Vagus nerve 331, 354
   testing 331
Valsalva ratio 262
Vascular lesions 243
Vasopressin 178
Vasovagal syncope 156
Velocity, calculation of 122
Venous blood 10, 10t
Venous occlusion, effect of 256
Venous pulse, examination of 296
Ventilation 206
   scan 214
   volume, maximum 207
Ventilatory function, tests of 206
Ventricular fibrillation 225
Ventricular muscle 125f
Vesicular breath sounds 292
Vessel
   stress relaxation of 178
   wall
      condition of 168
      defects 61
Vestibular functions, tests for 330, 354
Vestibular nerve 327

Vestibulocochlear nerve 327, 354
Vibration sense 350
   testing for 351f
Viral infections 36, 45
Viral influenza 45
Visceral reflexes 339, 341, 344
Visceral sensory fibers 331
Visible peristalsis 306
Visible pulsations 306
Vision, peripheral field of 231
Visual acuity 234, 317, 353
   factors affecting 317
Visual area, primary 232
Visual association areas 232
Visual axes, convergence of 321
Visual evoked potentials 251, 252
Visual field, factors affecting 234
Visual pathway 231, 232f
Visual reaction time 237, 237f, 238
Vital capacity 207, 208, 216, 218
   components of timed 208f
   measurement of 216
   slow 216
   timed 207, 216
Vital signs 285
Vitalograph 216
Vitamin 31
   K deficiency 62
   B12, deficiency of 74
Vocal fremitus 290
   eliciting 290f
Vocal resonance 292
   character of 292
Voltage current, low 237
Volume pulse, low 168
Volume transducer 109
Voluntary contraction 251
   maximum 255
Voluntary hyperventilation, effect of 201, 203
Voluntary ventilation, maximum 207
Vomiting 305
von Frey's esthesiometer 349, 349f
von Frey's hair esthesiometer 348
von Willebrand disease 61, 62

W

Waddling gait 338
Warfarin 13

Warm, latent periods of 118
Watch test 328
Water retention, loss of 94
Weber's compass 348, 349f
Weber's test 329, 329f
Weigh$t$
   loss of 305
   unit of 358
Wernicke's area 316
Westergren method 66, 67
Westergren pipette 67, 68f
Westergren stand 68f
Wheezing 288
Whisper test 328
Whispering pectoriloquy 292
White blood
   cell 39, 43t, 44, 80, 268
      pipette 24, 35f, 268
   corpuscles 34
White cell
   casts 313
   count 359
White coat hypertension 176, 177
White crescentic line 146, 154, 155f, 159
   stimulation, effect of 155f
Wintrobe method 66
Wintrobe tube 67f, 68, 69
   with stand 66
World Health Organization 184t
Wright's capillary glass tube method 61
Wright's peak flow meter 212, 212f
Wris$t$
   extensors of 336
   flexors of 336

X

Xylose 360

Y

Y descent 298
Yarn matching test 320
Young-Helmholtz theory 319

Z

Zinc 360
   traces of 312